DIABETIC NEPHROPATHY

DEVELOPMENTS IN NEPHROLOGY

Cheigh JS, Stenzel KH, Rubin AL eds: Manual of clinical nephrology of the
  Rogosin Kidney Center. 1981. ISBN 90-247-2397-3.
Nolph KD ed: Peritoneal dialysis. 1981. ISBN 90-247-2477-5.
Gruskin AB, Norman ME eds: Pediatric nephrology. 1981. ISBN 90-247-2514-3.
Schück O ed: Examination of the kidney function. 1981. ISBN 0-89838-565-2.
Strauss J ed: Hypertension, fluid-electrolytes and tubulopathies in pediatric nephrology. 1981. ISBN 90-247-
  2633-6.
Strauss J ed: Neonatal kidney and fluid-electrolytes. 1983. ISBN 0-89838-575-X.
Strauss J. ed: Acute renal disorders and renal emergencies. 1984. ISBN 0-89838-663-2.
Didio LJA, Motta PM eds: Basic, clinical and surgical nephrology. 1985. ISBN. 0-89838-698-5.
Friedman EA, Peterson CM eds: Diabetic nephropathy: strategy for therapy. 1985. ISBN 0-89838-735-3.

DIABETIC NEPHROPATHY

STRATEGY FOR THERAPY

EDITED BY

ELI A. FRIEDMAN
State University, Downstate Medical Center
Brooklyn, New York

AND

CHARLES M. PETERSON
Sansum Medical Research Foundation
Santa Barbara, California

SPRINGER-SCIENCE+BUSINESS MEDIA, B.V.

Library of Congress Cataloging in Publication Data
Main entry under title:

Diabetic nephropathy.

   Includes bibliographies.
   1. Diabetic nephropathies—Treatment.   2. Diabetes—
Complications and sequelae.   3. Diabetic retinopathy.
I. Friedman, Eli A., 1933–   .   II. Peterson, C. M.
[DNLM: 1. Diabetic Nephropathies—therapy.
W1 DE998EB / WK 835 D5357]
RC918.D53D53   1985   616.4'62   85–8990

ISBN 978-1-4612-9410-8   ISBN 978-1-4613-2287-0 (eBook)
DOI 10.1007/978-1-4613-2287-0

For Barry with admiration and respect for her marvelous ability to persist and prevail in the successful conduct of professional and personal life despite a handicap that would have stopped a less vital person.

CONTENTS

CONTRIBUTING AUTHORS

Linda S. Cohen, R.N., B.S.N.
Diabetes Research Nurse
Downstate Medical Center
Brooklyn, New York 11203

Thomas A. Einhorn, M.D.
Assistant Professor of Orthopedic Surgery
Department of Surgery
Downstate Medical Center
Brooklyn, New York 11203

Eli A. Friedman, M.D.
Professor of Medicine
Chief, Division of Renal Disease
State University of New York
Downstate Medical Center
Brooklyn, New York 11203

Mildred Friedman, B.S.
Diabetic Kidney Transplant Self-Help Group
Downstate Medical Center
Brooklyn, New York 11203

Lois Jovanovic, M.D.
Assistant Professor of Medicine
Cornell University Medical Center
New York, New York 10021

Ramesh Khanna, M.D.
Associate Professor of Medicine
University of Missouri Health Science Center
Columbia, Missouri

Franscis A. L'Esperance, Jr., M.D.
Associate Professor of Clinical Ophthalmology
College of Physicians and Surgeons
Columbia-Presbyterian Medical Center
New York, New York 10032

John S. Najarian, M.D.
Professor and Chairman
Department of Surgery
University of Minnesota
College of Medicine
Minneapolis, Minnesota

Dimitrious G. Oreopoulos, M.D.
Professor of Medicine
University of Toronto
Director, Peritoneal Dialysis Unit
Toronto Western Hospital
Toronto, Canada

Charles M. Peterson, M.D.
Director of Research
Sansum Medical Research Foundation
Santa Barbara, California 93105

Fred L. Shapiro, M.D.
Professor of Medicine
University of Minnesota
Chief, Division of Nephrology
Hennepin County Medical Center
Minneapolis, Minnesota

David E. R. Sutherland, M.D.
Professor of Surgery
University of Minnesota
College of Medicine
Minneapolis, Minnesota

Kathleen Y. Whitley, M.D.
Instructor in Medicine
University of Minnesota
Division of Nephrology
Hennepin County Medical Center
Minneapolis, Minnesota

Diabetic nephropathy is a tragic illness. Its often insidious onset in the insulin-dependent (type I) diabetic, typically a young adult, heralds the last act in the course of a disease that will increasingly become the dominant preoccupation in the patient's shortened life. For most type II diabetics, the beginning of clinical renal insufficiency is but a phase in a continuous deterioration that affects the integrity of job, marriage, and family.

The nephropathic diabetic is hypertensive, has worsening retinopathy, and more often than not, is also plagued by peripheral vascular insufficiency, heart disease, gastrointestinal malfunction, and deepening depression. Until the 1980's, few type I diabetics who became uremic (because of diabetic nephropathy) lived for more than two years. Hardly any attained true rehabilitation. This dismal prognosis is changing substantially for the better.

Research in diabetes has resulted in striking advances at both ends of the type I diabetic's natural history. In one exciting clinical trial now underway in London, Ontario, half of childhood diabetics treated with cyclosporine within six weeks of onset evince "permanent" disappearance of hyperglycemia and the need for insulin. At the other end of the natural history of diabetes for the nephropathic patient with worsening eye disease (renal-retinal syndrome), who receives a kidney transplant, patient and graft survival, two years after cadaveric kidney transplantation in type I diabetics is now equal to that of the nondiabetic.

It is widely appreciated that normalization of the blood glucose level and vigorous treatment of hypertension will retard the decline in renal reserve during the relatively clinically silent interval between onset of hyperglycemia and expression of vasculopathy in the eyes and kidneys (the in-between years). Impressive advances in ophthalmology and podiatry now make blindness and limb amputation no longer inevitable complications of long-duration diabetes.

This book provides a survey of the strides that have been made in converting diabetic nephropathy from a hopeless condition to a still difficult but manageable disorder. By utilizing a team consisting of nephrologist, transplant surgeon, ophthalmologist, endocrinologist, podiatrist, nurse educator, nutritionist, social worker, and psychologist-psychiatrist, useful life may be sustained for the majority of uremic diabetics for at least three years. Disregarding the necessity for more than renal care will, by contrast, lead to a functioning kidney, or technically adequate peritoneal or hemodialysis in a "failed" patient. Our intent is to share what we have learned from our collaborators about formulating a successful strategy for the nephropathic diabetic.

INTRODUCTION

ELI A. FRIEDMAN

During the past decade, uremic diabetics have increasingly been enrolled into long-term programs providing uremia therapy including peritoneal or hemodialysis, or kidney transplantation. Management of the uremic diabetic requires recognition and management of concurrent hypertension and retinal microvasculopathy. Formulating a successful treatment strategy for coincident failure of kidneys and eyes (and often limbs, heart, and central nervous system) poses a challenge to specialists who may be unaccustomed to working as components of a team. Forced to tolerate apparently unstoppable disintegration of multiple organs, the azotemic diabetic becomes desperate in, or (worse) detached from, the quest for a solution to his enormous medical, economic, and social problems. Although discomforted by gastropathy, peripheral vascular insufficiency, marginal cardiac compensation, motor and visceral neuropathy, and muscle wasting, it is most often the fear of impending blindness that induces the greatest despair and terror.

Uremic diabetics and their doctors have in the past interpreted loss of sight as a signal that death was imminent. The diabetic renal-retinal syndrome is defined as the coincident kidney and eye disease that results from microvasculopathy in retinal and glomerular arterioles and capillaries. Of uremic patients started on hemodialysis or peritoneal dialysis in 1983, in the United States, at least 25% developed renal failure because of diabetes. The majority of these patients manifested the renal-retinal syndrome.

The treated uremic diabetic, in fact, stands a reasonable chance of attaining at least several years of relatively comfortable life. Modern peritoneal dialysis, hemodialysis, or kidney transplantation are returning a growing proportion of diabetics to work, home, or school activities. Functioning as a team, uremic diabetics and their doctors are engaged in an exciting clinical trial based on the premise that, as is generally accepted for nondiabetics, there is life after the onset of renal failure.

This book is based on the belief that rehabilitation is a realistic objective for diabetics whose kidneys have failed. Its pages contain an approach to the diabetic renal-retinal syndrome derived from several hundred type I uremic diabetics managed in Minneapolis, Brooklyn, and Toronto. Recognizing that strict control of blood glucose levels has not yet been shown to prevent or reverse progressive eye and kidney disease in humans, the authors will nevertheless advocate such tight regulation of the blood glucose level. It is reasoned that the risks of inducing a near-normal blood sugar impose a lesser hazard (should tight control subsequently prove of no benefit in preempting eye and kidney damage) than hyperglycemia (if the thesis that hyperglycemia is the major cause of vascular damage in diabetes is sustained). Normalizing high blood pressure at every stage of progressive diabetic renal disease is stressed as an important component of the therapeutic program. There is no doubt that a lower blood pressure is kinder to the eyes and kidneys —as well as to the brain and heart.

Exploration of the renal-retinal syndrome in this text will review its presentation, pathogenesis, and treatment. Emphasis is placed on the necessity for converting the patient into a partisan in the struggle to retain vision and limbs. Once uremia has developed, a strategy for selecting peritoneal dialysis, hemodialysis, or a kidney transplant will be proposed. Chapters by a kidney transplant recipient and a nurse caring for diabetic kidney transplant recipients focus on the patient as a sick human being demanding emotional as well as physical therapy. The main focus throughout this book will be on the patient and his/her reaction to a devastating illness.

DIABETIC NEPHROPATHY

1. WHAT IS DIABETES? TYPES, DEFINITIONS, EPIDEMIOLOGY, DIAGNOSIS

CHARLES M. PETERSON

and

LOIS JOVANOVIC

TYPE I DIABETES MELLITUS

Diabetes mellitus is a heterogeneous group of disorders that are characterized by elevated blood glucose. At present it is not possible to classify these disorders by etiology, but the National Diabetes Data Group has provided guidelines for the classification of the various forms based on the pathophysiology of the hyperglycemia (see table 1–1). Type I diabetes mellitus is best conceptualized as total pancreatic failure in terms of ability to make insulin. This type of diabetes tends to occur before the age of 30. Since there is very little insulin available, persons with this type of diabetes have a vulnerability toward ketoacidosis, and often the diagnosis is made with the onset of the disease concomitant with an episode of ketoacidosis. The diagnosis of type I diabetes mellitus is generally not difficult. The young patient who presents with elevated blood glucose and ketonuria seldom needs further evaluation to determine the type of diabetes. Following treatment of the acute onset episode, there may be considerable return of pancreatic insulin output (the "honeymoon period"), but within five years insulin secretion will generally be undetectable.

There are two laboratory tests that are helpful in making the diagnosis of type I diabetes. The first is C-peptide (connecting peptide) determination. With each molecule of insulin secreted by the normal pancreas, a molecule of C-peptide is secreted as well. The secretion of insulin is summarized in figure 1–1. Both molecules are secreted into the portal circulation. Insulin is 50–70% cleared by the liver on the first pass, whereas C-peptide is not. Therefore measurement of C-

1

Table 1–1. Classification of diabetes mellitus
and other categories of glucose intolerance

Clinical classes
  Diabetes mellitus (DM)
    Insulin–dependent type (IDDM): type I
    Noninsulin-dependent type (NIDDM): type II
      Nonobese
      Obese
    Other types (includes diabetes mellitus associated with certain conditions and
      syndromes)
      Pancreatic disease
      Disease of hormonal etiology
      Drug- or chemical-induced condition
      Insulin receptor abnormalities
      Certain genetic syndromes
      Miscellaneous
  Impaired glucose tolerance (IGT)
      Nonobese
      Obese
    Impaired glucose tolerance associated with certain conditions and syndromes
      Pancreatic disease
      Disease of hormonal etiology
      Drug- or chemical-induced
      Insulin receptor abnormalities
      Certain genetic syndromes
      Miscellaneous
  Gestational diabetes (GDM)
Statistical risk classes (subjects with normal glucose tolerance but substantially increased
  risk of developing diabetes)
  Previous abnormality of glucose tolerance
  Potential abnormality of glucose tolerance

---

peptide can be helpful in the definition of the secretory status of the pancreatic beta cell mass. C-peptide can be measured in the fasting state or after a stimulus. Fasting levels tend to correlate well with stimulated values, but the latter tend to be preferred by clinical investigators. The stimulus given is generally either a mixed type meal such as SUSTACAL® or 1 mg of glucagon given intravenously. The SUSTACAL challenge is generally given in the fasting state with bloods drawn for glucose and C-peptide before and one hour after the SUSTACAL challenge. The diabetes Control and Complications Trial defined a one-hour value of 0.02 ng/ml C-peptide or below as type I diabetes mellitus eligible for the trial. Many investigators feel that values below 0.05 ng/ml are indicative of type I disease.

The glucagon test (1 mg given intravenously) need not be given in the fasting state. Blood for glucose and C-peptide is drawn before and six minutes after the glucagon injection. Glucagon injection is followed by nausea and/or vomiting in about 20% of patients. Marked hyperglycemia may result from both testing procedures, and therefore blood glucose levels should be monitored until they have returned to pretest levels.

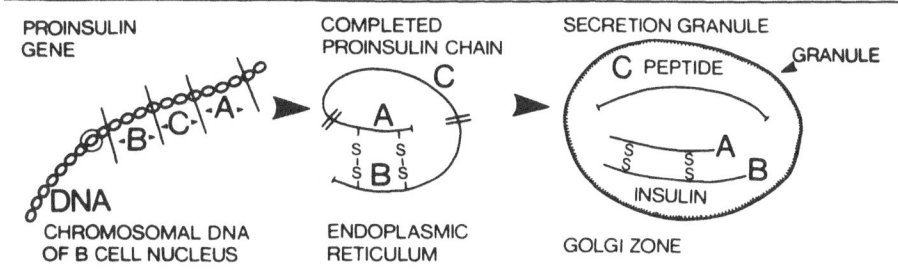

Figure 1–1. The formation of C-peptide and insulin in the Beta cell of the pancreas.

The second laboratory test that facilitates the definition of type I diabetes is the determination of islet cell antibody levels. It would appear that patients who have circulating antibodies to islet cells have an increased propensity to develop type I disease if followed for periods of up to 20 years. These observations, if confirmed, have exciting implications for disease prevention as well as diagnostic implications.

The best hypothesis for the genesis of type I diabetes follows. There is an inherited susceptibility to an environmental insult which initiates a process resulting in pancreatic islet destruction, insulinopenia, and diabetes mellitus. The genetic susceptibility appears to be linked to certain HLA types including DW3-DR3 and DW4-DR4 while a number of viral types, including coxsackie B, encephalomycarditis, rubella, and mumps, have been implicated as potential elicitors of the disease in susceptible strains of laboratory animals as well as humans.

TYPE II DIABETES MELLITUS

Type II diabetes mellitus does not lead to total loss of insulin secretory capacity as is seen in the type I variety. In type II diabetes, the pancreas is able to secrete insulin but there is a resistance to the circulating insulin. The nature of the defect appears to be complex, involving fewer receptors to the circulating insulin per cell as well as a postreceptor problem within the cell itself. Circulating insulin levels may even be high in the person with type II diabetes and yet the ability to clear glucose from the bloodstream is impaired.

Because the ability to produce insulin is still intact, the person with type II diabetes is not generally vulnerable to episodes of ketoacidosis, and the presentation of the disorder is generally not as dramatic as is seen with type I diabetes. For this reason, the diagnosis of type II diabetes becomes somewhat more problematic and relies on a glucose tolerance test. Again the National Diabetes Data Group has provided guidelines for the administration and interpretation of the glucose tolerance test. Table 1–2 gives the guidelines for glucose tolerance testing and interpretation. Three different criteria are included to illustrate the diversity of opinions that have surrounded the field of glucose tolerance as a diagnostic criteria for diabetes mellitus. In practice, the criteria of the National Diabetes Data Group have become most widely accepted. Nevertheless as is illustrated in figure 1–2, there is a gray zone of diagnosis that lies between the criteria of Fajans and Conn and those of

Table 1-2. Interpretation of the oral glucose tolerance test
as recommended by the National Diabetes Data Group

Procedure
1. 3 days of at least 100 gm a day of carbohydrate (carbohydrate loading)
2. Fast of at least 8 hours
3. Fasting blood sample drawn no later than 9 A.M.
4. 75 gm of oral glucose drink administered no later than 9 A.M.
5. Blood samples drawn at time 0, 30, 60, 120, 180 minutes

Interpretation
Plasma or serum glucose levels
1. Above 140 mg/dl at least twice in the fasting state and/or
2. A 2h or later plasma or serum glucose level greater than 200 mg/dl

the National Diabetes Data Group. Most clinicians agree that persons falling with
this intermediate area of "impaired glucose tolerance" warrant increased surveillance over time.

To be truly indicative of carbohydrate tolerance, the testing procedure must be
performed in the proper manner with the patient appropriately prepared. If the
pancreas is not "primed" with a high carbohydrate diet before the test, glucose
tolerance will be impaired. Therefore, for three days before testing the subject

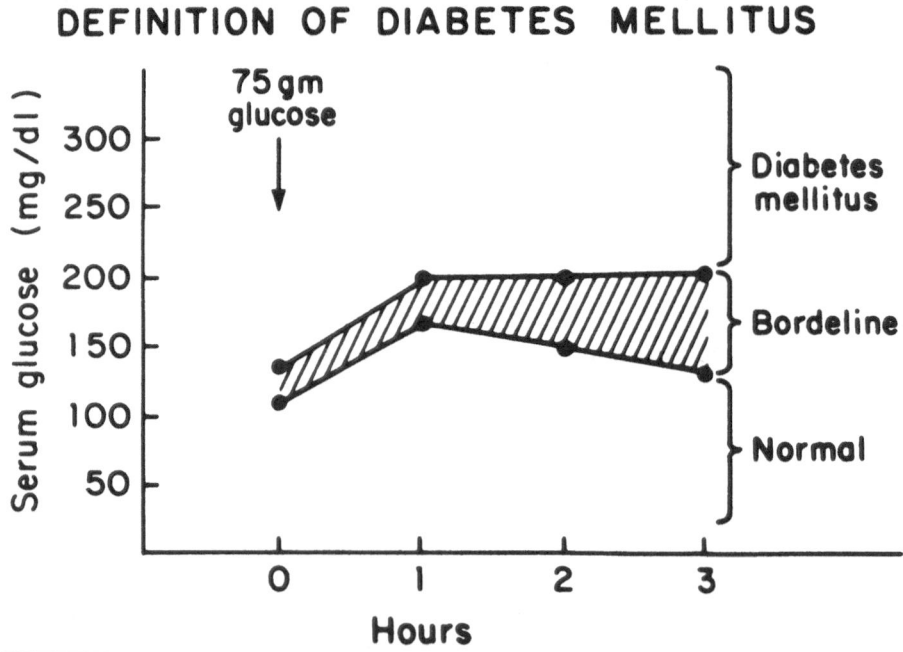

Figure 1-2. The glucose tolerance test as evaluated by the National Diabetes Data Group (top
dotted line) and Fajans and Conn (bottom dotted line).

should consume *and record* at least 100 grams of carbohydrate per day. No food is taken after 10 P.M. the day before the test procedure to ensure an overnight fast of at least 10 hours. The oral load is 1.75 grams of glucose/kg of ideal body weight as a 25% solution, up to a maximum of 75 grams. Blood samples for plasma glucose are obtained fasting and at 30-minute intervals after the first swallow of glucose solution for at least three hours. Although the National Diabetes Data Group requires values at fasting, one and two hours for diagnostic criteria, the pattern of response at the intervening points and at three hours is often helpful in interpreting the test. Since the test is cumbersome and expensive, the above approach is best strictly adhered to, as a poorly performed test will only lead to confusion and probable repetition.

The genetic propensity toward the development of type II diabetes is a little more defined than that of type I. There is a very high concordance (> 80%) in twins to develop this type of diabetes—if one twin has the disease—and the concordance is almost as high with first-degree relatives. While type I diabetes tends to be a disease primarily of Caucasian populations, type II diabetes is found in high prevalence in American Pima Indians, migrant populations from the Indian subcontinent, Pacific Island populations, and Micronesians. Obesity and a sedentary lifestyle are highly associated with the expression of the disorder; environmental factors play a major role for expression of the gene. The differences are summarized in table 1–3.

Table 1–3. Evidence of heterogeneity in diabetes

	Type I	Type II
Clinical onset	Abrupt, symptoms severe	Mild; incidental finding
Insulin dependence	Virtually always	Rare (except after many years of diabetes)
Pathology	Insulitis, mononuclear cell infiltration in early onset cases; eventual virtually complete destruction of B cells	Hypertrophy in early stages; atrophy and hyaline degeneration late on
Immunity		
islet-cell antibodies	Present	Absent
cell-surface antibodies	Present	Absent
cell-mediated immunity	Present	Absent
Genetics	Familial aggregation HLA-associated	Strong familial aggregation; no HLA association
Other autoimmune diseases present (or in close relatives)	Frequent, particularly in older onset cases	Absent
Possible initiating events	Virus infection (? chemical toxins)	Overnutrition and obesity

GESTATIONAL DIABETES

A type of diabetes which is analogous to type II diabetes is that seen during pregnancy: gestational diabetes. This form of diabetes occurs during pregnancy and tends (95%) to disappear after delivery. About 2–4% of normal pregnancies will be complicated by gestational diabetes. It is important that all women be screened for diabetes during pregnancy. Screening is especially indicated if the woman is over 30 years old, obese, was a large baby at birth herself (over nine pounds), has a family history of diabetes, or has a poor obstetrical history including previous fetal losses, urinary tract infections, toxemia, congenital anomalies, or a history of a previous baby weighing over 4,000 grams.

The screening test for gestational diabetes involves administration of 50 grams of glucose as an oral challenge. There is no need to prepare or fast the woman in advance of the glucose challenge. About 20% of those screened will have plasma glucose values at one hour greater than 140 mg/dl and will require a formal three-hour glucose tolerance test following a 100-gram glucose load administered in the fasting state. The approach to gestational diabetes is summarized in tables 1–4. Since pregnant women have lower blood glucose values than nonpregnant women, criteria for interpreting the glucose tolerance test are stricter during pregnancy; the goals of treatment are more stringent as well. Blood glucose levels during pregnancy are about 20% lower than outside pregnancy.

Gestational diabetes is a window into the metabolic future. Fully 65% of women who have had gestational diabetes will develop type II diabetes within 20 years

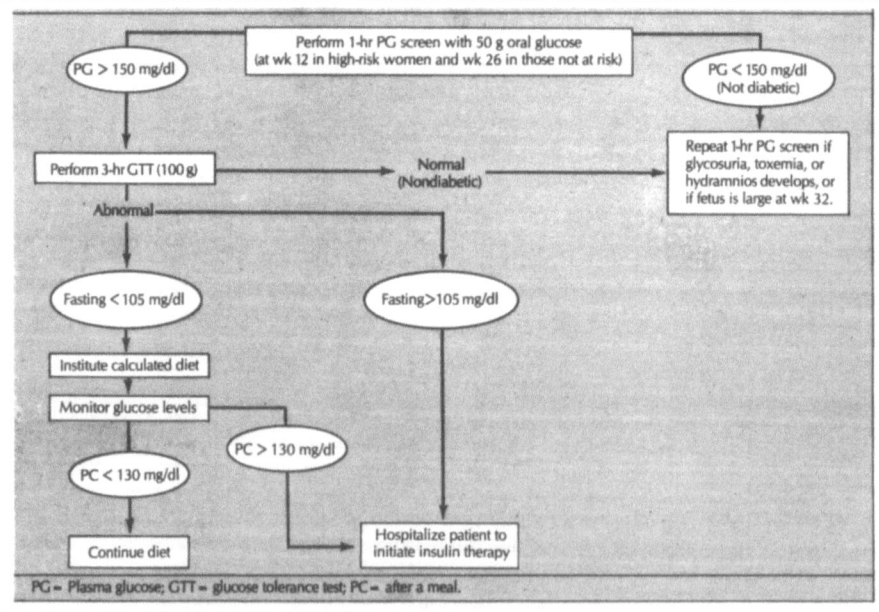

Figure 1–3. Triage procedure for gestational diabetes.

Table 1–4. O'Sullivan (Diabetes 13:278–85, 1964) criteria for diagnosis of diabetes in pregnancy

	Plasma glucose[1] (mg/dl)	Whole blood glucose equivalent[1] (mg/dl)
Fasting	105	90
1	190	165
2	165	145
3	140	125

1. Values represent two standard deviations above the mean.
Note: An elevated fasting or two elevated subsequent values = gestational diabetes.

of their pregnancy. The prevalence of type II diabetes among this risk group decreases to 25% when these women become lean and stay fit into their mature years. Because the 50-year-old woman with type II diabetes 20 years after her gestational diabetes may, due to diabetic nephropathy, become a renal dialysis patient at age 65, every effort should be made to urge that women who have had gestational diabetes lose and maintain weight loss postpartum.

It is important to remember that persons with renal disease and both type I and II diabetes are also becoming pregnant in greater numbers because of the more hopeful outlook for pregnancy complicated by diabetes. It is vital for all diabetics to normalize blood glucose before pregnancy because of the increased risk of congenital malformations associated with hyperglycemia during organogenesis (the first eight weeks of pregnancy). Type I diabetes can also be first manifested during pregnancy. In this instance, the woman usually presents in ketoacidosis, and prognosis tends to be guarded for mother and fetus.

GLYCOSYLATED PROTEINS

It has been suggested that glycosylated proteins might be useful for the diagnosis of diabetes mellitus since levels of glycosylated hemoglobin and albumin reflect average blood glucose values over the previous six to eight weeks and two weeks, respectively. The advantage of measuring glycosylated proteins is such testing requires no patient preparation and only one venipuncture. An elevated blood glucose combined with an elevated glycosylated protein measurement indicates that there is a problem at the moment with hyperglycemia, and the hyperglycemia has been present for at least a number of weeks, i.e., diabetes mellitus. While attractive as an alternative, the fact that at present there are no references or standards for glycosylated protein measurements makes it impossible for the potential clinical utility of these measurements as a diagnostic tool to be realized. Finally, the lack of sensitivity of glycosylated protein measurements to acute hyperglycemia and glucose intolerance makes provocative glucose challenges the approach of choice for the diagnosis of gestational diabetes.

OTHER TYPES OF DIABETES

As can be seen from table 1–1, there are a number of less common causes of diabetes which should be mentioned. Several toxins can lead to diabetes, including a rat poison (Vancour) and excessive alcohol intake. Severe stress may result in hyperglycemia which may be transient or may persist. Stress with its excess secretion of a number of hormones which impair insulin action can make the treatment or preexisting diabetes more difficult as well. These factors may play a role in the vulnerability of patients with renal insufficiency to diabetes mellitus in any of its forms.

GLUCOSE METHODS

The diagnostician working with patients with renal disease and diabetes should have a working knowledge of the blood glucose method used in his/her laboratory. Key information required includes: (1) what the actual name is of the method; (2) whether the method measures true glucose (it should); (3) whether whole blood, plasma, or serum is analyzed; and (4) what the normal ranges are for the method. Although a detailed description of each of the available methods is beyond the scope of the present text, the information obtained by asking these basic questions of the laboratory will facilitate interpretation of the diagnostic procedures utilized, though distinguishing the carbohydrate intolerance of uremia from type II diabetes may be difficult.

In summary, there are many ways by which an individual can develop diabetes mellitus or an elevated blood glucose. There are tests by which most diabetics can be classified as to which form of the disease they have. Nevertheless, until etiologic diagnostic criteria are available, the classification of diabetes mellitus is somewhat arbitrary. As will be shown in chapter 4, hyperglycemia per se is potentially toxic regardless of the etiology of the disorder; and the lack of a precise cause should not serve to impede a thorough therapeutic approach toward establishing euglycemia, thereby returning the internal milieu to normal.

SELECTED BIBLIOGRAPHY

1. Craighead JE. Viral diabetes in man and experimental animals. Am. J. Med. 70:127–136, 1980.
2. Ellenberg M, Rifkin H. Diabetes mellitus. New Hyde Park, New York: Medical Examination Publishing Co., 1983.
3. Faber OK, Bender C. C-peptide response to glucagon: a test for residual beta-cell function in diabetes mellitus. Diabetes 26:605–10, 1977.
4. Montague W. Diabetes and the endocrine pancreas. New York: Oxford University Press, 1983.
5. National Diabetes Data Group Classification and diagnosis of diabetes mellitus and other categories of glucose intolerance. Diabetes 28:1039–1057, 1979.
6. O'Sullivan JB, Mahan CM. Criteria for the oral glucose tolerance test in pregnancy. Diabetes 13: 278–285, 1964.

2. INSULIN, ORAL AGENTS, AND MONITORING TECHNIQUES

CHARLES M. PETERSON
and
LOIS JOVANOVIC

RATIONALE FOR EUGLYCEMIA

In the normal individual, glucose is perhaps the metabolic substrate least subject to deviation from the "norm." This metabolite is highly regulated and has minimal alternatives for metabolic conversion. Glucose may be entered into enzymatic degradation through glycolysis, glycogen formation, or the pentose shunt. In general, the initial enzyme steps in these reactions are rate-limiting and, therefore, they have little influence on substrate concentration. Gluconate and sorbitol pathways are also possible, although these latter pathways have high km values and therefore probably play a small role in biology during periods of extremely high glucose concentrations. Another alternative to substrate utilization of glucose is through the nonenzymatic glycosylation of proteins. These reactions, known as the Maillard Reaction, occur in two forms: (1) nonenzymatic glycosylation and (2) nonenzymatic browning resulting from rearranged products of the glycosylation reaction itself.

Because of the observation that hemoglobin Alc levels are increased in the blood of patients with diabetes mellitus, these types of reactions have drawn an increasing amount of attention regarding their potential role in causing diabetic sequelae especially in tissues which are non-insulin dependent for their intracellular glucose concentrations. Glycosylation reactions have been implicated in the secondary sequelae of diabetes in the lens, collagen structures, and the nerve.

In addition to providing impetus to the hypothesis that glycosylation reactions

9

initiate or propagate the secondary sequelae of diabetes, the observation that hemoglobin Alc results from a nonenzymatic glycosylation of normal hemoglobin gave rise to the utilization of this molecule as a measurement of control, and also generated the hypothesis that many sequelae of diabetes might not only be preventible but also reversible if glycosylation were an underlying mechanism, depending on the rate of repair or regeneration of the altered protein. This latter hypothesis has in turn generated a number of studies to determine whether certain sequelae of diabetes might not improve when glucose control improved as measured by hemoglobin Alc levels.

HEMOGLOBIN ALC

As shown in figure 2–1, hemoglobin is classically separated on cation exchange chromatography. An elution profile is obtained which includes peak 1 (or hemoglobins Ala+b), peak 2 (or hemoglobin Alc); hemoglobin Ao which comprises of about 95% of adult human hemoglobin and a shoulder, (hemoglobin A2) which is elevated in beta thalassemia minor. Hemoglobin Alc results from glycosylation of the N-terminus of the beta chain. This specific glycosylation undergoes rearrangement through an Amadori-type process resulting in a stable ketoamine from an unstable aldiamine or Schiff-base configuration. This rearrangement accounts for the stability of the adduct and its clinical utility (figures 2–2 and 2–3).

Early studies were designed to evaluate whether hemoglobin Alc levels would

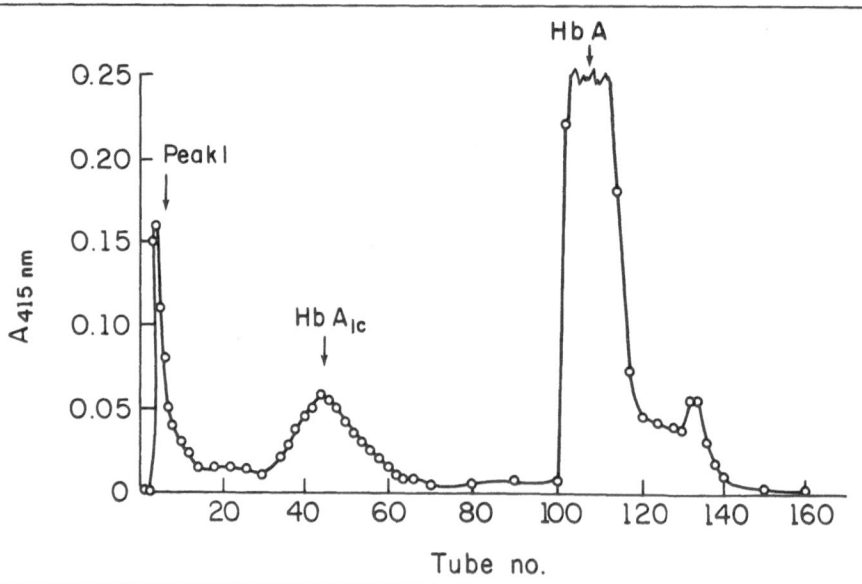

Figure 2–1. Cation exchange chromatography of adult hemoglobin on Biorex 70 resin. Peak 1 contains hemoglobins Ala+b. Peak 2 is hemoglobin Alc while hemoglobin A or Ao comprises 90–95% of adult hemoglobin. The shoulder to the right of hemoglobin A is hemoglobin A2 useful in the diagnosis of β-Thalassemia.

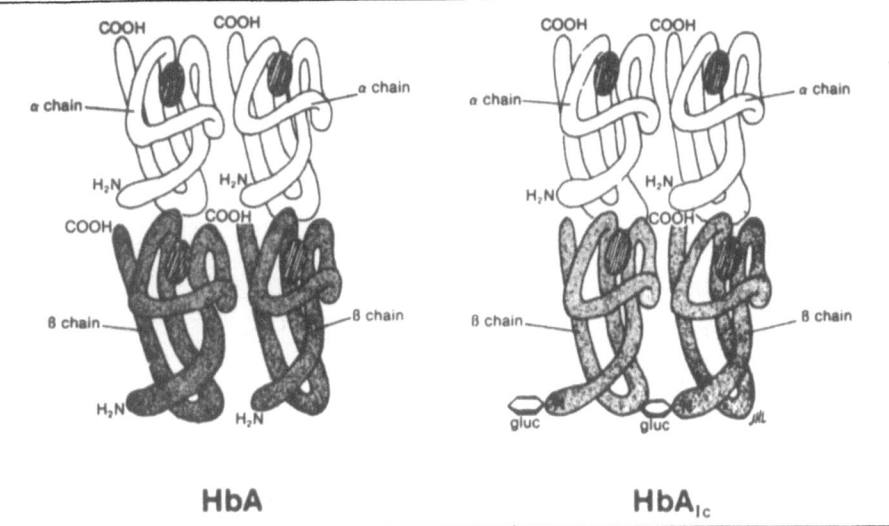

HbA   **HbA$_{1c}$**

Figure 2–2. The difference in hemoglobin A1c is hemoglobin A is the attachment of a glucose molecule to the N-terminus of the B chain of hemoglobin A1c.

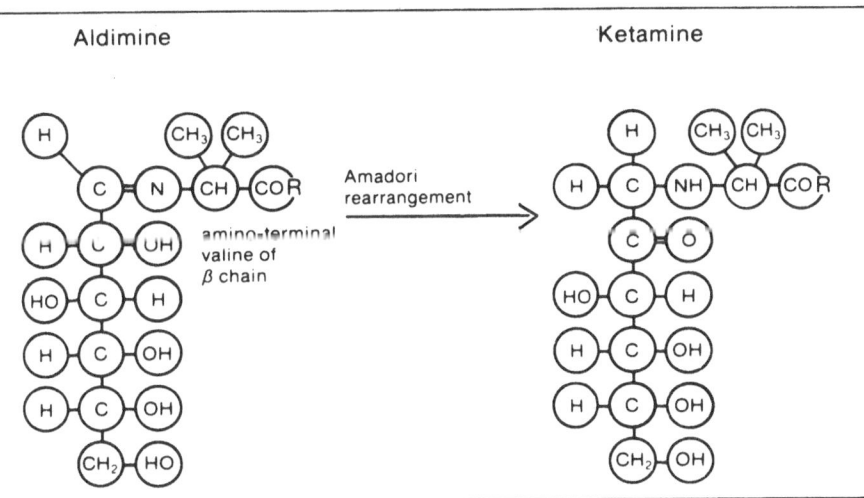

Aldimine   Ketamine

Figure 2–3. Stabilization of the glucose attachment occurs via the Amadori rearrangement. Further nonenzyamtic browning reactions are possible through rearrangements classified under the Maillard reaction.

correlate with standard assessments of glucose control, including a glucose tolerance test or serial urinary glucose excretion. As shown in figure 2–4, hemoglobin A1c levels do correlate with the maximum value of a glucose tolerance test and also the area under the curve. These provide the best correlations, although correlations have been documented with any point on the tolerance test. In adult onset diabetics,

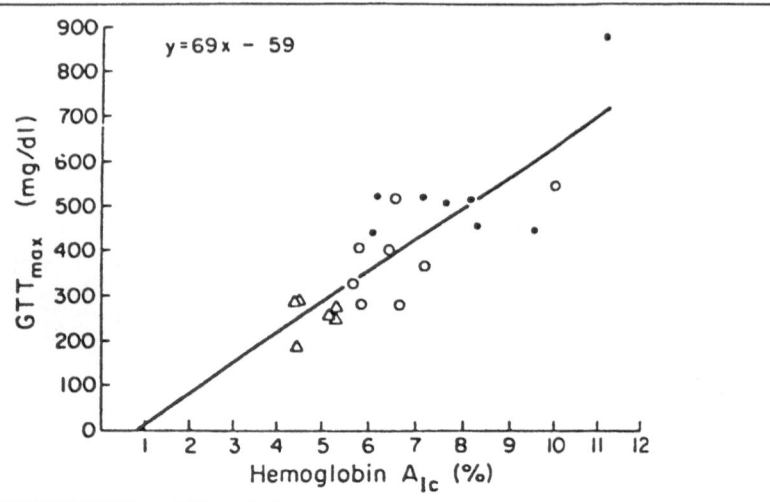

Figure 2–4. Correlation of hemoglobin Alc with a maximum glucose value following a glucose tolerance test of 100 gms of oral glucose.

the fasting blood glucose itself correlates quite well with hemoglobin Alc determinations.

When patients were hospitalized and more rigid control was established through the introduction of insulin therapy, hemoglobin Alc levels (figure 2–5) as well as hemoglobin Ala+b (figure 2–6) decreased. These observations provided the rationale for the utilization of the whole fast fraction or total glycohemoglobin determination which has, in many laboratories, replaced the more tedious but specific hemoglobin Alc determination. A number of methods are now being utilized to measure these glycosylated hemoglobins including standard chromatographic

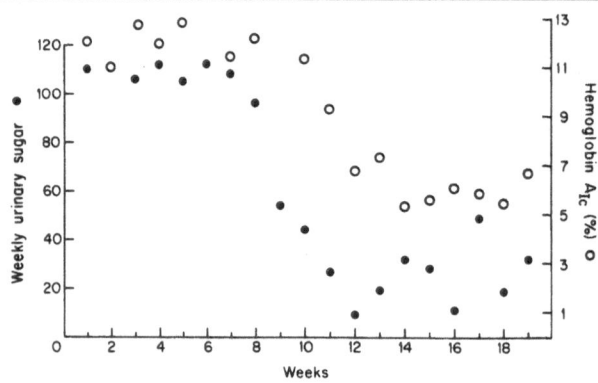

Figure 2–5. The lag phase between summed weekly urinary glucoses and hemoglobin Alc values in about four weeks while a new plateau is reached in about six weeks following the institution of improved therapy on a metabolic word.

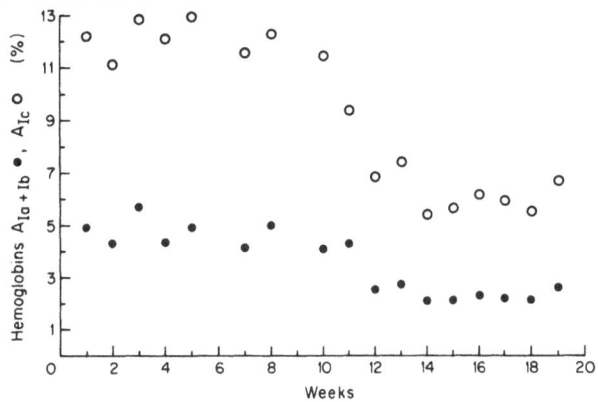

Figure 2–6. Hemoglobin Ala+b fall in a manner parallel to hemoglobin Alc following the institution of strict metabolic control. These minor hemoglobins comprise about 30–35% of the total fast eluting fraction on cation exchange chromatography. Commercial laboratories report hemoglobin Ala−c as the "Total glycohemoglobin," "fast fraction," or hemoglobin Al (from N. Engl J of Med 295:417–420, 1976; with permission).

procedures, high pressure liquid chromatographic procedures, isoelectric focusing techniques, electrophoresis on agar, colorimetric, and affinity chromatography methodologies.

IN-HOSPITAL STUDIES OF REVERSIBLE LESIONS

When diabetics are hospitalized in a metabolic ward for careful glucose control, as shown in figure 2–7, both cholesterol and triglyceride levels improve as glucose control is improved. Triglyceride levels actually fall into the normal range antecedent to the drop in hemoglobin Alc levels, whereas cholesterol levels may take as long as 6 to 10 weeks to reach a more stable plateau.

A number of hematologic variables also improve when blood glucose levels are normalized. Early senescence of the erythrocyte in hyperglycemic individuals is corrected if hemoglobin Alc levels are improved. In general, hyperglycemic individuals with hemoglobin Alc levels of about twice the normal range show a 10% decrement in red cell survival which is corrected following achievement of normoglycemia.

Defects in polymorphonuclear leukocyte function have been documented in diabetics. Normal leukocytes must be able to migrate to the site of inflammation, migrate toward specific chemical stimuli (chemotaxis), engulf organisms, and also effect killing. Abnormalities in each of these leukocyte properties have been documented in diabetics. However, most of the above properties depend in turn upon adherence which has been documented to be abnormal in hyperglycemic diabetics. As shown in figure 2–8, abnormal adherence corrects as euglycemia is achieved with improved glucose control.

The platelet has also been demonstrated to behave abnormally in vitro when

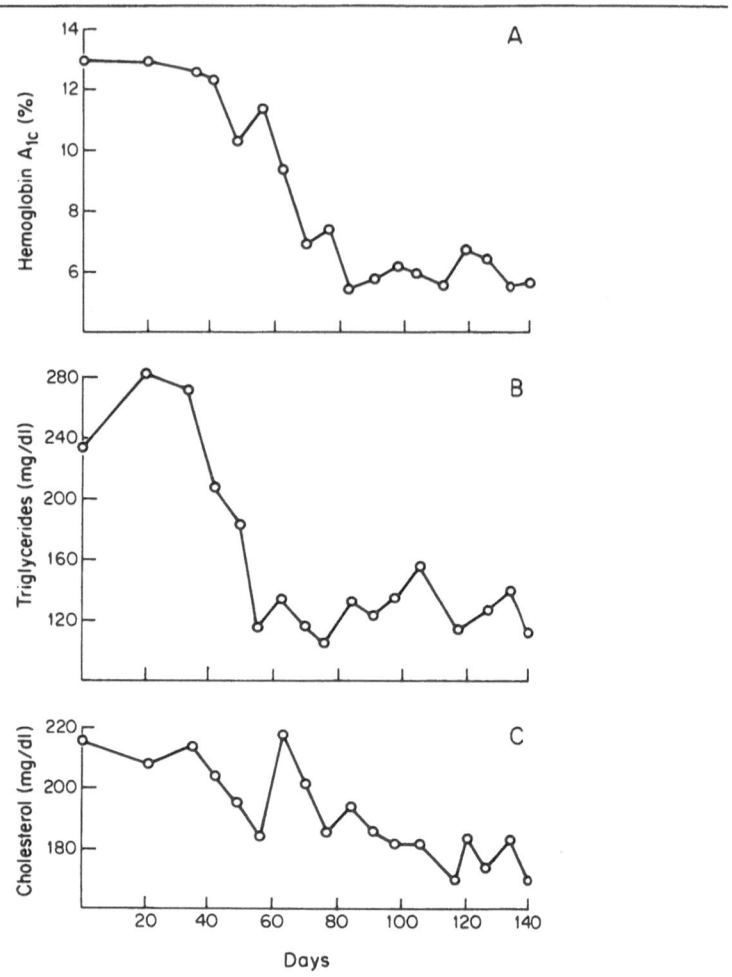

Figure 2–7. Decrease in hemoglobin Alc, serum triglycerides, and cholesterol in a patient following the institution of improved insulin delivery and metabolic control (from Peterson et al. Diabetes 26:507–509, 1977; with permission)

obtained from hyperglycemic diabetics. Hyperaggregation of platelets in vitro returns to normal if hyperglycemia (reflected by hemoglobin Alc levels) is corrected. Whether these in vitro observations reflect in vivo pertubations and whether the platelet contributes to either genesis or propagation of vascular lesions in diabetes remains controversial. Recent studies of in vivo platelet survival in diabetic patients detected no difference between platelet survival between hyperglycemic diabetic patients and euglyemic diabetic patients or in normal age-matched controls. On the other hand, diabetics with proliferative retinal disease requiring photocoagulation have decreased platelet survival (figure 2–9) as do normal nondiabetics who smoke.

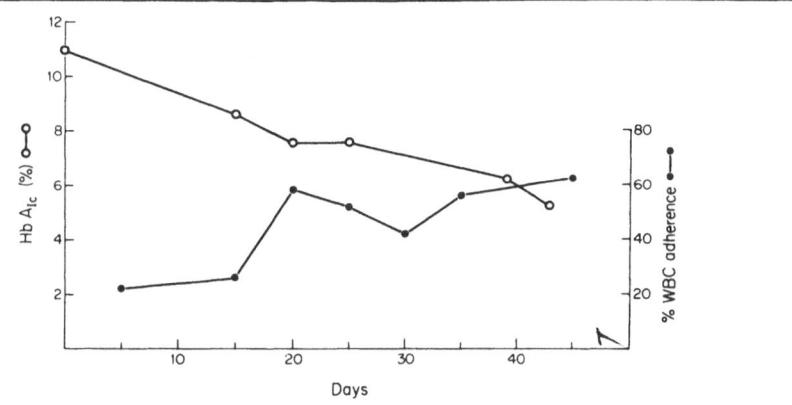

Figure 2–8. White cell adherence improves (normal > 50%) while hemoglobin Alc returns to normal (nl 3–6%) (from Annals Int. Med. (Peterson and Jones, Ann of Internal Med 297:4104, 1977; with permission).

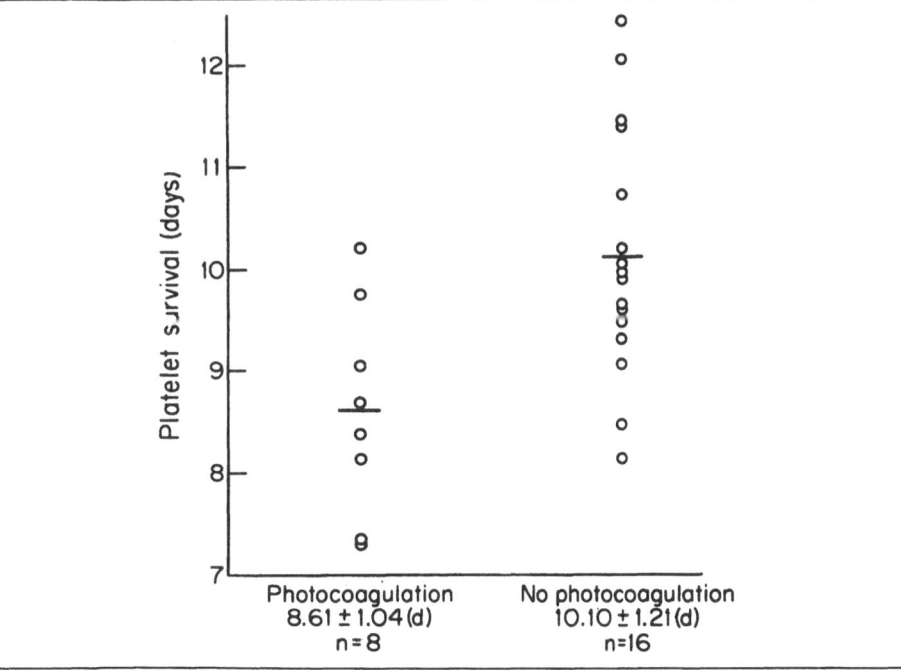

Figure 2–9. Diabetics with retinopathy of sufficient severity to require laser photcoagulation have shortened platelet survival *(left)* as compared with diabetics with more benign fundi *(right).*

Studies of fibrinogen survival demonstrated (figure 2–10) that fibrinogen survival is markedly shortened in the hyperglycemic diabetic. In this instance, the patient's own fibrinogen was labelled and reinfused. Following establishment of euglycemia, a similar study was performed using a second radioactive label: an

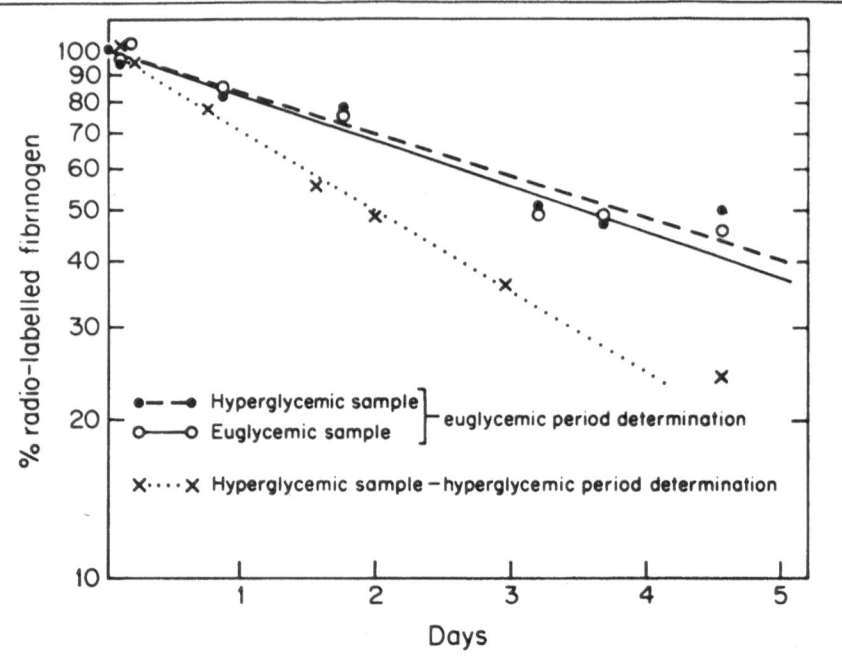

Figure 2–10. Fibrinogen survival in markedly shortened in patients who are hyperglycemic as shown by the dotted line. This abnormality corrects when hyperglycemia is corrected (Jones and Peterson, J of Clin Investigation 63:485–493, 1979; with permission).

aliquot from the hyperglycemic period was infused labelled with [131]iodine, and an aliquot from the euglycemic period infused utilizing [125]iodine. Simultaneous survival studies demonstrated that the decrement in fibrinogen survival was corrected during euglycemia. This experiment indicated that the defect in fibrinogen function was induced by the diabetic environment and not a faulty fibrinogen molecule. Subsequent studies showed that the abnormality in fibrinogen survival could be corrected by heparin but not by aspirin and dipyridamole. These observations implicate the thrombin-antithrombin axis in the documented abnormalities. Noteworthy is the fact that the fibrinogen abnormality appears to be relatively quickly reversible as shown in figure 2–11. When patients had hyperglycemia sustained by an artificial pancreas (BIOSTATOR®) at 300 mg/dl, fibrinogen kinetics were markedly shortened. At a blood glucose of about 100 mg/dl, fibrinogen kinetics were normalized, but after the program was subsequently increased to a mean blood glucose of 300 mg/dl, fibrinogen kinetics shortened again. These observations have definite therapeutic implications for the person with diabetes who undergoes intraoperative or postoperative care or parturition.

OUTPATIENT STUDIES UTILIZING HOME MONITORING PROGRAMS
Since a number of pathophysiologic changes in diabetics correct if euglycemia is established in hospitalized patients, we initiated an outpatient program to determine

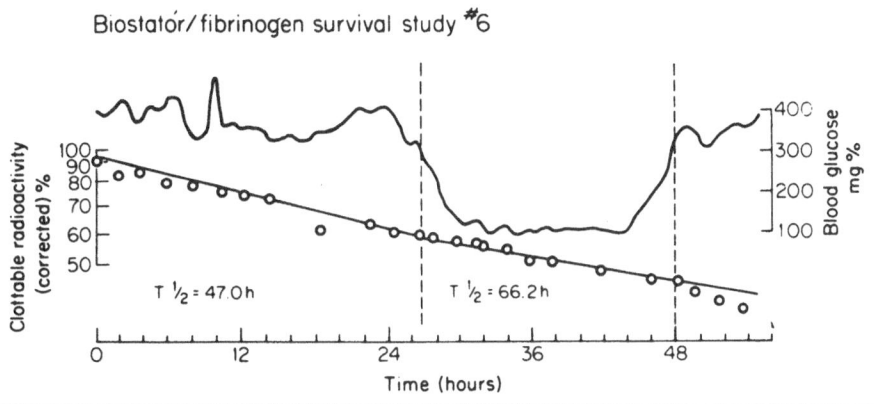

Figure 2–11. The changes in fibrinogen survival occur rapidly concomitant with changing blood glucose values. The clottable radioactivity values have been corrected for vascular volume shifts by red cell labelling techniques.

whether certain variables might improve over a longer period of glucose control. Measurement of glycemic control was performed by patient-monitored blood glucose determinations before and one hour after meals as had been performed in the hospital, and hemoglobin Alc levels were performed monthly. As shown in figure 2–12, hemoglobin Alc levels and mean blood glucose levels dropped markedly during the period of observation. In addition, there was a good correla-

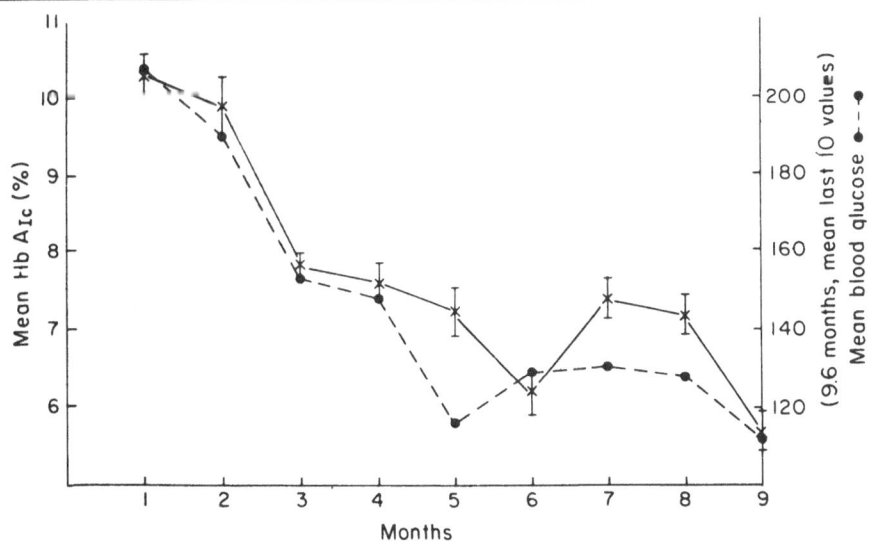

Figure 2–12. Changes in hemoglobin Alc values and blood glucose values over time in the outpatient department in 10 patients placed on a program of home blood glucose monitoring and self-adjusted calibrated insulin administration (Peterson et al., Diabetes Care, 2:329–335, 1979; with permission).

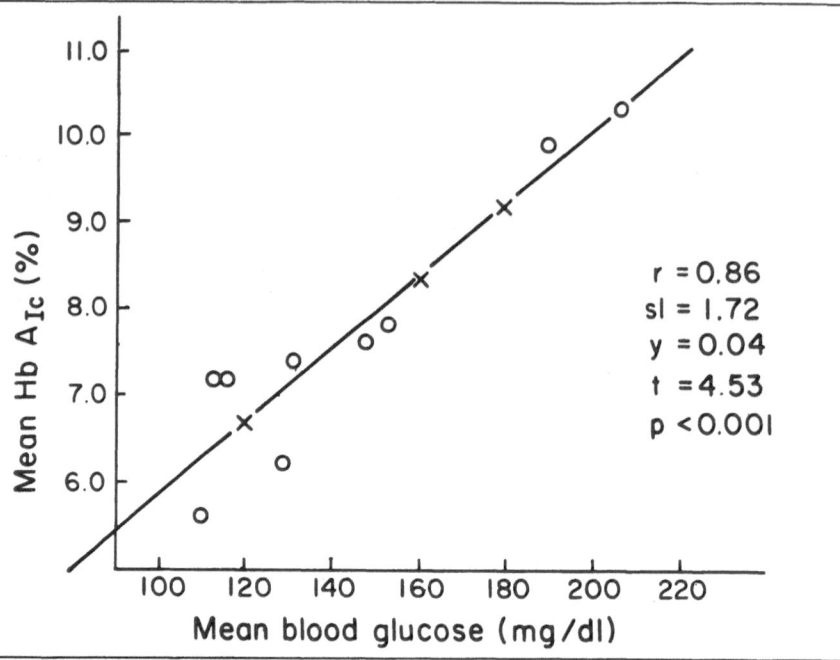

Figure 2–13. Correlation of hemoglobin Alc and mean blood glucose. As can be seen, a mean blood glucose of 200 mg/dl (11.1 nM) corresponds to a hemoglobin Alc value of about 10% (ml 3–6%) (Peterson et al., Diabetes Care, 2:329–335, 1979; with permission).

tion between the two variables as shown in figure 2–13. The regimen, in addition to home glucose monitoring and a split-dose insulin delivery system, demanded rigorous exercise consisting of 30 minutes of cardiovascular-type exercise performed under the supervision of a trainer three times per week. Compliance for this exercise program over the 10 months of observation was 86%. Within three months of starting this program (figure 2–14), systolic blood pressure significantly decreased in the group. There was an associated increase in ankle pressures as measured by pulse volume recordings and a marked increase in the ankle arm index for the group. This increase in flow was actually accompanied by an increase in vascular compliance as reflected by the decreasing ankle pressure curves.

Quadriceps capillary basement membrane thickening was measured at the beginning and after approximately 10 months of observation. In each patient in whom successful biopsy could be obtained, basement membrane thickening decreased except for one patient who was unable to maintain her hemoglobin Alc levels below 10% (table 2–1).

Other variables also corrected with improved blood glucose control. Sensory and motor nerve conduction values improved in the group, and there was a 50% normalization of nerve conduction abnormalities by nine months of followup. Alkaline phosphatase values were slightly elevated at the beginning of the study but corrected to normal during the course of the study (figure 2–15).

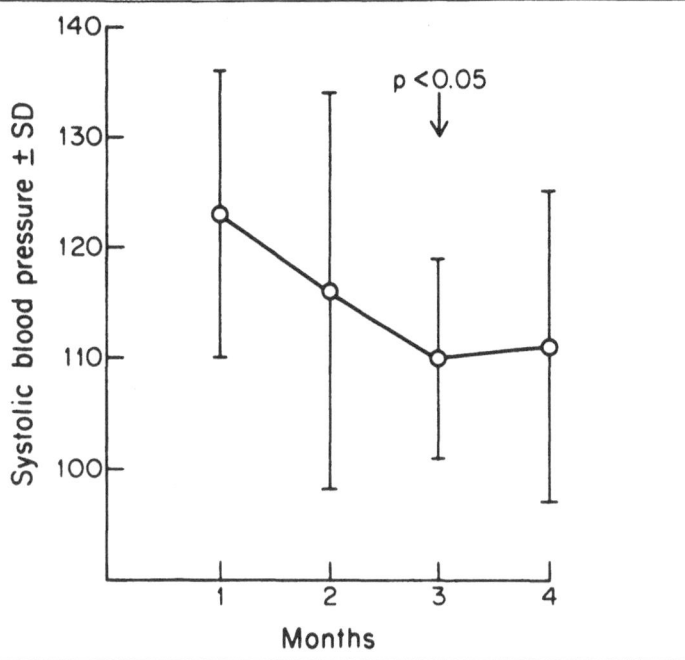

Figure 2–14. Fall in systolic arm pressure following the institution of a program of home glucose monitoring and improved, calibrated, self-administered subcutaneous insulin administration and exercise (from Diabetes Care; with permission).

One of the more striking observations during the course of the study was the high degree of depression found in patients entering the program. Table 2–2 demonstrates depression as measured by the Hamilton Rating Scale for depression versus hemoglobin Alc levels on entry into the program. Several of the patients were significantly depressed as reflected by Hamilton Rating Scale values of 20 or greater. It was also noteworthy that there was a correlation between hemoglobin Alc levels and the Hamilton Rating Scale for depression ($r^2 = 0.7$). This observation raises the question of whether glucose levels per se may influence mood or affect. Although many patients enrolling in the program were clinically depressed, this did not prevent their participation in the program which improved both their hemoglobin Alc levels and their followup evaluations for depression. These observations suggest that rather than being a contraindication to an intensive management regimen, depression may be an indication for an intensive management program.

STUDIES IN PREGNANCY
Perhaps one of the best models for evaluating the role of elevated glucose levels in the secondary problems associated with diabetes is the diabetic pregnant women. Figure 2–16 shows the correlation between mean blood glucose during pregnancy

Table 2–1. Muscle biopsy following euglycemia

Patient no.	Age (yr)	Duration diabetes (yr)	Basement membrane thickening (Å)	SD	Coefficient of variation	HbA$_{1c}$ (%)	Patient mean HbA$_{1c}$ (%)	SD HbA$_{1c}$
1 (M), initial	23	11	1618.3	±587	36	11.9	9.14	±3.06
10 mo			884.5	±192	21	7.4		
3 (M), initial	16	02	1331.0	±228	24	8.6	6.75	±1.98
8 mo			767.9	±132	17	4.4		
4 (F), initial	21	08	1094.2	±615	56	10.6	7.94	±2.28
10 mo			942.0	±200	21	6.4		
5 (F), initial	26	01	756.0	±114	15	9.9	7.63	±2.49
10 mo			731.0	±233	31	6.5		
7 (F), initial	19	05	868.0	±193	22	9.8	8.45	±2.38
10 mo			746.8	±256	24	4.4		
8 (F), initial	37	18	1648.9	±1088	66	8.1	5.79	±2.18
10 mo			803.5	±100	12	2.3		
10 (F), initial	19	02	1071.0	±221	26	11.3	10.90	±2.25
9 mo			1584.5	±604	38	10.2		
Normal (N = 95)			824	±125		3–6%		

and infant morbidity from a number of studies performed in the insulin era. The correlation is striking. Also noteworthy in this model system is the fact that the X — intercept is at 84 mg/dl or the normal mean blood glucose for the normal pregnant person. Therefore, it would appear from these data that even minimal glucose elevation portends an increase in infant mortality.

The hormonal profiles of early gestation have been shown to be abnormally low

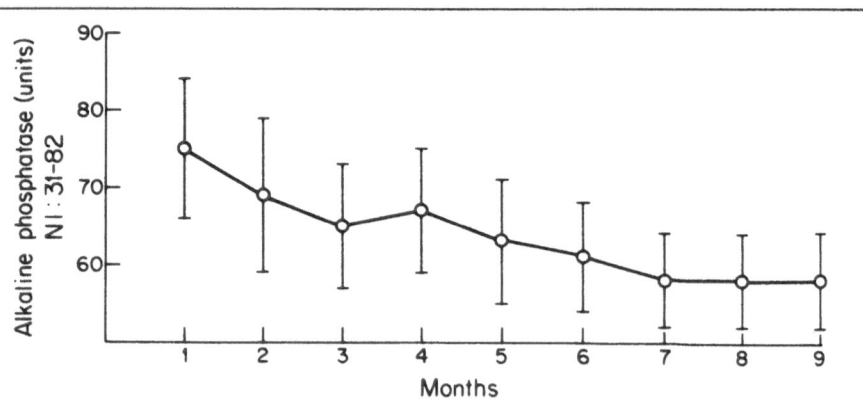

Figure 2–15. Decrease in serum alkaline phosphatase values over time during the same program (Peterson et al., Diabetes Care 2:329–335, 1979; with permission).

in diabetic women who are hyperglycemic. Prolactin, estradiol, and human chorionic gonadotrophic levels will correct to normal in these women if blood glucose levels are corrected as well (figures 2–16 & 2–17).

It has recently been shown that infant morbidity associated with maternal diabetes such as hypoglycemia, hypocalcemia, hyperbilirubinemia, respiratory distress, and macrosomia can be eliminated if blood glucose levels are maintained within the normal range during gestation. Thus, it appears that the glucose molecule itself is a teratogen and toxin during gestation, and that these deleterious effects are eliminated if euglycemia is maintained in the diabetic pregnant women.

The studies cited above indicate a number of variables associated with hyperglycemia not only may be amenable to prevention but also may be reversible if therapeutic intervention is initiated at an early stage. Certain hematologic abnormalities, biochemical parameters, and variables associated with microvascular and macrovascular disease have been documented to improve in programs of improved glucose control and exercise. Whether there is a critical threshold below which a given patient can be reassured that his glucose control is adequate to prevent diabetic sequelae is a question that remains unanswered. Many abnormalities appear to be corrected at glucose levels which are still somewhat in excess of euglycemia. Nevertheless, others may not be corrected, and therefore the present aim of therapeutics should be establish normoglycemia inasmuch as it is possible. Certainly during pregnancy, normal glucose levels must be maintained or pathological consequences appear likely.

Table 2–2. Hamilton depression scores and hemoglobin A1c levels

	At onset of study		After 8 months	
Patient	Depression scores[1]	Hb A1c[2]	Depression scores	Hb A1c[2]
		(%)		(%)
1	36	11.9	22	4.3
2	35	15.0	21	9.4
3	30	11.0	16	3.5
4	24	8.1	18	4.4
5	19	11.3	4	6.9
6	16	9.8	6	5.7
7	16	10.6	4	5.2
8	14	9.9	7	4.8
9	10	6.5	2	4.2
10	7	8.6	2	6.0
Mean	20.7[3]	10.3	10.2[3]	5.4

1. Total score obtained by adding individual scores of each of the 19 items. Total score < 10 is nonsignificant.
2. Hemoglobin A1c (Hb A1c) levels represent percent of total hemoglobin. Normal values: 3%–6%.
3. Depression scores at the start and after eight months differ statistically, $P < .005$ by paired f-test, one tailed.

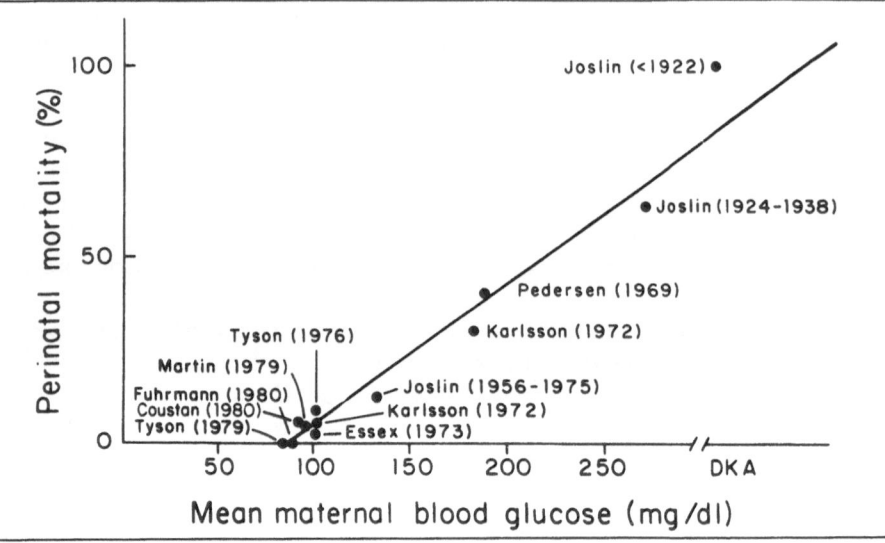

Figure 2–16. A review of the results of pregnancy in diabetics since the introduction of insulin. The horizontal axis represents mean maternal blood glucose level reported for pregnant women in each series. The vertical axis represents perinatal mortality.

STEPS TO DIABETIC CONTROL, MEASUREMENTS OF INTEREST

Blood glucose:

Urine testing is an inadequate means of clinical assessment in the management of diabetics. Furthermore, in the uremic diabetic, urine testing is totally unreliable. Therefore, to manage a diabetic patient optimally, reliance must rest on the blood glucose. Home glucose monitoring programs have been successful in aiding both patient and physician in diabetic control. Patients can be taught to obtain a drop of blood by fingerstick and to test the blood glucose level with the use of visual strips or a reflectance meter. It is recommended that patients check their blood glucose in the fasting state, just before and one hour after meals and at 3 A.M., until adjustments in treatment have been made. After that, and as long as glucose control is stable, individualized schedules are continued. In general, glucose levels of 50–150 mg/dl are acceptable.

HEMOGLOBIN ALC

Measurements of hemoglobin Alc (HbAlc) have been found to correlate well with mean serum glucose determinations over time, thus providing an excellent tool for the evaluation of long-term control of diabetes. HbAlc is one of several minor adducts of HbA. HbAlc is formed from HbA by the addition of a molecule of glucose to the N-terminal valine of one or both of the B chains. HbAlc is formed at a rate dependent on the glucose concentration to which the erythrocyte is exposed. Although HbAlc comprises 3–6% of the total hemoglobin in normal

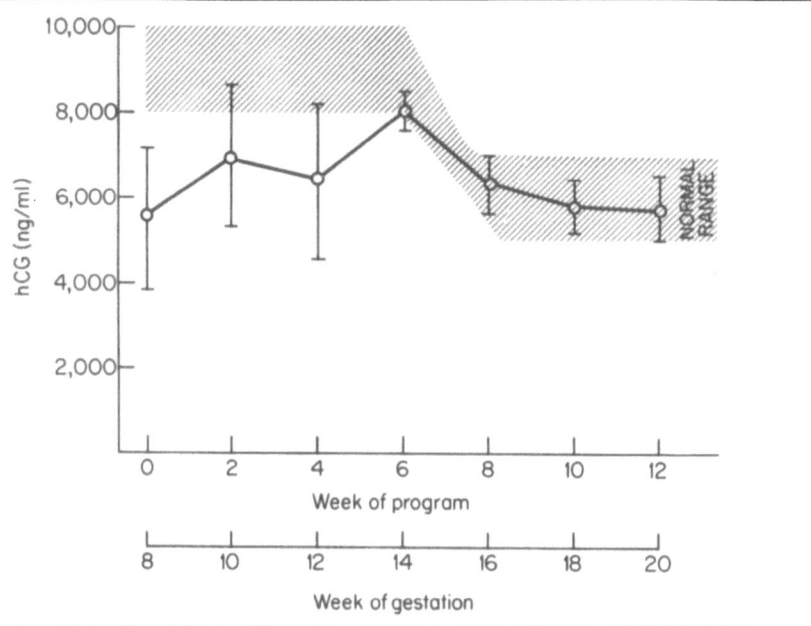

Figure 2–17. Human chorionicgonadotropin (hCG) levels in 10 insulin-dependent diabetics at the start of a program to normalize blood glucose level. The time course of normalization of hCG is shown. The hatched area represents 596 normal control patients (Reprinted with permission from Amer J Med 68:105–112, 1980).

persons, it generally accounts for over 6% of the hemoglobin in patients with diabetes. Therefore, a low HbAlc value (closer or equal to that of the normal control—3% to 6%) would reflect excellent glucose control over the last 120 days (the average lifetime of the human erythrocyte). Conversely, high HbAlc levels would reflect poor glucose control over the last several weeks. A HbAlc level should be obtained initially and within four weeks after implementation of home blood glucose monitoring. Thereafter, HbAlc levels are monitored monthly, or as indicated, in order to follow up the degree of long-term glucose control.

In the uremic patient, however, interpretations of levels of modified hemoglobin components are complicated by the presence of a shortened red-cell life span and the need for transfusions in hemodialyzed patients. In uremia both HbAlc and HbAl levels have been reported to be elevated or decreased. Furthermore, in uremic patients HbAlc levels have been found not to correlate as well with glucose levels. It has been suggested that in addition to measuring hemoglobin glycosylation one could measure hemoglobin carbamylation which permits assessment of the uremic state in a way analogous to the use of hemoglobin glycosylation to monitor glycemia in nonuremic patients. Measurement of glycosylated albumin or serum proteins may prove to be a more useful means of monitoring glycemia in the uremic individual since these proteins do not have altered turnover in uremia, and their measurement relies on structural rather than physical principles of analysis.

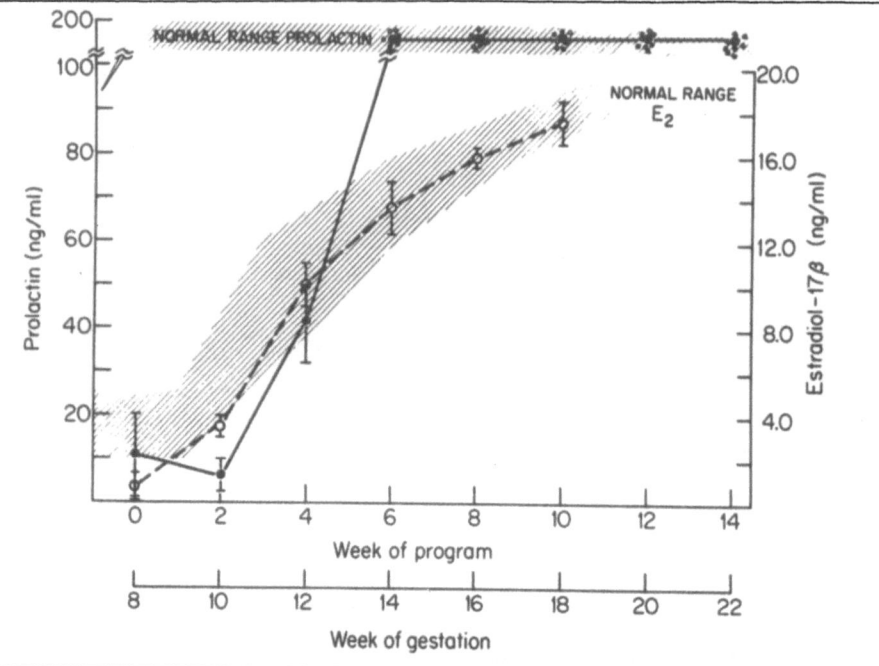

Figure 2–18. Estradiol and prolactin levels in the same subjects shown in figure 2–17. The hatched area represents the normal range for both estradiol and prolactin compared to the same controls used in figure 2–17 (Reprinted with permission from Amer J Med 68:105–112, 1980).

Lipids

Diabetes is estimated to double the risk of arteriosclerotic-related events, and as a result, 75% of deaths in diabetics are believed to be due to macrovascular disease. One risk factor appears to involve high cholesterol levels. Elevation of very low–density lipoproteins (VLDL) and their major lipid component—triglycerides —is a frequent finding in hyperglycemic diabetics. Strict diabetic control reduces both plasma triglycerides and cholesterol with subsequent increase in high–density lipoproteins (HDL). It is advisable, therefore, that all diabetic patients have plasma cholesterol, triglyceride, and HDL determinations during their initial assessment and at three-month intervals after the initiation of a glucose control program. If these variables should remain elevated, then more specific treatment should be considered.

Cardiovascular status

Many studies have shown that exercise in the diabetic results in improved glucose tolerance, a normalization of serum lipids, and a normalization of work capacities. The possibility of cardiovascular disease should be assessed in the routine evaluation of patients with diabetes. Exercise testing may be useful. With the exception of hypertensive patients, most type I and type II diabetics have an intact response to physical stress. Exercise electrocardiogram (EKG) testing may, therefore, define the patients with reduced cardiovascular reserve and at the same time provide guidelines for initiation of a cardiovascular training program.

MODES OF TREATMENT

Type II diabetes mellitus

Endogenous insulin production can be assessed by measuring C-peptide levels in diabetic patients even if they are injecting exogenous insulin. If the C-peptide level is found to be normal or high, the patient can be placed on a diet (weight-reducing or isocaloric) and exercise protocol. If, after a period of four to six weeks, normalization of blood glucose levels has not been achieved, oral hypoglycemic agents may be added. If the patient still shows no or an insufficient response in two to four weeks, then insulin therapy should be initiated.

At present the oral agents available include only the sulfonylureas with the general chemical structure represented below:

$$R_1 \langle 0 \rangle SO_2 - NH - \underset{\underset{0}{\parallel}}{C} - NH - R_2$$

The potency of these agents is modified depending on the lipid solubility of the substitutions at R_1 and R_2, but the mechanism of action remains essentially the same. These drugs lower blood glucose initially by increasing insulin output in response to a given glucose stimulus. Their mechanism of action appears to alternate with time and becomes supplemented by an enhancement of insulin action at the cell receptor or postreceptor levels.

Hence, oral sulfonylurea administration is associated with lower blood glucose levels if there is sufficient insulin present in the bloodstream. Most sulfonylureas are relatively equivalent in their toxic/therapeutic ratio, although chlorpropamide may exhibit a worrisome antidiuretic hormone-like effect with water retention. The differences between agents lies more with relative potency or duration of action.

Upon initiating oral hypoglycemic treatment, the physician should have previously documented pancreatic reserve and warned the patient of the following: (1) oral drug treatment may not work and hence insulin may still be necessary; (2) hypoglycemia may occur at unpredictable times; and (3) blood lipid (risk factors for vascular disease) may not correct despite a drop in blood glucose levels.

The patient is instructed to measure blood glucose before and after meals. If normal values are achieved within one week, glucose values are then measured at 3 A.M. Drug dose is adjusted until normal values of blood glucose are achieved, or when it is apparent that blood glucose is not responding to the oral agent (two to four weeks) and insulin therapy is required.

Type i diabetes mellitus

These patients have low or absent endogenous insulin production as reflected by low C-peptide levels. Exogenous insulin is the appropriate therapy. Different types of insulin delivery systems are discussed below.

INSULIN DELIVERY SYSTEMS

The normal state

The goal of management of the diabetic patient is normalization of blood glucose with total correction of all metabolic abnormalities. "Normal" insulin production is usually defined by the profile of peripheral plasma insulin concentration observed throughout the day. Such peripheral venous insulin profiles, however, reflect only a fraction of the original amount secreted by the pancreas, since a large proportion of insulin is removed from the portal circulation by the liver. It is quite difficult to simulate normal insulin delivery by subcutaneous, intramuscular, or intravenous administration, which cannot achieve higher portal vein levels than those attained peripherally. Of all methods of insulin delivery, only the intraperitoneal route may achieve normal portal levels of insulin, while avoiding excessive peripheral levels. This approach, for the present, is experimental.

NPH/regular insulin—three-injection schedule

This is our favorite insulin scheme at the moment since it can readily be calculated and appears to be successful in most patients. Initial total 24-hour insulin requirements for nonpregnant patients with Type I diabetes are calculated at 0.6 units/kg/24 hr. Pregnant patients are begun on a dose of insulin which is based not only on present pregnant body weight but also the gestational week of the pregnancy. The insulin requirement is 0.7 units/kg for the first 18 wks, 0.8 units/kg for weeks 18–26, 0.9 units/kg for weeks 26–36, and 1.0 u/kg for weeks 36–41. In the case of progressive renal failure, the total insulin requirement per 24 hours remains at the expected requirement for metabolic needs (growth, pregnancy, stress) until the creatinine clearance drops below 30 ml/min. The insulin requirement is then divided into three injections whose peak levels are timed to cover three meals and three snacks. Two-thirds of the total daily insulin dose is given in the morning. Two-thirds of the morning dose—or, in other words, $8/18$ of the total daily dose—is given in the form of NPH insulin; the remaining one-third of the morning dose—$4/18$ of the daily total—is given in the form of regular insulin. This fractioning of the total dose is shown in table 2–3. One-sixth of the total dose is given before dinner as regular insulin, and the final one-sixth before bedtime as NPH insulin. Further individual adjustments are almost always necessary.

The regimen shown in table 2–4 can serve as a guideline by which adjustments can be made. Momentary blood glucose rises are normalized by the adjustment protocol shown in table 2–5. This allows calibration of insulin dosage according to insulin needs at the moment. Each patient should be encouraged to determine

Table 2–3. Insulin dose distribution when beginning insulin therapy

	Total insulin requirement/24 h = I		
	8:30 A.M.	5:00 P.M.	11:00 P.M.
NPH	8/18 I		3/18 I
Regular	4/18 I	3/18 I	
or	2/3 I	1/6 I	1/6 I

Table 2–4. Insulin titration procedure

1. Fix fasting blood glucose. If fasting blood glucose is > 100 mg/dl, add 2 units of NPH to bedtime dose of NPH. If fasting blood glucose is < 60 mg/dl, decrease bedtime NPH by 2 units.
2. Normalize 10 A.M. blood glucose. If 10 A.M. blood glucose is > 140 mg/dl today, add 2 units of regular to the 7:30 A.M. injection of regular.
3. Normalize 4:30 P.M. blood glucose. If 10 A.M. blood glucose is > 100 mg/dl, add 2 units of NPH to 7:30 A.M. dose of NPH. If 4:30 P.M. blood glucose is < 60, decrease the 7:30 A.M. dose of NPH by 2 units.
4. Normalize 6:30 P.M. blood glucose. If 6:30 P.M. blood glucose is > 140 mg/dl today, add 2 units of regular to 4:30 P.M. injection of regular.

Table 2–5. How to make an immediate correction of abnormal blood glucose

7:30 A.M. and 4:30 P.M. doses of regular insulin should be given according to the following sliding scale:

7:30 A.M.

glucose < 100 = calculated dose of regular ($4/18$ I_R)
100–140 = calculated + 2 units regular ($4/18$ I_R + 2)
> 140 = calculated + 4 units regular ($4/18$ I_R + 4)

4:30 P.M.

glucose < 100 = calculated dose of regular ($3/18$ I_R)
100–140 = calculated + 2 units regular ($3/18$ I_R + 2)
> 140 = calculated + 4 units regular ($3/18$ I_R + 4)

If the blood glucose is ever > 140 mg/dl, the next meal or snack should not be eaten until the blood glucose is less than 100 mg/dl. Insulin should be taken as usual. No insulin other than the dose shown above should be added.

how much a given unit of insulin lowers blood glucose from a given level. From two to four units of regular insulin can be added at times of hyperglycemia to lower blood glucose acutely. Should such extra doses of regular insulin be required for more than two days in a row, then appropriate changes in NPH dosage may be required. NPH insulin injected in the morning determines the 4 P.M. blood glucose level, and NPH injected at night determines the morning blood glucose level. It has been found most helpful to deal with and "conquer" the fasting blood glucose level first, since once this is normalized, the remaining levels tend to stabilize more readily. If lunch remains a problem with postprandial elevated blood glucose, then the procedure outlined in table 2–6 is employed.

Ultralente/regular system

Some physicians prefer to use long-acting ultralente insulin to cover metabolic needs and regular insulin to cover meals. In this case, the basal need or insulin requirement while fasting (0.4u/kg/24 hours) is given as ultralente. One-third of the ultralente dose is given before breakfast and two-thirds before dinner. Regular insulin to cover meals is given as 0.12 u/kg before breakfast, 0.1 units/kg before lunch, and 0.1 u/kg before dinner. In most cases, these insulin doses will have to be titrated according to the individual needs of the patient and to the meal pattern selected based on blood glucose measurements.

MATCHING INSULIN TO FOOD AND BLOOD GLUCOSE

Once insulin is adjusted to an appropriate range and variations in levels of blood glucose are minimized, patients can be told to adjust their diet in a way to help keep these levels normal. The optimal dose of regular insulin for the patient with renal insufficiency matches the carbohydrate content of the meal about to be consumed. Although total insulin requirements may be less than the needs of a patient without severe renal insufficiency, insulin still should be injected 30–45 minutes before the meal. The lag time for insulin to peak is not altered in renal failure because the onset and peak of insulin is not changed; it is only the duration of insulin which is prolonged. For example, if the preprandial blood glucose level is > 120 mg/dl, the patient is asked to postpone a meal until the blood glucose is lowered to 120 mg/dl following the preprandial insulin dose. In addition, patients learn to estimate the amount of regular insulin needed to cover a given food intake. In general 1.5 units/10 Gm ingested carbohydrate are required at breakfast, and 1.0 unit/10 Gm ingested carbohydrate at lunch and dinner.

PREVENTION OF HYPOGLYCEMIA

It is important for each patient to have a protocol for preventing hypoglycemia. Blood glucose should be documented before hypoglycemia is treated. We use milk as the primary treatment for hypoglycemia. Patients are taught to respond to blood glucose values of less than 70 mg/dl; at this level 240 ml or 8 oz of whole milk is consumed (150 kcal). The patient waits 15 minutes and rechecks the blood glucose. If the blood glucose is greater than 70, then the daily routine can be continued; if the blood glucose is still less than 70, then another 8-oz glass of milk is consumed, and the blood glucose is measured again 15 minutes thereafter. If this is not successful, the patient may then consume another glass of milk and a bread exchange (15 grams carbohydrate). The bread is included for psychological reasons,

Table 2–6. Normalizing postlunch blood glucose

If, one hour after lunch, the blood glucose is > 140 either (1) decrease the carbohydrate content of the lunch or (2) add a prelunch injection of regular insulin.

---

since a patient will very rarely need three glasses of milk to correct any given hypoglycemic episode. Other foods may be calibrated in an analogous fashion, and patients will wish to calibrate other foods that are more portable than milk. However, milk is useful because it contains not only carbohydrate but also fat and protein, which will maintain blood glucose for a longer time than a simple carbohydrate. All patients and their families should be instructed on the use of glucagon. A subcutaneous injection of 0.15 mg of glucagon elevates blood glucose levels 30–40 mg/dl within 20 minutes and will maintain blood glucose levels for about three hours.

EXERCISE

Exercise has long been recognized and recommended as integral to the management of diabetes. Every uremic patient entering an exercise program should be pretested in order to determine their level of cardiovascular conditioning, flexibility, and strength training. Unless medically contraindicated, an optimum program would be a supervised exercise session three times a week, including a period of cardiovascular conditioning lasting for at least 20 minutes, during which the heart rate is kept at 70% of the maximum predicted rate. Such a program should be reevaluated after about 6–10 weeks. Improvement can be documented and the patient given psychological reinforcement and reports of improvements in laboratory tests and in the physical examination.

Patients should be warned, however, that exercise-induced hypoglycemia may occur due to the potentiation of insulin-mediated suppression of hepatic glucose production. This complication may be avoided by: (1) increasing carbohydrate intake before exercise; (2) exercising at times that do not overlap with peak periods of insulin action; (3) using nonexercised injection sites; and (4) lowering insulin dose when necessary.

SPECIAL CONSIDERATIONS/PROBLEM SITUATIONS
Menstrual irregularities

Most women find that the insulin requirement increases just prior to the onset of the menstrual period. The timing of this increase may change from individual to individual, as may the amount of insulin required. But once this increased need is documented, it tends to repeat itself each cycle. It has also been our experience that menses are more regular once normoglycemia is achieved; therefore, with time, the onset of menses and the change in insulin requirements become more predictable.

Viral syndromes, nausea, vomiting, and fasting

One of the benefits of self-monitoring of blood glucose is that a patient need not be hospitalized for nausea, vomiting, or the inability to eat. As a rule, blood glucose levels will tend to increase with illness of any kind. If, however, the patient is on an infusion system or a monitored, calculated insulin system, the basal insulin dosage can be covered by long-acting insulin or low-dosage continuous infusion. A constant infusion of about 0.3 units/kg/24 hr generally maintains normoglycemia without the ingestion of calories. Calculated insulin can be used in the same manner. The calculated dose of NPH to carry the patient through the night (as delineated above) can be given every eight hours; most patients will maintain euglycemia with this regimen.

Patients can be encouraged to monitor their blood glucose and may take regular insulin in small doses at three- to four-hour intervals or as needed to lower glucose to 100 mg/dl. This will ensure that patients do not develop ketoacidosis and that they avoid hypoglycemia. This approach is also useful for hospitalized, presurgical patients. An intravenous solution may be administered at the rate of about 100 ml per hour. If the blood glucose is less than 100 mg/dl, the solution should be 5% dextrose in water. If the blood glucose is greater than 120 mg/dl, the solution should be normal physiologic saline; and if the blood glucose is less than 80 mg/dl, then the solution should be 10% dextrose in water. In general, most patients require normal saline or 5% dextrose in water if the insulin has been administered by one of the above systems. Blood glucose levels should be monitored every hour in the preoperative or postoperative situation.

INSULIN REQUIREMENTS IN RENAL FAILURE
During renal insufficiency, insulin, C-peptide, and proinsulin are elevated 2.5-, 4.9-, and 7.5-fold, respectively, probably because of decreased clearance and increased secretion accompanied by insulin resistance. Insulin secretion in nondialyzed uremic patients is higher than in dialyzed patients. Secondary hyperparathroidism associated with renal insufficiency has been associated with enhanced insulin secreting responses thought to be due to elevated calcium levels, since normocalcemic patients secrete less insulin than hypercalcemic individuals.

As kidney failure progresses, it is not unusual for a decrease in insulin dose to be noted because of diminished catabolism of endogenous and exogenous insulin by diseased kidneys. After diabetic patients begin maintenance hemodialysis, daily insulin requirements nearly double and a single dose of long-acting insulin alone will not afford satisfactory control. Better control is achieved with a split-dose insulin regimen. We observed a young type I diabetic patient who had undergone a successful cadaveric renal transplant and was well controlled on a constant insulin infusion pump with a steady daily insulin requirement, who suddenly had frequent hypoglycemic attacks. No apparent reason for this glucose level change was found until one month later when his transplant showed signs of rejection with renal function deterioration and its eventual surgical removal. Thus, a decrease in insulin requirements may be the first sign of clinically inapparent renal function deterioration presumably because of decreased clearance of insulin.

PSYCHOLOGICAL ASPECTS
Diabetes mellitus is a chronic disease that confronts the patient on a daily basis with the constant attention to disease management, as well as the threat of the long-term complications. The behavioral responses to diabetes encompass a wide spectrum, ranging from overwhelming preoccupation with the details of treatment, to com-

plete denial and disregard, leading to poor control and its consequences. The latter pattern of behavior is more commonly observed in the adolescent diabetic. It should be noted, however, that within this response range one finds a large number of patients who attain a satisfactory balance between the therapeutic requirements of diabetes and the demands and satisfactions of everyday life.

Programs of self-monitoring of blood glucose allow interesting observations regarding patient adjustment to their disease and this treatment method. Initially, patients are upset and overwhelmed by the task. However, as they achieve successes along the way, they become increasingly confident and less dependent on physicians and health professionals. This phase is accompanied by a shift from an external locus of control and dependence to an internal locus of control, with increased self-reliance and decreased depression (decreased helplessness and hopelessness).

In our study, a correlation was found at the beginning of the program with blood glucose levels, reflected by hemoglobin Alc determinations, and depression evaluation reflected by the Hamilton Rating Scale for depression. When patients initiated a program of home blood glucose monitoring, their mood improved with the improvement in blood glucose. The symptoms of depression that were most accentuated in patients with diabetes and that showed the most improvement with the home glucose monitoring program included somatic and psychic anxiety, hypochondrias, worthlessness, insomnia, and those symptoms related to work and activities.

The situation of the diabetic patient with end-stage renal disease is more complex. Avram and others have shown that the rate of suicidal behavior among dialysis patients is higher than the suicide rate in the normal population. Similarly the suicide rate appears much higher than normal among transplant patients. Diabetic patients are likely to have many handicaps at the time that they require dialysis. Simonds reported that poorly controlled diabetic patients have an increased frequency of anxiety and depression as well as both intrapersonal and nonintrapersonal conflicts when compared with a group of well-controlled diabetic patients. As these patients experience greater expectations and aspirations for an improved lifestyle following transplantation, they become vulnerable to severe and sometimes suicidal depression if there is subsequent failure of the transplant. Thus it seems that well-controlled diabetic patients may be able to accept the added burden of renal care more easily, and once offered with a successful kidney transplant, they may be able to enjoy a better lifestyle with the hope of ultimately avoiding the development of diabetic nephropathy in the transplant.

SELECTED BIBLIOGRAPHY

1. Abram HS, Moore GL, Westervelt FB. Suicidal behavior in chronic dialysis patients. Am J Psych 127:1199–1207, 1971.
2. Amair P. Khanna R, Leibel B, et al. Continuous ambulatory peritoneal dialysis in diabetics with end stage renal disease. N Engl J Med 306:225–330, 1982.
3. Avram MM. Natural history of diabetic renal failure and paradoxical insulin requirements in uremia. In: Diabetic Renal-Retinal Syndrome, Friedman EA, L'Esperance FA (eds). New York: Grune and Stratton, 1980, p. 175.

4. Cahill FG, McDevitt HD. Insulin–dependent diabetes mellitus: the initial lesion. N Engl J Med 304:1454–1465, 1981.
5. Dupuis A. Assessment of the psychological factors and responses in self-managed patients. Diabetes Care 3:117–120, 1980.
6. Dupuis A, Jones RL, Peterson CM. Psychological effects of a program of strict carbohydrate control through self-monitored blood glucose determinations on insulin dependent diabetics. Psychosomatics 21:581–591, 1981.
7. Eaton RP, Schade DS. "Normal" human insulin secretion: the goal of management of the diabetic patient. In: Diabetes Management in the 80's, Peterson CM (ed). Philadelphia: Praeger, 1982, pp. 82–89.
8. Fluckiger R, Harmon W. Meier W, et al. Hemoglobin carbamylation in uremia. N Engl J Med 304:823–827, 1981.
9. Guthrow CE, Morris MA, Day JF, et al. Enchanced non-enzymatic glycosylation of human serum albumin in diabetes mellitus. Proc Nat Acad Sci 76:4258–4261, 1979.
10. Jovanovic L, Peterson CM. The clinical utility of glycosylated hemoglobin. Am J Med 70:-331–338, 1981.
11. Knowles HC. Magnitude of the renal failure problem in diabetic patients. Kidney Int. 6 (Suppl. 1):2–7, 1974.
12. Levin ME, Bonink I, Anderson B, Avioli LV. Prevention and treatment of diabetic complications. Arch Intern Med 140:691–696, 1980.
13. McVerry BA, Hopp A, Fisher C, Huehns ER. Production of pseudodiabetic renal glomerular changes in mice after repeated injections of glucosylated proteins. Lancet 1:738–740, 1980.
14. National Diabetes Data Group. Classification and diagnosis of diabetes mellitus and other categories of glucose intolerance. Diabetes 28:1039–1057, 1979.
15. Peterson CM (ed). Proceedings of a conference on non-enzymatic glycosylation and browning reactions: their relevance to diabetes mellitus. Diabetes 31 (Suppl. 3): 1982.
16. Peterson CM, Jones RL. Minor hemoglobins, diabetic "control" and diseases of postsynthetic protein modification. Annals Int Med 87:489–491, 1977.
17. Peterson CM, Jones RL, Esterly JA, et al. Changes in basement membrane thickening and pulse volume concomitant with improved glucose control and exercise in patients with insulin-dependent diabetes mellitus. Diabetes Care 3:586–589, 1980.
18. Peterson CM, Jones RL, Koenig RJ, et al. Reversible hematologic sequelae of diabetes mellitus. Ann Intern Med 86:425–429, 1977.
19. Peterson CM, Jones RL, Koenig RJ, Melvin ET, Lehrman ML. Reversible hematologic sequelae of diabetes mellitus. Ann Intern Med 86:359–364, 1977.
20. Peterson CM, Koenig RJ, Jones RL, Saudek CD, Cerami A. Correlation of serum triglyceride levels and hemoglobin Alc concentrations in diabetes mellitus. Diabetes 26:507–509, 1977.
21. Pickup JC, Keen H, Viberti GC, Bilons RW. Patient reactions to long-term outpatient treatment with continuous subcutaneous insulin infusion. Br Med J 282:347–350, 1981.
22. Pietri A, Dunn F, Raskin P. The effect of improved diabetic control on plasma lipid and lipoprotein levels: a comparison of conventional therapy and continuous subcutaneous insulin infusion. Diabetes 29:1001–1005, 1980.
23. Rupp WM, Barbosa JJ, Blackshear PJ, et al. The use of an implantable insulin pump in the treatment of type II diabetes. N Engl J Med 307:265–270, 1982.
24. Saltin B, Lindgarde F, Houston M, Horlin R, et al. Physical training and glucose tolerance in middle-aged men with chemical diabetes. Diabetes 28 (Suppl 30): 1979.
25. Stein RA, Goldberg N, Lundin P, Kapelners, Rubin J. Exercise EKG testing in diabetic patients. In: Diabetic Renal-Retinal Syndrome, Friedman EA, L'Esperance FA (eds). New York: Grune and Stratton, 1980, pp 229–237.
26. Tamborlane WV, Sherwin RS, Genel M, Felig P. Outpatient treatment of juvenile-onset diabetes with a preprogrammed portable subcutaneous insulin infusion system. Am J Med 68:190–196, 1980.
27. Tchorbroutsky G. Relation of diabetic control to development of microvascular complications. Diabetologia 15:143–152, 1978.
28. West KM. Epidemiology of diabetes and its vascular lesions. New York: Elsevier, 1978, p. 357.

3. INSULIN PUMPS: FOR WHOM, WHEN, WHY?

CHARLES M. PETERSON
and
LOIS JOVANOVIC

In view of increasing knowledge of the function of the normal human pancreas, it is not surprising that there are now an increasing number of technical innovations that attempt to mimic pancreatic endocrine function. The normal pancreas secretes insulin constantly at a rate based on the metabolic needs of the individual. The basal rate of insulin secretion is relatively constant and comprises about one-half the total 24-hour insulin output, or about 0.3 units/kg/24 hours in the normal individual who is within 80–120% ideal body weight. The normal pancreas also senses blood glucose continuously and gives insulin or initiates counterregulatory activity depending on the absolute value of blood glucose and the rate of change of blood glucose. In addition, through neural input, the pancreas can anticipate ingestion of calories with insulin secretion so that the liver is "primed" to metabolize caloric intake. Finally, insulin is secreted in response to food based not only on the caloric and carbohydrate intake but also on the blood glucose at the moment of eating. Such a system is known as a "closed loop system" since it has the capability to sense glucose and respond appropriately. An open loop system provides only one limb of a closed loop system—either sensing glucose or infusing glucose.

CLOSED LOOP INSULIN DELIVERY

Figure 3–1 depicts the only closed loop insulin delivery system now on the market. Two varieties of this instrument are now available through Miles Laboratories, Elkhart, Indiana: the Biostator glucose-control insulin-infusion system (GCIIS)

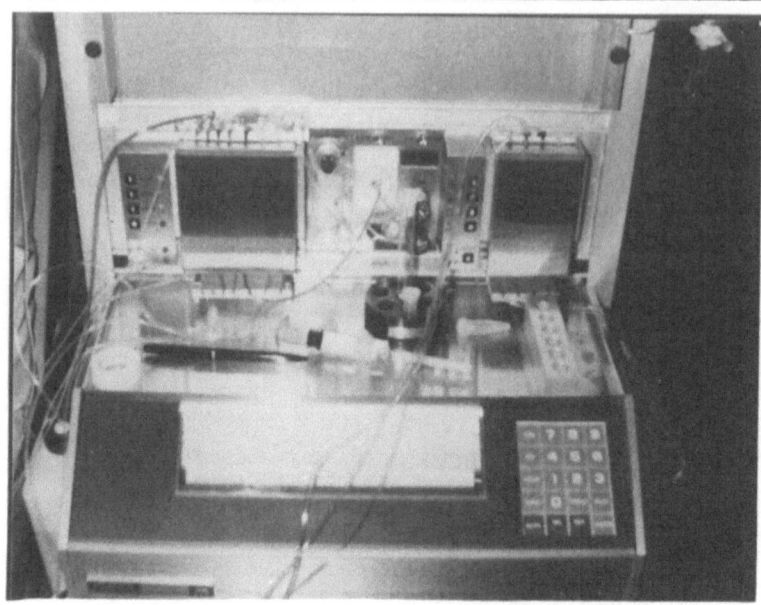

Figure 3–1. The glucose-controlled insulin infusion device (Biostator).

and the Biostator Controller. These systems rely on a set of roller pumps whereby blood is sampled and glucose, insulin, or other solution is infused. The sampling side relies on continuous sampling of blood through a double lumen catheter with continuous heparin anticoagulation in the tubing. The blood is diluted and passed through a membrane with immobilized glucose oxidase. The potential difference generated across the membrane allows the continuous measurement of blood glucose via a double lumen catheter placed in either an artery or vein. The infusion side is then programmed to infuse insulin or glucose (and/or other solutions) based on the glucose values obtained via a second in-dwelling catheter.

The GCIIS allows the operator more freedom in choosing algorithms, while the Controller is preprogrammed. The rate of blood withdrawal can be adjusted but requires 1–3 ml/hour. The time from sampling of blood to response by the machine in terms of insulin or glucose infusion adjustment is approximately 90 seconds, which compares favorably with normal pancreatic performance. These systems have been used throughout the world for over 10 years. They have been extremely useful for research and in some clinical situations. Nevertheless the systems are bulky and heavy. They are also quite expensive with the GCIIS costing about $55,000, and the Biostator Controller about $30,000. Furthermore, the systems require constant supervision by trained personnel since the lines are subject to clotting, the glucose oxidase membrane may become exhausted (they usually last about 48 hours), and the machine needs constant attention to calibration due to drift. The devices are burdensome to patients since they require access to two sources of blood (one for infusion and one for withdrawal) and require that the patient be relatively immobile for the entire run due to the short tubing, size of the equipment, and the need for an electrical source.

OPEN LOOP DEVICES

The evolution of open loop devices is summarized in figure 3–2. In the mid-1970s, it was found that improved blood glucose control for up to several days could be achieved with continuous intravenous infusions of insulin without continuous monitoring of blood glucose values. It subsequently was found that alternate routes of insulin delivery such as intraperitoneal or subcutaneous infusion could result in equally improved blood glucose values without the need for continuous vascular access. Nevertheless, the term "open loop" is something of a misnomer since even the most sanguine of investigators follows blood glucose in some manner and it is only with the advent of solid-phase reagent strip systems for glucose monitoring that it has been possible to establish surveillance systems so that open loop systems became feasible or popular.

All of the open loop infusion systems rely on the same principle. There is the capability for basal infusion at one or more rates. There is also the capability to "pulse" insulin before meals or as needed for acute insulin adjustment. To work well with an open loop system, the patient generally must be given approximately 40 hours of education to familiarize himself with the equipment, the matching of

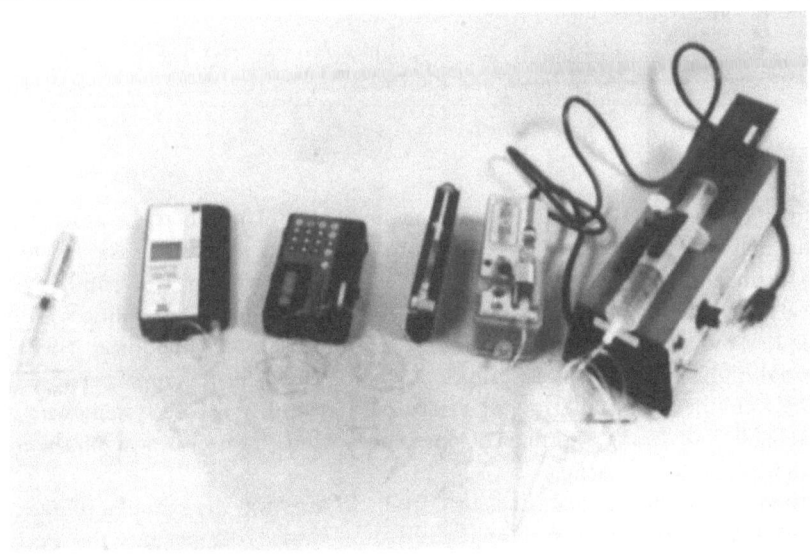

Figure 3–2. The development of the insulin infusion pump.

Table 3–1. Matching insulin with food utilizing an insulin delivery pump

---

1. Calculation of the 24–hour insulin requirement
   Total insulin requirement = (constant) × Wt in Kg
   The "constant" depends on
   a. Metabolic needs
      1. Growth
      2. Puberty
      3. Pregnancy
      4. Lactation
      5. Menses
      6. Menopause
   b. Stress needs
      1. Psychological
      2. Physical
         a. Infectious
         b. Traumatic
         c. Inflamatory
   c. Renal status
   d. Exercise program
      1. Acute
      2. Chronic
   For a normal adult male the constant = 0.6 units
2. Calculation of basal metabolic insulin requirement
   The basal need = ½ of the total insulin requirement. For the hours of 4 A.M. to
   10 A.M., a time of insulin resistance, an extra amount of insulin over the basal may
   be necessary.
3. Calculation of insulin mealtime needs.

$$\frac{[\text{total calories for day}] \times 40\%}{4\text{Kcal/gm CHO}} = \text{gm CH0 per day}$$

In general, 1.5 units of insulin are required per 10 gm. CHO at breakfast, and 1.0
unit per 10 gm CHO at lunch and dinner.

---

insulin to his metabolic condition in the steady state(s), and to be able to match
insulin delivery to food, activity, or acute changes in mood. A basic formula for
these insulin delivery systems is shown in Table 3–1. It cannot be emphasized too
strongly that the potential user of an open loop system must be willing to monitor
his or her own blood glucose at times of potential lows (including 3 A.M.) and
potential highs in order that insulin delivery may be adjusted appropriately. Thus,
the total number of blood glucose checks per day to keep these systems safe equals
6–10. Table 3–2 details a number of open loop infusion systems now on the market
and the attributes of each.

When evaluating a system, it is important to question the manufacturer regarding safety features and service availability. Section 510K permits the Food and
Drug Administration (FDA) to allow the sale of new devices for insulin infusion
if they are demonstrated by the manufacturer to be substantially equivalent to

Table 3–2. Some commercial devices for continuous subcutaneous insulin infusion

Pump model	Weight (oz)	Basals #	Range	Comments
Mill Hill Infuser 2703	10.6			Used predominantly in Europe; uses diluted insulin
Auto-Syringe AS6C–U100 MP	10.1			Uses U100 Insulin; has several alarms
Cardiac Pacemaker 9100	12.9			Uses any insulin; has several alarms
Medix Corp. 209/100	6.00			Uses U100 Insulin; has several alarms
PYE Dynamics MS 16	6.20			Not available in the United States
SIEMENS Corp. Promedos El	6.70			Not available in the United States
Delta Medical Industries Accu-Rynge	5.80			Uses U40 or U100 Insulin; introduced in USA in 1983
Cardiac Pacemaker Betatron 9205	3.80			Uses U100 Insulin; became available in 1983
Nordisk Infuser	5.30			Uses U100 Insulin; made by Mill Hill Group
Pacesetter-Parker Hannifin Micromed	3.50			Uses U40 or U100 Insulin; available since 1983
New generation pumps				
Beta 1 Orange Medical	8.00	3	0.1–6 U/hr	Has keyboard lock; temporary infusion stop; 2 alarms
Betatron 1	5.75	1	1–150 U/day	Has temporary infusion stop; accumulated dose readout
Betatron 11 (CPI)	5.75	2	1–500 U/day	Has temporary infusion stop; dose limit protection
Eugly (Travenol Autosyringe)	5.60	4	0.1–8 U/hr	Has two alarms; fully enclosed syringe/tubing link
Mark 1 Windsor Medical	5.00	4	0.5–6.4 U/hr	Has runaway alarm; must use attachable programmer; water resistant, accumulated dose readout
Minimed Pacesetter	3.10	4	0.1–7.5 U/hr	Has three alarms; readout of remaining insulin
Provider U-100 Pancretec	7.00	2	0.1–5.0 U/hr	Has back-lit LCD display; readout of remaining insulin; three alarms
Delta Pump Healthdyne	5.50	1	0.28–28 U/hr	Has three alarms; uses standard 9V battery
Medix Medivix	5.30	1	12–42 U/day	Has three alarms; uses standard 9V battery
Micropump Parker	3.10	2	0.1–2 U/hr	Water-resistant; has accumulated dose readout
Nordisk Infuser Nordisk	6.30	1	7.2–96 U/day	Uses insulin cartridges prefilled with Nordisk insulin

devices available prior to 1976. Current FDA authorization for sale does not provide a guarantee that a device will work as advertised so that caution on the part of the consumer is advised when evaluating one of the many new systems coming to market. The newer pump control systems will undoubtably respond to patient demands for convenience, smaller size, and portability—hopefully without compromising reliability.

FUTURE DEVELOPMENTS

Future technology will continue to respond to patient wishes for more portable equipment which is easier to use, safer, and more cosmetic. One of the earliest innovations will be computer-assisted insulin delivery programs. Figure 3–3 illustrates a hand-held computer that assists in insulin delivery. The patient must still enter the appropriate data in terms of daily weight, and calories and carbohydrate ingested as well as blood glucose measurements. Nevertheless, computers with memory capability and programmed with self-adjusting algorithms provide great potential to the individual not in only adjusting insulin therapy but also in maintaining accurate records for problem-solving.

While the computer can help in facilitating more physiologic delivery of insulin, the major unsolved requirement to date is the development of a sensor device. A quantatative blood glucose sensor is the goal of these researchers, but a qualitative alarm system for hypoglycemia will also add a dimension of safety which is now unavailable to open loop systems. Figure 3–4 illustrates a "perspira-

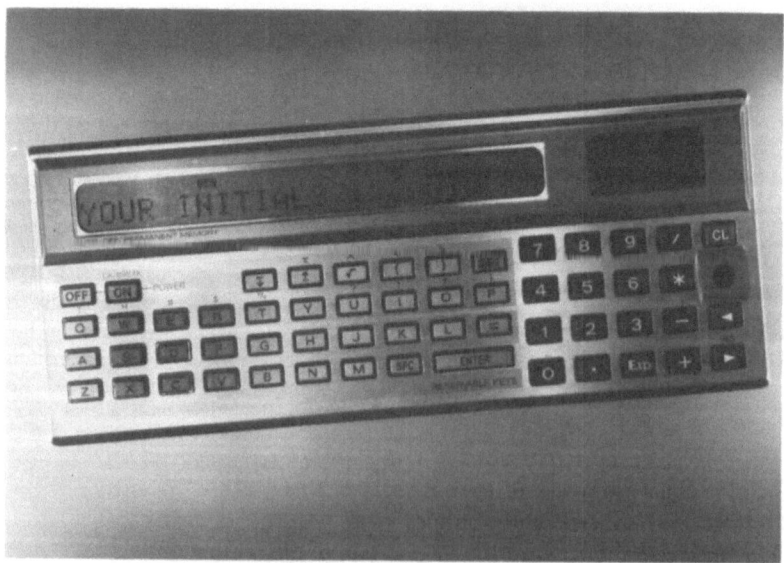

Figure 3–3. The hand-held computer for suggesting insulin adjustments.

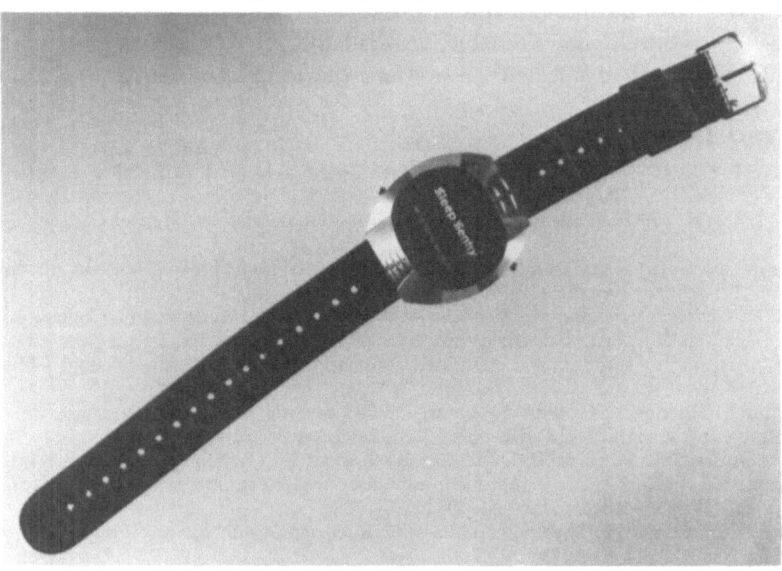

Figure 3–4. The insulin reaction sensor.

tion sensor" that alarms if the skin becomes moist. The problem with this type of device is that it requires a relatively intact counterregulatory system to activate the alarm. Those patients with impaired sympathetic nervous system function—in other words, those who need it most—are not aided by these types of devices. The concept, however, is a good one, and other devices to aid in the detection of hypoglycemia are under development.

The ultimate technological goal would be an implantable closed loop system. As noted above, the main stumbling block at present for the development of such a system remains the sensor. Nevertheless a number of advances have been made in implantable pumps in terms of biocompatability, size, pump design, and insulin reservoirs. The pump itself runs on batteries. The insulin reservoir can be filled through a port which is located under the skin. Finally the unit can be controlled through a remote electronic controller. A major requirement of such a device is that the batteries be reliable and long-lived. Therefore, the power requirements of the pump need to be minimal. In addition, the remote controller needs to be designed so that it is safe from interference. Otherwise a trip past the microwave oven might result in an insulin bolus! Obviously the attention to safety features is no less important in future implantable pumps than in the open loop systems now available.

In summary, the technologies for physiologic insulin delivery will continue to improve rapidly. Features which improve safety, portability, reliability, and cosmetics are already being developed through several generations. Computer-assisted insulin delivery for the individual is now a reality. The major problem to be solved remains that of developing a reliable, implantable, safe, long-term glucose sensor. With the advent of such a device, "closing the loop" will be relatively simple.

SELECTED BIBLIOGRAPHY

1. Brunetti P, Alberti K, Albisser M, Hepp KD, Massi Beneditti M (eds). Artificial systems for insulin delivery. New York: Raven Press, 1982.
2. Clark L Jr, Duggan C. Implanted electroenzymatic glucose sensors. Diabetes Care 5: 174–180, 1982.
3. Peterson CM. Diabetes management in the 80's: the role of home blood glucose monitoring and new insulin delivery systems. New York: Praeger, 1982.
4. Rizza R, Gerich J, Haymond M, Westland R, Hall L, Clemens A, Service FJ. Control of blood sugar in insulin-dependent diabetes: comparisons of an artificial endocrine pancreas, continuous subcutaneous insulin infusion, and intensified conventional insulin therapy. N Engl J Med 303: 1313–1318, 1980.
5. Santiago J, Clemens A, Clarke, W, Kipnis D. Closed-loop and open-loop devices for blood glucose control in normal and diabetic subjects. Diabetes 28: 71–81, 1979.
6. Schade D, Eaton R, Edwards W, Doberneck R, Spencer W, Carlson G, Bair R, Love J, Urenda R, Gaona J Jr. A remotely programmable insulin delivery system. Successful short-term implantation in man. J Am Med Assoc 247: 1848–1853, 1982.
7. Schade DS, Santiago JV, Skyler JS, Rizza RA. Intensive insulin therapy. Princeton: Excerpta Medica, 1983.
8. Chanoch L, Jovanovic L, Peterson CM. Hand held computer programs to assist patients with type I diabetes to make insulin delivery decisions. Presented at the International Diabetes Educator Meeting, Australia, 1984.

4. CLINICAL EVALUATION AND MANAGEMENT OF DIABETIC RETINOPATHY

FRANCIS A. L'ESPERANCE, JR.

CLINICAL EVALUATION

Ophthalmoscopic evaluation with either the direct or indirect ophthalmoscope has been the principal method of assessing the diabetic retina. Slip–lamp examination with a contact lens has proven highly valuable for studying more minute defects in the retinal structures. Photography of the retina, both regular and stereoscopic, has proven useful for carefully documenting retinal changes over long intervals of time.

Fluorescein angiography, introduced in 1961 [1], has been the one laboratory test that has dramatically increased our knowledge of the diabetic retinal process and our ability to implement rational treatment procedures (figure 4–1). Ultrasonography has permitted the ophthalmologist to document the structural relationship of various parts of the eye even though direct visualization is clouded by blood, debris, or membranes. Electrophysiologic aids, such as electroretinography, permit one to assess the functional capabilities of the retina in order to determine whether surgical intervention, such as cataract extraction or vitrectomy, would prove useful in a particular eye. The adaptation of modern and recent technologic advances in other scientific disciplines has proven most rewarding in the field of ophthalmology, and particularly in the study of diabetic retinal disease.

Fluorescein angiographic evaluation

Intravenous fluorescein angiography has been available for the study of posterior segment diseases, such as diabetic retinopathy, macular degeneration, and various

I would like to acknowledge the invaluable assistance of Beth Ann Hughes, Ruth J. Helmich, and Paul Saivetz.

41

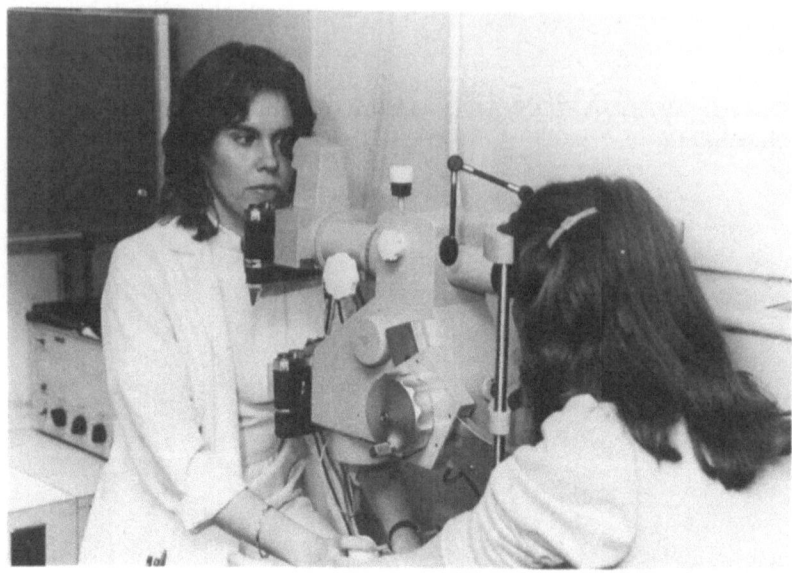

Figure 4–1. A typical fluorescein angiography camera used to document, by rapid-sequence photography, the passage of fluorescein dye through the retinal vessels of the diabetic eye. The enlarged photographs can assist in the identification of microaneurysms, leaking retinal vessels, neovascularization, and areas of microinfarction.

vasculopathies. With this technique it has been possible to study various chorioretinal diseases with the use of advanced photoelectrical devices and rapid-sequential photography. This particular technique has been extremely useful in all phases of nonproliferative and proliferative diabetic retinopathy (figures 4–2 and 4–3).

The technique involves the rapid injection of 5 ml of a 10% solution of sodium fluorescein into the antecubital vein and recording the results photographically on black and white film at intervals of 0.6–0.8 sec. In this manner the entire transit of the fluorescein-blood mixture can be documented as it enters the retinal and choroidal circulation. All abnormalities of the retinal circulation present in diabetic retinopathy can be visualized and identified with precision, and the appropriate therapeutic steps taken.

In nonproliferative diabetic retinopathy, fluorescein antiography can easily demonstrate the irregularity and dilation of the retinal veins and can show the presence of multiple microaneurysms, areas of patchy retinal edema, hemorrhages, zones of capillary closure, and intraretinal microvascular abnormalities (figures 4–4 and 4–5). Usually exudates fail to appear on a fluorescein angiogram, and hemorrhages can be identified by the areas of blocked transmittance of the fluorescent dye from the choroidal circulation. Perhaps the most important use of this technique in nonproliferative diabetic retinopathy is the assessment of the leakage of the retinal vessels in the macular area with the subsequent pooling of fluorescein in the perifoveal space, the disruption of the circumfoveolar capillary network, and the

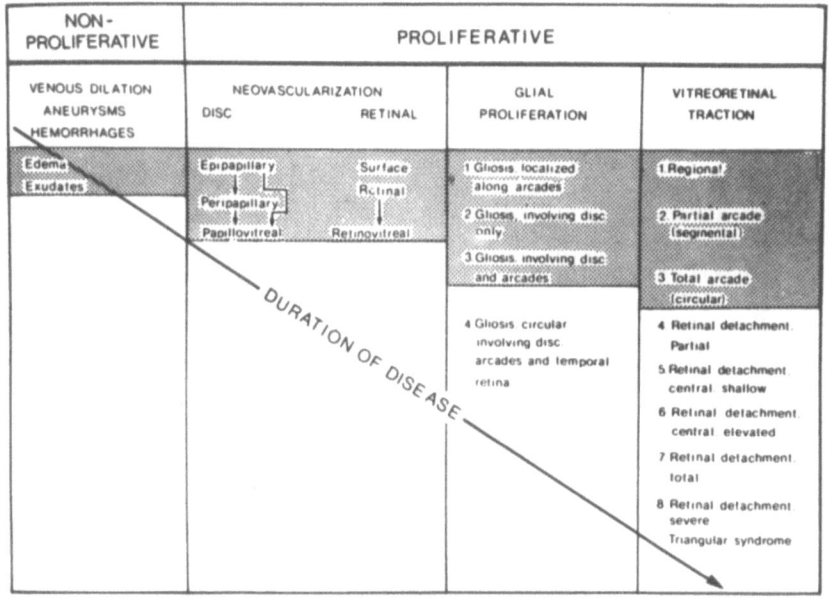

NON-PROLIFERATIVE	PROLIFERATIVE			
VENOUS DILATION ANEURYSMS HEMORRHAGES	NEOVASCULARIZATION		GLIAL PROLIFERATION	VITREORETINAL TRACTION
	DISC	RETINAL		
Edema Exudates	Epipapillary Peripapillary Papillovitreal	Surface Retinal Retinovitreal	1 Gliosis localized along arcades 2 Gliosis, involving disc only. 3 Gliosis, involving disc and arcades 4 Gliosis circular involving disc, arcades and temporal retina	1 Regional 2 Partial arcade (segmental) 3 Total arcade (circular) 4 Retinal detachment. Partial 5 Retinal detachment central shallow 6 Retinal detachment central elevated 7 Retinal detachment total 8 Retinal detachment severe Triangular syndrome

DURATION OF DISEASE

Figure 4–2. The various stages of nonproliferative diabetic retinopathy include venous dilatation, microaneurysm formation, hemorrhages, edema, and exudate formation which progress to the various stages of neovascularization, glial proliferation, and vitreoretinal traction. The shaded area indicates those conditions and stages of the diabetic retinopathy process that are treatable by laser photocoagulation.

presence of large areas of microinfarction and capillary closure. With the correct evaluation of fluorescein angiograms, the proper treatment technique can be selected and the various photocoagulation parameters adjusted for the degree of retinopathy.

With proliferative diabetic retinopathy, fluorescein angiography has been shown to be indispensable in identifying not only all of the factors previously discussed and demonstrated to exist in the nonproliferative phase of retinopathy but also the presence of small areas of retinal or optic nerve neovascularization (figure 4–6). The extent of the neovascular complexes and their leakage capabilities are important to analyze in conjunction with the degree of capillary closure and other hemodynamic and vascular pathology in the posterior pole of the eye. The various types of neovascularization can be documented, and the amount of background retinopathy and pathologic alterations can be assessed in order to implement the panretinal photocoagulation or focal photocoagulation approach in the proper manner.

Ultrasonography and electroretinography

Ultrasonography and bright-flash electroretinography (ERG) should be used as complementary tests when evaluating a patient being considered for vitrectomy.

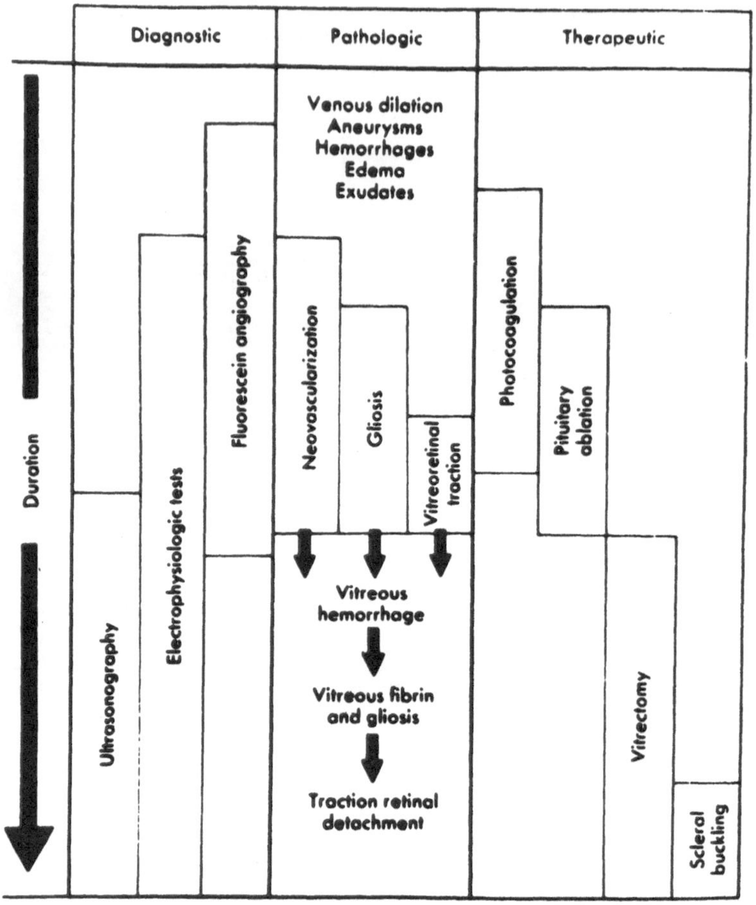

Figure 4–3. The progressive stages of diabetic retinopathy (pathologic column) and the appropriate diagnostic and therapeutic modalities used during the various phases of the diabetic process.

Ultrasonography can provide excellent information regarding the anatomy of the eye with an opaque vitreous or severely opacified lens (figure 4–7). The presence and distribution of membranes in the vitreous or traction retinal detachments can be detected by ultrasonography, and these factors can be used to determine the feasibility of vitrectomy intervention. The bright-flash ERG can indicate if the retina is attached and capable of some visual function. When there is a poor response to bright-flash ERG, ultrasonography can be of assistance in clarifying whether the decreased ERG is due to a retinal detachment or to a poorly functioning attached retina. In eyes with a retinal detachment, the visual potential depends on the technical possibility of surgical reattachment of the retina and the potential of the retina to function once it is reattached.

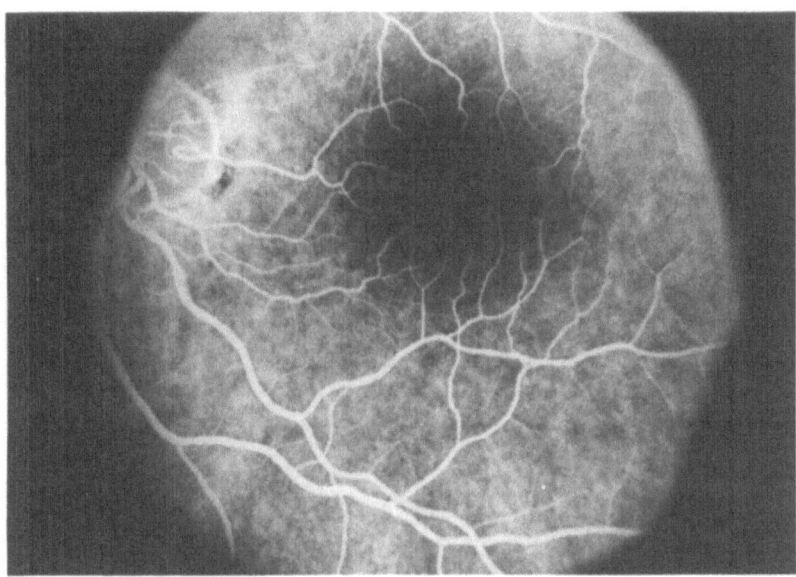

Figure 4–4. Fluorescein angiography photograph showing the normal configuration of the optic nerve, retinal arterioles and venules as well as the darkly pigmented central macular region. No leakage or structural defects can be seen in this normal fluorescein angiograph.

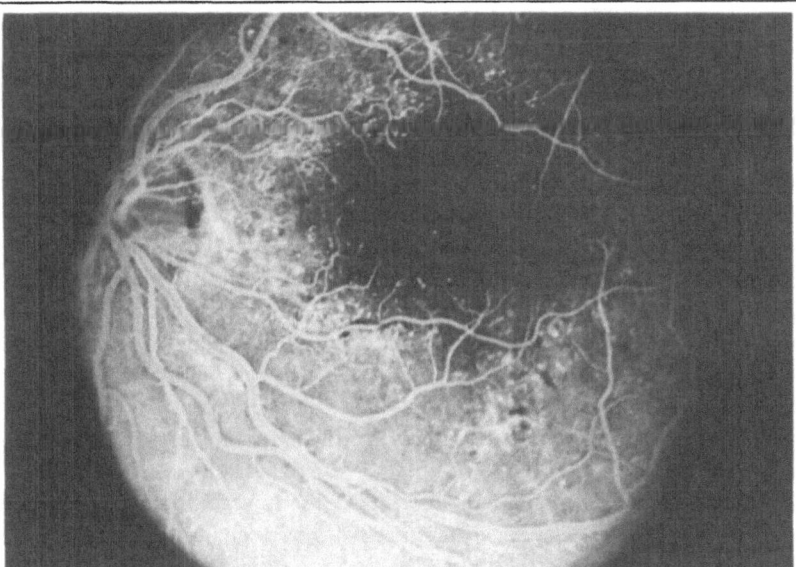

Figure 4–5. Fluorescein angiography photograph showing the optic nerve, macula, microaneurysms, intraretinal shunts, intraretinal hemorrhages, and areas of microinfarction and capillary closure, in the left eye of a patient with moderately severe nonproliferative diabetic retinopathy.

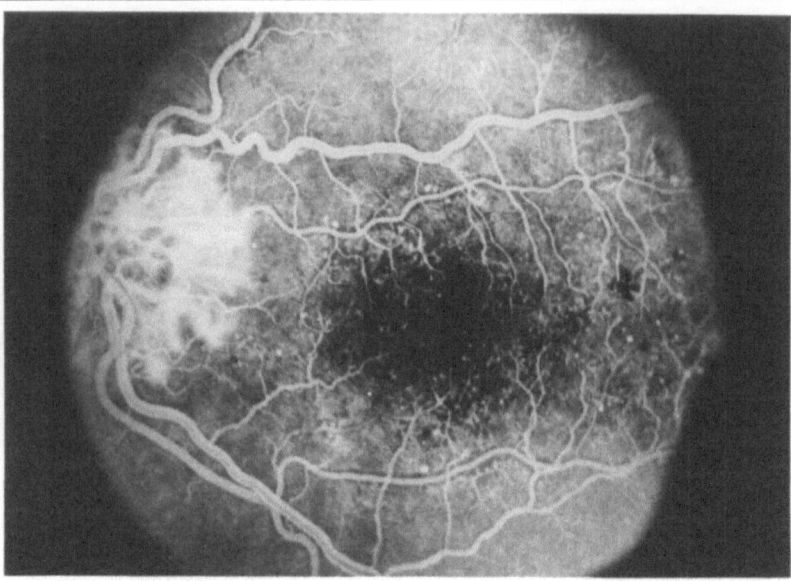

Figure 4–6. Fluorescein angiography photograph showing areas of intraretinal shunting, microaneurysm formation, and multiple hemorrhages in the macular area of the left eye of a patient with moderately severe proliferative diabetic retinopathy. Most striking is the neovascularization growing from the optic nerve *(left)* into the vitreous body.

MANAGEMENT

The increasing incidence of diabetic retinopathy in recent decades is a sober reminder that medical therapy for diabetic retinopathy has not proven very successful. For centuries prior to insulin, dietary restriction, often severely imposed, was the only means of coping with diabetes. Such strict measures painfully improved the life expectancy of diabetics.

Insulin lessened the necessity for harsh diets in the treatment of diabetes. Diabetics now enjoy a more normal life, but microvascular complications have only increased as patients live longer. Today there remains significant controversy as to whether or not strict control of blood sugar alleviates complications such as retinopathy [2–34]. At the heart of this issue is the need for more physiologic methods of insulin administration and blood sugar regulation. Until this is achieved, weight reduction and low-fat diets, although seemingly old-fashioned, probably do not receive adequate emphasis in the medical treatment of diabetes and diabetic retinopathy.

Numerous drugs have been used to treat diabetic retinopathy, a fact that only emphasizes how ineffective such treatment has proven. However, better understanding of the pathogenesis of diabetic retinopathy will hopefully create new opportunities for successful drug therapy. The need for careful and controlled clinical trials, so often overlooked in the past, is now recognized. This, in itself, is an important step in the search for more effective drugs to treat retinopathy.

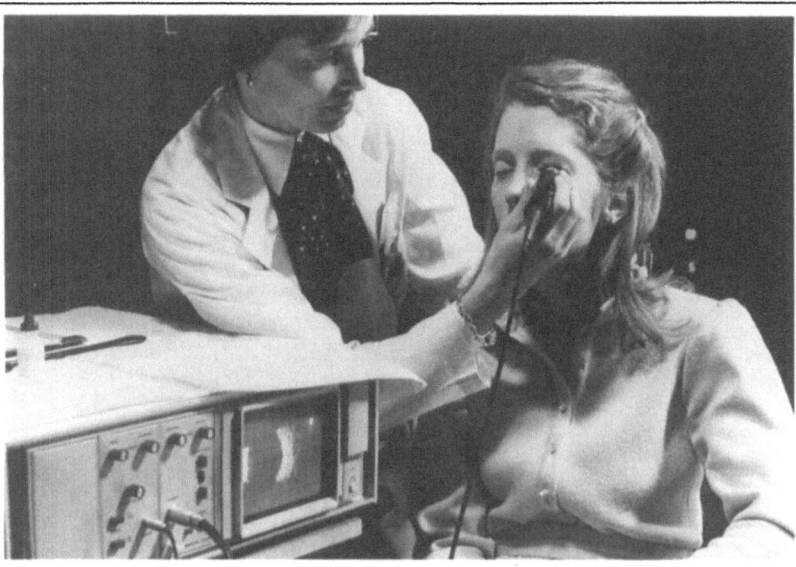

Figure 4–7. A typical ultrasonography unit showing the console (oscilloscope tracing) and the hand-held transducer used for identifying posterior ocular structures obscured by opacification of the central or anterior portions of the eye. In this case, a relatively normal ultrasonographic scan can be visualized on the oscilloscope screen.

Photocoagulation

During the last decade, diabetic retinopathy has been proven to be treated effectively in controlled clinical trials by photocoagulation intervention [35–37] Photocoagulation therapy involves the channeling of an incandescent or laser light beam to the retina of the eye through a dilated pupil (figure 4–8). As the light energy strikes the retina, it is absorbed by melanin, xanthophyll, or oxy- and reduced-hemoglobin. These treatments convert the light energy to heat with varying efficiency but with sufficient heat production to raise the temperature of the retina from 37° C to 65–70° C, thereby producing a coagulum. This coagulum can be produced in strategic areas of the retina in order to destroy microaneurysms, leaky retinal vessels, patches of retinal or vitreal neovascularization, and areas of retinal edema or capillary microinfarction. In this way, the incidence of hemorrhage as well as glial proliferation can be markedly reduced, and, in some cases, can be nearly normalized.

Practical photocoagulation was introduced by Meyer-Schwickerath in 1959 utilizing an incandescent xenon-arc high-pressure bulb source [38]. Although not a laser source, the intense white light produced by this instrument contains all the wavelengths of the visible and near-infrared spectrum. It is still being used effectively as a photocoagulation device in certain circumstances. Argon laser photocoagulation introduced by L'Esperance [39] in 1968 has gained wide accept-

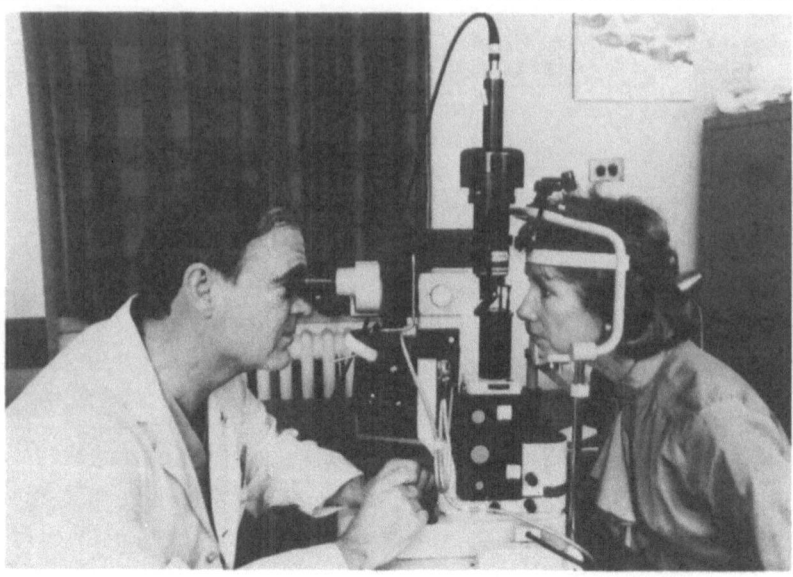

Figure 4–8. Argon laser photocoagulation instrument with the laser beam channeled to the microscope through a fiberoptic cable. Photocoagulations as small as 50 microns, at exposures of one fiftieth of a second or longer can be produced and visualized with magnifications of up to 40x in order to coagulate and destroy leaking retinal vessels, neovascularization, and other areas of potential hemorrhagic activity.

ance in ophthalmic practice because the absorption characteristics of the argon laser beam can be readily determined, an extremely small coagulation spot can be produced, the blue-green beam is highly absorbed by the abnormal red retinal vasculature, and the procedure can be performed without anesthesia other than topically applied drops. Krypton laser photocoagulation introduced by L'Esperance in 1972 [40] has also been utilized by ophthalmologists to photocoagulate extremely hemorrhagic areas of diabetic retinopathy, to coagulate abnormal vasculature through a hazy blood-filled vitreous, and to produce pan-retinal photocoagulation ablative retinal procedures in areas where the fragile diabetic neovascularization might be ruptured by the more highly absorbed argon laser beam. Very recently, photocoagulation by the frequency–doubled neodymium-YAG green beam and the organic liquid dye red or yellow laser beam, both introduced by L'Esperance in 1971 [41] and 1983 [42], respectively, have been shown to be highly absorbed by critical elements of the retina so that each individual case of diabetic retinopathy can be treated precisely with respect to the particular underlying vascular, hemodynamic, or metabolic defect.

Rationale

The basic rationale of photocoagulation is to destroy neovascular complexes, to obliterate areas of microinfarction or capillary closure, to destroy leaking vessels in the macular and paramacular region, and ultimately to produce a chorioretinal adhesion that will resist the later ravages of increasing vitreoretinal traction.

The proliferation of neovascular tissues is probably a result of localized hypoxia in the region of the retinal vessels near the internal limiting membrane. It would seem obvious that these blood vessels are proliferating in a response to some biochemical stimulus, and neovascularization seems to be an appropriate defense for the reparative mechanism of the body. However, the in-growth of neovascularization with the support of glial tissue, as well as the attendant leakage of damaged vessels into the surrounding retinal spaces, the transport of high molecular weight lipoproteinaceous material throughout the neovascular walls into the retina, the resulting hemorrhages, and the dynamic changes occurring from the interposition of the fibrovascular membranes, can irreparably damage the retina.

Panretinal photocoagulation appears to obliterate successfully or cause the regression of neovascularization by one of four mechanisms: (1) the reduction or destruction of areas of hypoxic retina that are producing the vasoformative factor that is calling forth neovascularization from more healthy areas of the retina; (2) the creation of a closer apposition of the inner layers of the retina to the choriocapillaris by the multiple scattered photocoagulation scarring around the entire posterior polar region, thereby allowing greater oxygen perfusion from the choroidal layers to the inner retinal layers that have undergone a relatively high degree of microinfarction; (3) the destruction of unhealthy microinfarcted areas of retina and sluggishly perfused capillaries, thereby allowing the available retinal blood to increase nourishment to the remaining retina; and (4) the destruction of leaking blood vessels and other abnormal vascular complexes that are creating an abnormal hemodynamic situation in the diabetic retina, thereby more nearly normalizing the vascular supply of the macular region of the eye. The entire concept of the vasoformative factor being elaborated by hypoxic retina, secondary to microinfarction and capillary closure, is a most inviting explanation for the beneficial effect of panretinal photocoagulation. If the vasoformative factor emanating from the hypoxic areas of retina can be reduced in the posterior vitreous, the neovascular stimulus is thereby decreased, and the new vessels tend to regress or become obliterated. Certainly the better nutrition of the inner portions of the retina by the closer apposition of the inner layers to the choriocapillaris and the choroidal blood supply would also appear to be a beneficial result of the panretinal photocoagulation technique [43].

Photocoagulation results

The application of photocoagulation is divided either into the focal type of treatment or panretinal photocoagulation [44–46]. Focal argon laser or xenon-arc photocoagulation of isolated patches of neovascularization involves the coagulation of zones of retinal vessels, leakage, or herniation. The photocoagulation is not extensive, but serves to contain the retinopathy and to destroy those more localized regions of retinal vascular abnormalities [47]. Panretinal photocoagulation involves the systematic photocoagulation of the retina from the region several disc diameters

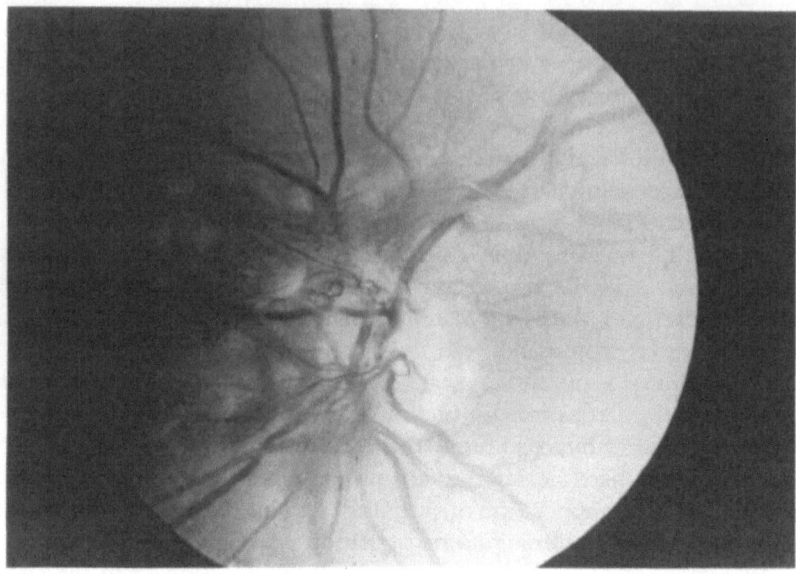

Figure 4–9. A typical confluent papillovitreal frond of neovascularization extending from the optic nerve into the vitreous cavity prior to photocoagulation therapy.

outside the macula to the equator of the eye in six to eight photocoagulation sessions, spaced at weekly intervals [45]. By coagulating approximately 20–30% of the retina in these areas, the demand for oxygen and nutrition is decreased along with the areas of hypoxic retina, thereby theoretically decreasing the vasoformative factor which calls forth and supports neovascular growth and perhaps the glial proliferation process in diabetic retinopathy. This indirect application of photocoagulation, usually away from the neovascularization, by panretinal photocoagulation leads to the partial ablation of the peripheral retina and to the regression or obliteration of the neovascularization in the central retina in more than 80% of cases [44]. L'Esperance recently analysed 256 cases of proliferative diabetic retinopathy during an eight-year period following argon laser panretinal photocoagulation and found that 90–95% of insulin-dependent diabetics and 84% of non-insulin dependent diabetics retained useful vision (greater than $20/400$) [48] (figures 4–9 to 4–13).

The results of the Diabetic Retinopathy Study (DRS) sponsored by the National Eye Institute have shown that during recent years, various configurations of diabetic vitreoretinal neovascularization were treated with considerable effectiveness by the panretinal photocoagulation technique. Because of the clinical importance of diabetic retinopathy and the increasing use of photocoagulation in its management, the DRS was begun in 1971. This randomized, controlled, clinical trial involved more than 1,700 patients enrolled in 15 medical centers. The primary eligibility criteria for this trial were: (1) diabetic retinopathy in both eyes, with

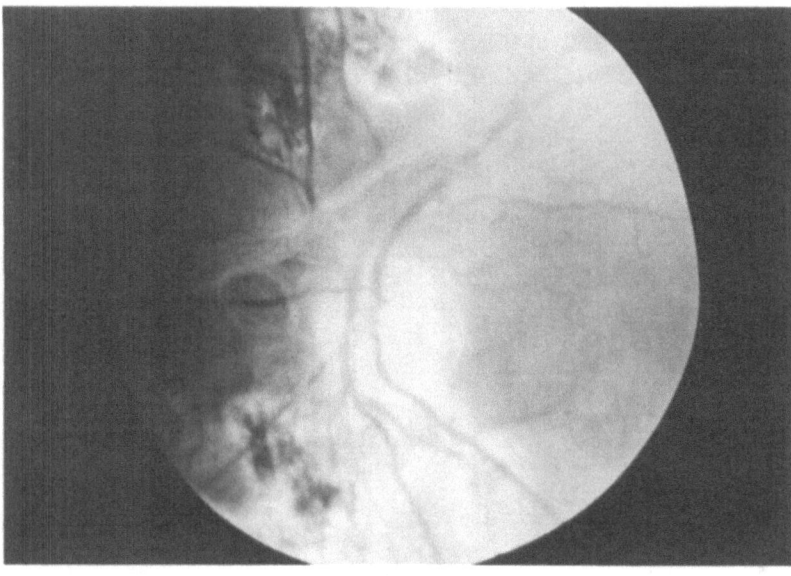

Figure 4–10. The same eye as noted in figure 4–9 six weeks following panretinal photocoagulation with disappearance of all of the neovascularization, but with the retention of the supportive glial tissue.

proliferative changes in at least one eye or severe nonproliferative changes in both eyes; and (2) visual acuity of $^{20}/_{100}$ or better in both eyes. One eye of each patient was randomly selected for treatment, and the other eye was observed without treatment. One of the two treatment modalities, xenon-arc or argon laser, was also chosen randomly. Both treatment techniques included extensive scatter photocoagulation (panretinal photocoagulation, retinal ablation) and focal treatment of new vessels on the surface of the retina. Focal treatment of new vessels on the disc was required in the argon-laser-treated eyes [49].

The results of this report provided evidence that photocoagulation treatment as carried out in the DRS (extensive scatter photocoagulation and focal treatment of new vessels) is of benefit in reducing, but not entirely eliminating, the occurrence of severe visual loss over a two-year period, at least for eyes with certain characteristics. The occurrence of visual acuity less than $^{5}/_{200}$ for two consecutive, completed four-month followup visits was reduced from 16.3% in all untreated eyes to 6.4% in all treated eyes, a change of 61%. There was evidence that loss of two to four lines of visual acuity occurred in some treated eyes as well as loss of peripheral visual field, more so in xenon-arc-treated eyes. The location of new vessels relative to the optic disc, severity of new vessels, and the presence of hemorrhage (vitreous or preretinal) have proven to be important prognostic factors. It was recommended by the DRS that photocoagulation treatment should be considered in eyes with any one of the following criteria: (1) moderate or severe new vessels on or within

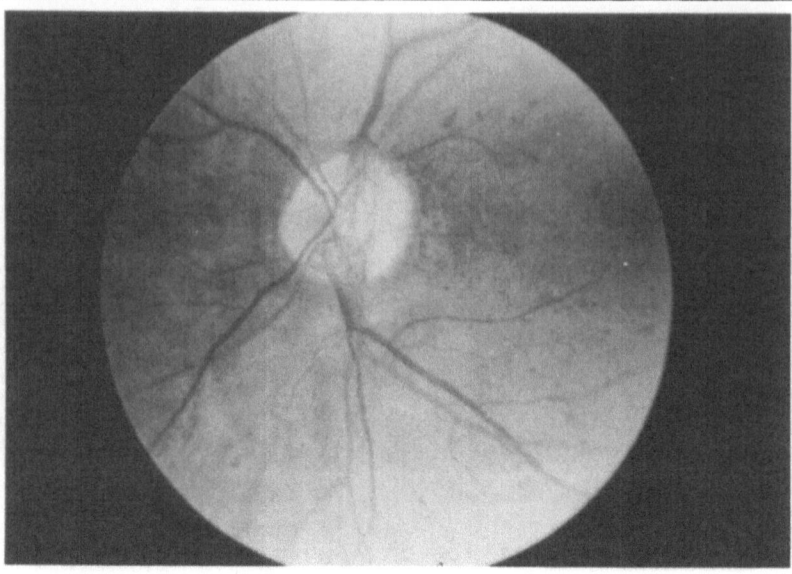

Figure 4–11. Wide-angle photograph showing epipapillary neovascularization extending off the optic nerve along the superotemporal vascular arcade of the left eye prior to photocoagulation.

one-disc diameter on the optic disc; (2) mild new vessels on or within one-disc diameter of the optic disc if a hemorrhage is present; and (3) moderate or severe new vessels elsewhere if a fresh hemorrhage is present [48].

In a recent communication, the DRS emphasized that: (1) the presence of vitreous or preretinal hemorrhage, (2) the presence of new vessels, (3) the location of new vessels on or near the optic disc, and (4) the severity of the new vessels increased the risk of developing severe visual loss; and photocoagulation was indicated earlier if these particular factors were present [50]. The occurrence of visual acuity less than 5/200 for two consecutive, completed four-month followup visits, when determined over a four-year period, was reduced approximately 50% in all treated eyes in the study as compared with the untreated group. Further analysis and followup of these patients will continue, and the efficacy of photocoagulation therapy will be evaluated more completely, although this modality has been shown to be of definite benefit in the treatment of most forms of diabetic retinopathy [51].

VITRECTOMY AND VITREOLYSIS

A promising new therapy for eyes previously blinded from vitreous hemorrhage is pars plana vitrectomy. Vitrectomy involves a technique whereby a needle-like cutting and aspiration device is introduced into the central cavity of vitreous in the eye, and blood, membranes, and fibrin are delicately removed from that region and replaced with clear Ringer's solution (figure 4–14). Vitrectomy has been

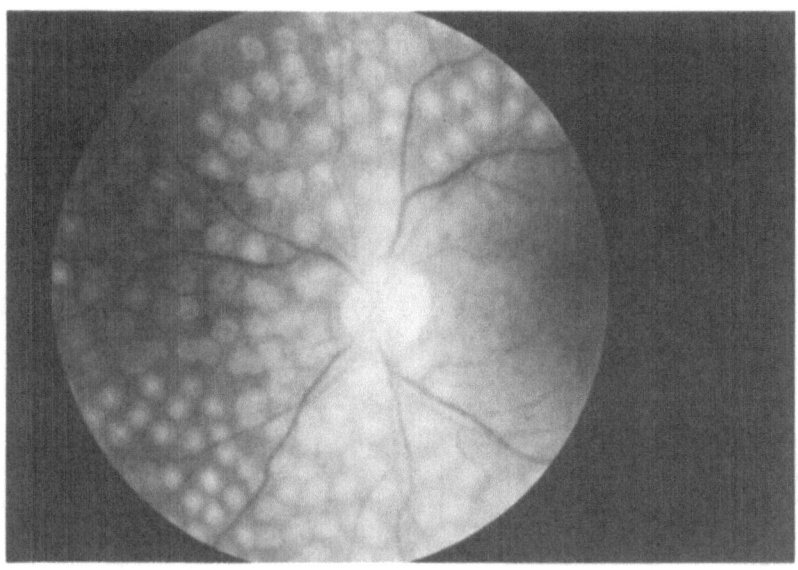

Figure 4–12. A wide-angle photograph showing the same eye as noted in figure 4–11 immediately after panretinal photocoagulation.

proven to be useful in cases in which blindness is due primarily to vitreous opacification from fibrin or vitreous membranes, and it has not been as useful if the retina has been previously severely damaged by advanced retinopathy, fibrosis, and degeneration. Mandelcorn and his co-workers [52] have reported major visual improvements in over one-half their cases. Unfortunately, many blind diabetics are not candidates for this operation because of concurrent retinal deterioration as noted by electrophysiologic tests, advanced traction retinal detachments as documented by ultrasonography, or the development of diabetic neovascular glaucoma.

Indications

The following conditions have been considered as the optimal requirements in order for an eye to be selected for pars plana vitrectomy [53]. Rarely are all of the *ideal* conditions present at the time of vitrectomy. Repeated vitreous hemorrhages, a progressively enlarging retinal detachment, known zones of neovascularization that could be photocoagulated, rapid visual and electrophysiologic deterioration of the eye, or marked debilitation of the fellow eye may all be indications for earlier vitrectomy intervention. These conditions and the following more ideal indications should be integrated with the Diabetic Retinopathy Vitrectomy Study (DRVS) criteria as soon as they have been firmly established:

1. Absence of recurrent hemorrhage or new red blood in the vitreous during the preceding six-month period.

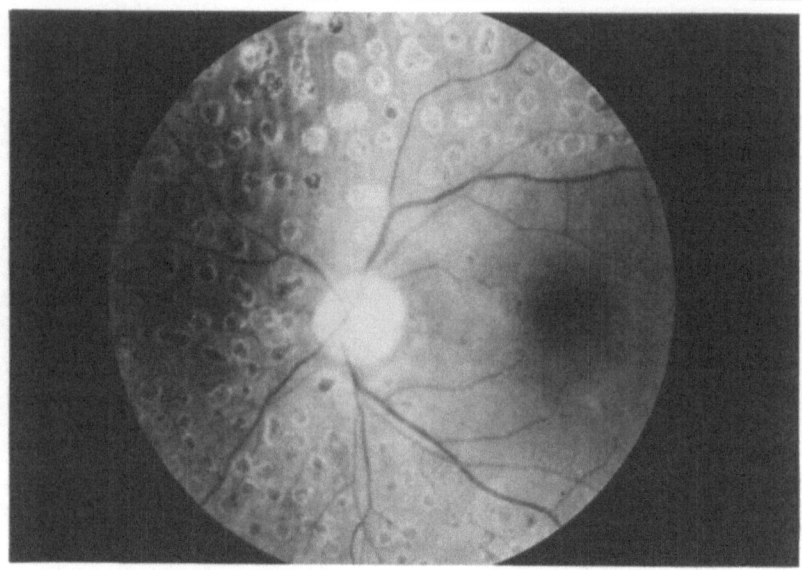

Figure 4–13. The same eye as noted in figures 4–11 and 4–12, two months after panretinal photocoagulation with complete disappearance of the neovascular component near the optic nerve.

2. No evidence of clearing of the opacified vitreous during the preceding six-month period.
3. Presence of light perception and, ideally, the presence of an accurate light projection in two or more fields.
4. No definite ultrasonographic evidence of retinal detachment in eyes with questionable light projection.
5. No previously documented evidence of long-standing retinal gliosis or detachment.
6. Ideally, an ERG response that is present, although possibly diminished in intensity.
7. Complete understanding of the purpose of the procedure by the patient with totally informed patient consent.

Traction retinal detachments often complicate proliferative diabetic retinopathy. In these cases the posterior vitreous is attached to sites of epiretinal proliferation, and they result in a traction detachment of the underlying retina. Characteristically, a retinal detachment occurs along the course of the superotemporal vascular arcade, but other areas may be involved. Although extensive detachment along the vascular arcades often spares the macular region and because of the operative risks associated with these eyes, vitreous surgery is usually not recommended before the macular region has been threatened. However, vitreous surgery should be considered if the macula is partially detached, particularly if the detachment is of recent onset [43].

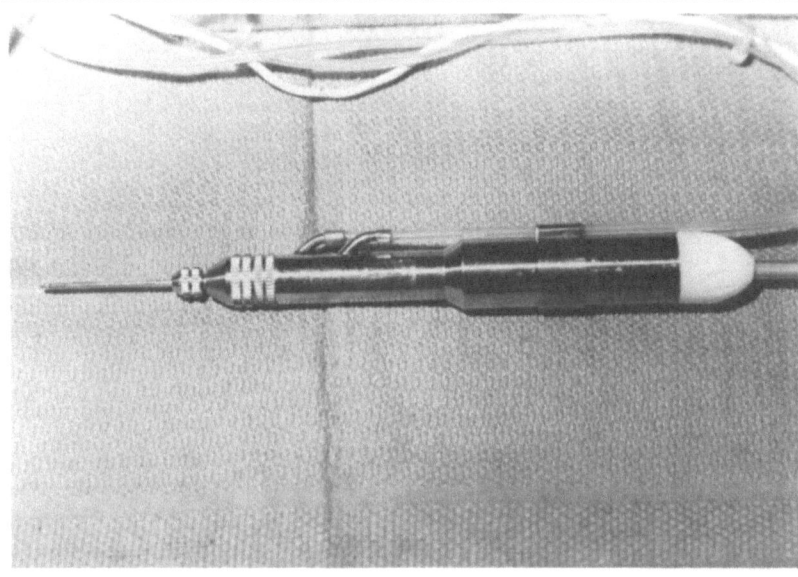

Figure 4–14. A typical vitrectomy instrument with small tip in place. The needle-like cannula tip performs the functions of cutting, infusion, and suction of debris away from the operated eye. The handle of the instrument houses the small motor which drives the cutting tip.

Vitrectomy results

The Diabetic Retinopathy Vitrectomy Study (DRVS) is a randomized, controlled trial now being conducted by 14 cooperating medical centers. Patterned after the Diabetic Retinopahy Study, the DRVS is supported by contracts from the National Eye Institute. The study acknowledges the value of vitrectomy in eyes in which vitreous hemorrhage has been present for a year or more (figures 4–15 and 4–16). The DRVS is now attempting to determine if better visual results can be achieved by operating earlier on eyes that have sustained a severe vitreous hemorrhage due to proliferative diabetic retinopathy.

In a review of 120 consecutive vitrectomies performed by Okun, 60 eyes with opacified vitreous showed a visual improvement in 70% of the eyes [54]. Douvas [55], Kloti [56], Ryan and Michels [57], and Shea and Young [58] have reported an improvement in vision ranging from 60–85% after vitrectomy for a variety of conditions that included opacification of the vitreous, severe membrane formation, and diabetic traction retinal detachments. Machemer recently reported a large series of cases in which vitrectomy was performed for diabetic vitreous hemorrhage [59]. In those cases in which the retina was found to be attached, 59% experienced an improvement in vision within six months following surgery, whereas only 25% of the eyes with a retinal detachment showed any increase in the visual acuity. Six months following vitrectomy, 60% of the eyes undergoing vitrectomy showed an increase in visual acuity if proliferative diabetic retinopathy was not present,

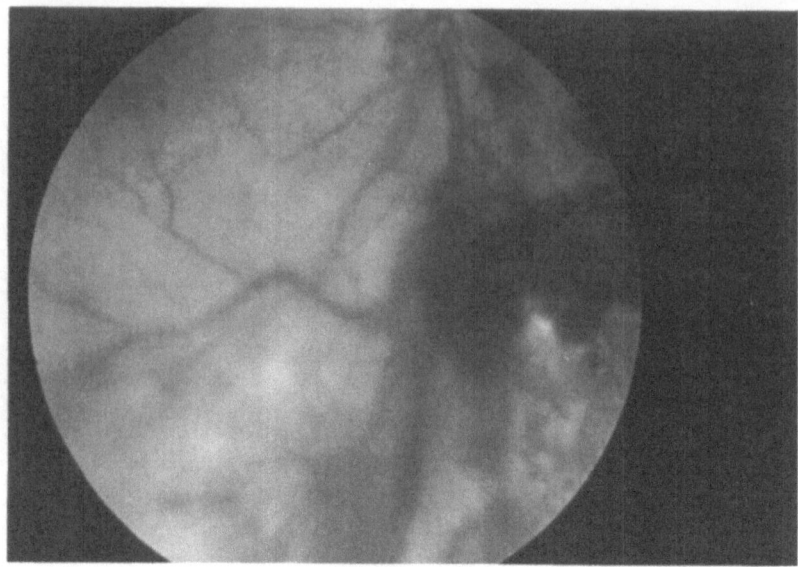

Figure 4–15. Marked vitreous fibrin, blood, and membranes obscuring visualization of the retina prior to vitrectomy.

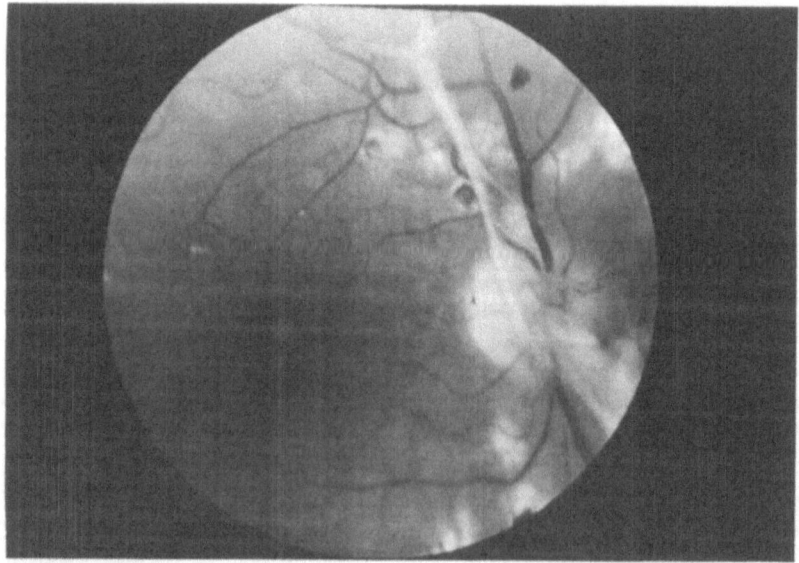

Figure 4–16. Visualization of the optic nerve, macular region, and posterior pole of the same eye as shown in figure 4–15 two weeks following pars plana vitrectomy.

whereas only 21% of the eyes with proliferative diabetic retinopathy at the time of surgery sustained an increase in visual acuity during the same interval. In this series of 663 cases, those eyes with preoperative neovascularization of the iris retained this neovascularization in 71% of the eyes six months after vitrectomy, whereas eyes without rubeosis iridis preoperatively developed neovascularization in 32% of the cases during this interval. Of the eyes with neovascularization six months after vitrectomy, 23% of the total series went on to develop moderate to severe neovascular glaucoma.

Aaberg reported a series of 125 cases in which the vitreous was clear, but vitrectomy was performed in order to properly treat severe traction retinal detachments [60]. One year following surgery, 72% of his cases had sustained an improvement in visual acuity of at least two Snellen lines, while 28% remained unchanged and 17% experienced worse visual acuity than previously documented. Thirteen percent of the phakic eyes and 21% of the aphakic eyes undergoing vitrectomy for traction retinal detachment developed neovascular glaucoma during the one-year followup period, an increase in the aphakic population of 62% over the phakic group. Aaberg's overall statistics for cases reviewed over an interval of 39 months showed that approximately 80% of eyes sustained an improvement in vision during that period, with 18% showing an increase in visual acuity from the immediate postoperative period, 44% maintaining their postoperative vision, and 16% becoming worse during the 39 months. L'Esperance analysed 117 cases over an eight-year period following vitrectomy and showed that 66% of eyes maintained useable vision (greater than $^{20}/_{400}$) [61]. The rapid introduction of new technological improvements in the vitrectomy procedure has permitted the precise evacuation of fibrin, blood clots, and the excision of vitreal as well as preretinal membranes. These improvements in surgical instrumentation in conjunction with the newly developed photocoagulation approaches to diabetic retinopathy have allowed the ophthalmologist to deal effectively with most of the advanced stages of the diabetic retinopathy process.

Pituitary ablation

Pituitary surgery was tried in many centers throughout the world following Luft and Poulsen's publications [62, 63]. Many authors assessed the results only in terms of better, worse, or no change, although 75% of the patients were reported to have improved to some degree or extent. Bradley and associates [64] reviewed about 400 treated cases in 1965, and Kohner reviewed the literature of over 1,000 patients treated by surgical removal of the pituitary gland, stalk section, stereotactic cryosurgery, implant of radioactive isotopes, or external irradiation [65]. Pituitary ablation has been shown to be most effective in the treatment of rapidly progressive, severe, proliferative (florid) retinopathy. Recent controlled clinical trials of pituitary ablation versus no treatment [66] and versus photocoagulation [67] have both shown significantly better retention of vision in the hypophysectomized patients. However, in view of the acknowledged occasional severe side effects of hypophysectomy [68], it has been recommended that this procedure should be reserved for florid retinopathy. Despite good results in certain cases following utilization of hypophysectomy, the technique has been abandoned in many centers [67].

GENERAL PATIENT MANAGEMENT

The most frequently asked questions, by both physicians and patients, will be answered as simply as possible. The answers to these questions should provide an overall pattern that has been discussed more completely in the previous pages of this chapter.

1. **When should the diabetic patient be seen or referred to an ophthalmologist?** Every patient should be seen by an ophthalmologist when diabetes mellitus has been first diagnosed. Particularly type II diabetic patients who may have some degree of diabetic retinopathy requiring immediate treatment.
2. **How frequently should the diabetic patient be seen by an ophthalmologist?** If the patient is newly diabetic and has no obvious retinopathy ophthalmoscopically, the patient is usually observed at yearly intervals. If retinopathy is progressing or is far advanced, patients may be seen as frequently as every two to three months.
3. **When are fluorescein angiographic or ultrasonographic evaluations performed on the diabetic patient?** *Fluorescein angiography* is usually not performed until ophthalmoscopic evidence of the early stages of diabetic retinopathy can be detected. Thereafter, fluorescein angiographic evaluations can be performed at 6- to 12-month intervals, or more frequently, in order to document closely any retinal vascular changes. *Ultrasonography* should be done in some cases in order to produce a baseline study and also is used during later stages of diabetic retinopathy when vitreous hemorrhage, cataract, or corneal changes obstruct the view of the retina which can only be evaluated, at that point in time, by ultrasonographic examination.
4. **What restrictions does the diabetic patient have after photocoagulation?** All of these directions should be followed for at least two weeks after photocoagulation unless advised otherwise.
    1. Keep your head up and move slowly. Do not bend over or move suddenly.
    2. Remain calm. Do not worry about the treatment or anything else, if possible. Contact your physician if you feel you are overly anxious or overly disturbed about your condition or other problems.
    3. Do not strain at anything. Do not lift any object heavier than 20 pounds or hold your breath for any reason. Do not strain during bowel movements and try not to get constipated. Try not to engage in any strenuous or "surge" type activities (athletics, sex, heavy housework, furniture moving, etc.).
    4. Your vision may be blurry and blotchy for two to three weeks, or longer, after treatment. Nearly always, but not invariably, vision will return to the pretreatment level.
    5. You may have some discomfort around your treated eye. Aspirin is sufficient to relieve the pain in most cases. Also, the eye may be bloodshot, a common

occurrence following photocoagulation. Your nose may "run" on the treated side for a few days.

The following directions should be followed indefinitely.

1. Sleep with the head of your bed raised 15–20 degrees. This is best accomplished by placing a foam rubber wedge seven inches high and one-third the length of the mattress under your mattress. If this wedge is not available, use several pillows to elevate your head. This will decrease the blood pressure in the tiny blood vessels in your eyes.
2. Control coughing and sneezing by cough syrup or other medications. However, do not stifle a sneeze since this raises the blood pressure in your eyes.
3. Continue to avoid bending, straining, and heavy lifting.
4. Do not rub eyes since this may disrupt blood vessels inside the eyes.
5. Try not to use those nose drops, sprays, or inhalators which contain ephedrine or adrenalin. These may raise your blood pressure and predispose to hemorrhage. Ask your physician about this.
6. Use a stool softener, one or two capsules of Colace each bedtime, if constipated.
7. Avoid altitudes over 8,000 feet; e.g., mountain passes, private plane flying. Scheduled commercial aircraft are pressurized to this altitude and are permissible.

5. **What exercise can a diabetic patient with nonproliferative diabetic retinopathy do?** Excessive exercise can result in severe retinal, preretinal, or vitreal hemorrhages due to a momentary or sustained increase in systemic hypertension or an extended Valsalva maneuver. A combination of vitreo-retinal adhesions, vitreo-retinal traction, and vitreous movement during exercise may cause a *stress* hemorrhage or retinal tear. The combination of hypertension, hypoglycemia, and the Valsalva maneuver will, in many cases, cause a *hypertensive* or "blow-out" hemorrhage. It is recommended that the patient with nonproliferative diabetic retinopathy engage in non-Valsalva maneuver exercises such as swimming, jogging, bicycling, and racket sports.
6. **What exercise should a diabetic patient with nonproliferative diabetic retinopathy *not* do?** It is imperative that the patient with any phase of retinopathy refrain from excessive Valsalva maneuvers, such as holding one's breath while lifting or exercising, particularly if the diabetic individual has mild or moderate systemic hypertension. The exercises to be avoided are bowling, yoga, weight-lifting and advanced Nautilus or similar type exercises.
7. **What exercises can a diabetic patient with proliferative diabetic retinopathy do?** The patient with proliferative diabetic retinopathy has developed new diabetic retinal blood vessels which may extend from the retina into the vitreous body. These areas of neovascularization do not have sufficient muscular or other reinforcement to withstand increases in blood pressure much above normal day-to-day activity. Therefore, it is recommended that exercise and muscular toning, important to all diabetic patients, be limited to swimming,

light jogging or bicycling, passive exercise machines, walking briskly, and mild nonisometric toning.

8. **What exercises should a diabetic patient with proliferative diabetic retinopathy not do?** The patient with proliferative diabetic retinopathy runs the risk of producing a disabling intraocular hemorrhage with one or a combination of: (1) an increase in systemic blood pressure; (2) a decrease in the blood sugar level; or (3) a modified Valsalva maneuver. The exercises that should not be attempted by a patient with proliferative diabetic retinopathy include diving, bowling, yoga, Nautilus and similar type workouts, pushups, situps, head–below–the–waist exercises, strenuous jogging, bicycling, strenuous racket sports, or any advanced isometric exercises.

9. **What can internists do to help stabilize diabetic retinopathy?** The most important factors appear to be to stabilize, as much as possible, the patient's blood pressure and blood glucose level; closely monitor the renal and retinal condition; and to be certain that the patient is being seen at regular intervals by his ophthalmologist. Patients with late nonproliferative or proliferative diabetic retinopathy should be controlled in such a way that hypoglycemic shocks should be minimized or eliminated due to the devastating effect that they can have on retinal vessels.

10. **What appears to be the most detrimental to diabetic patients with diabetic retinopathy?** The Valsalva maneuver, where external muscles contract against a lungful of air in order to lift or cough, etc., raises the pressure in the vessels of the head and the retina causing hypertensive or blow–out hemorrhages into the vitreous cavity. Therefore, as documented previously, constipation should be avoided, lifting of any object over 20–30 pounds should be avoided, as well as bending at the waist with the back held horizontally. Vomiting, excessive coughing, frequent bouts of hypoglycemia with or without frank "shocking" all can lead to severe retinal problems. In addition, extreme surge exercises, as noted previously, can be disastrous. Any combination of the multitude of physical states that can dilate or increase the pressure within the retinal vessels can lead to immediate hemorrhaging from the tiny retinal vessels.

11. **Do diabetic patients have an increased problem in cataract extraction?** Although a few special precautions should be taken with diabetic patients during a cataract extraction, the actual operation, postoperative healing, and eventual recovery (providing retinal damage is not present) is similar to the nondiabetic population.

12. **Can diabetic patients have intraocular lenses as a replacement for the cataractous lens after its removal?** An intraocular lens implant should not be placed in a diabetic eye with advanced retinopathy or in a younger person with less retinopathy but with a greater lifespan in which to develop advanced retinopathy. However, intraocular lens implants can be considered for most diabetic patients without significant retinopathy.

13. **Do diabetic patients have an increased incidence of glaucoma?** The incidence of glaucoma in diabetic patients without retinopathy or with early

retinopathy is not essentially different from the nondiabetic population. However, the incidence of glaucoma, especially diabetic neovascular glaucoma, increases with the duration of diabetes and, therefore, with the duration and severity of the diabetic retinopathy process. Ophthalmologists and internists should be constantly aware of the potential for their patients to develop an elevation in intraocular pressure.

14. **Can diabetic neovascular glaucoma be treated?** Until recently it was difficult to treat diabetic neovascular glaucoma successfully with any assortment of medications and, in many cases, destructive surgery was finally recommended. However, various types of laser therapy to the anterior portion of the eye have proved successful in a number of patients, and this therapy appears to be promising.

15. **Can diabetic patients expect to retain usable visual function during their lifetimes?** The diabetic individual can expect to retain usable visual acuity during his or her lifetime provided he or she is willing to follow the lifestyle and regulations recommended by their internist, nephrologist, neurologist, and other medical care personnel. On the other hand, it is imperative that the internist, nephrologist, and ophthalmologist work closely together to integrate their treatment, so that individual recommendations coordinate with other physicians' recommendations to maximally benefit the patient with regard to their vision and to other organs attacked by the diabetic process.

SUMMARY

The only methods of treatment for severe diabetic retinopathy that have been proven effective by controlled clinical trials are photocoagulation [35, 36] and pituitary ablation [69, 70]. It must be noted that photocoagulation and pituitary ablation impede, but do not cure, diabetic retinopathy. Pars plana vitrectomy can be highly effective for removing blood from the vitreous of the eye, allowing better vision, particularly if the retina has been shown to be functional by electrophysiologic testing and ultrasonography. In addition, vitrectomy allows the ophthalmologist to visualize, evaluate, and treat the diabetic retina by photocoagulation or other methods.

Attempts at better regulation of blood sugar have reduced the development of microangiopathy in experimental animals [71] and recently in man [72].

The benefits of rigorous regulation of the blood sugar have been noted in a policy statement by the American Diabetes Association [73]. The development of a practical, beneficial pancreas has been undertaken and may be required in order to reap the full benefits of rigorous blood sugar control. It has been recommended that all patients be evaluated by an ophthalmologist as soon as they have been found to have diabetes, that all diabetics be examined ophthalmologically on an annual basis, and that patients with significant retinopathy be seen at six-month or shorter intervals by their ophthalmologist.

The evaluation and treatment of diabetic retinopathy has progressed enormously during the past decade. It is hoped that the cause of diabetic microangiopathy and retinopathy will be discovered in the near future so that treatment will ultimately cure rather than control the process of diabetic retinopathy.

REFERENCES

1. Novotny H, Alvis DL. A method of photographing fluorescence in circulating blood in the human retina. Circulation 24:82–86, 1961.
2. Brown JK, Jones AT. Retinopathy and diabetic control. Br J Ophthalmol, 48:148–153, 1964.
3. Colwell JA. Effect of diabetic control on retinopathy. Diabetes 15:497–499, 1966.
4. Hardin RC, Jackson RL, Johnston TL, Kelly HG. The development of diabetic retinopathy: effects of duration and control of diabetes. Diabetes 5:397–405, 1956.
5. Jackson RL, Hardin RC, Walker GL, Hendricks AB, Kelly HG. Degenerative changes in young diabetic patients in relationship to level of control. Pediatrics 5:959–971, 1950.
6. Keiding NR, Root HF, Marble A. Importance of control of diabetes in prevention of vascular complications. JAMA 150:964–969, 1952.
7. Schlesinger FG, Franken S, van Lange LTP, Schwartz F. Incidence and progression of retinal and vascular lesions in long-term diabetes: a follow-up of a group of patients over 7 years. Acta Med. Scand 168:483–488, 1960.
8. Spoont S, Dyer WW, Day R, Blazer H. Incidence of diabetic retinopathy relative to the degree of diabetic control. Am J Med Sci 221:490–494, 1951.
9. Dolger H. Clinical evaluation of vascular damage in diabetes mellitus. JAMA 134:1289–1291, 1947.
10. Larsson Y, Sterky G. Long-term prognosis in juvenile diabetes mellitus. Acta Paediatr 51 (Suppl 130):1–76, 1962.
11. Oakley WG, Pyke DA, Tattersall RB, Watkins PJ. Long-term diabetes: a clinical study of 92 patients after 40 years. Q J Med 43:145–156, 1974.
12. Taylor E., Adnitt PI. Factors relating to the progression of diabetic retinopathy. Am Heart J 82:425–427, 1971.
13. Knowles HC. Long-term juvenile diabetes treated with unmeasured diet. Trans Assoc Am Physicians 84:95–101, 1971.
14. Knowles HC, Guest GM, Lampe J, Kessler M, Skillman TG. The course of juvenile diabetes treated with unmeasured diet. Diabetes 14:239–273, 1965.
15. Balodimos MC, Aiello LM, Gleason RE, Marble A. Retinopathy in mild diabetes of long duration. Arch Ophthalmol 81:660–666, 1969.
16. White P. Childhood diabetes. Its course, and influence on the second and third generations. Diabetes 9:345–355, 1960.
17. Caird FI, Garrett CJ. Progression and regression of diabetic retinopathy. Proc R Soc Med 55:477–479, 1962.
18. Szabo AJ, Stewart AG, Joron GE. Factors associated with increased prevalence of diabetic retinopathy: a clinical survey. Can Med Assoc J 97:286–292, 1967.
19. Parving HH, Noer I, Deckert T, Evrin PE, Nielson SL, Lyngsoe J, Mogensen CE, Rorth M, Svendsen PA, Trap-Jensen J, Lassen NA. The effect of metabolic regulation on microvascular permeability to small and large molecules in short-term juvenile diabetics. Diabetologia 12:-161–166, 1976.
20. Miki E, Fukuda M, Kuzuya T, Kosaka K, Nakao K. Relation of the course of retinopathy to control of diabetes, age, and therapeutic agents in diabetic Japanese patients. Diabetes 18:773–780, 1969.
21. Pirart J. Diabete et complications degeneratives presentation d'une etude prospective portant sur 4400 cas observes entre 1947–1973. Diabete Metab 3:97–107, 1977.
22. Job D, Eschwege E, Guyot-Argenton C, Aubry JP, Tchobroutsky G. Effect of multiple daily insulin injections on the course of diabetic retinopathy. Diabetes 25:463–469, 1976.
23. Askikaga T, Borodic G, Sims EAH. Multiple daily insulin injections in the treatment of diabetic retinopathy. The Job study revisited. Diabetes 27:592–596, 1978.
24. Constam GR. Zur spatprognose des diabetes mellitus. Helv Med Acta 32:287–306, 1965.
25. Caird FI. Control of diabetes and diabetic retinopathy. In Symposium on the Treatment of Diabetic Retinopathy, Goldberg, MF, Fine, SL (eds.). PHS Pub. No. 1890. Health, Education and Welfare, 1968, Washington, DC: U.S. Department of 1968, pp. 107–114.
26. University Group Diabetes Program. A study of the effects of hypoglycemic agents on vascular complications in patients with adult-onset diabetes. Diabetes 19 (Suppl. 2):789–830, 1970.

27. University Group Diabetes Program. A study of the effects of hypoglycemic agents on vascular complications in patients with adult-onset diabetes. Diabetes 19 (Suppl. 2):789–830, 1970.
28. University Group Diabetes Program. Effects of hypoglycemic agents on vascular complications in patients with adult-onset diabetes. JAMA 218:1400–1410, 1971.
29. University Group Diabetes Program. Effects of hypoglycemic agents on vascular complications in patients with adult-onset diabetes. JAMA 217:77–784, 1971.
30. University Group Diabetes Program. A study of the effects of hypoglycemic agents on vascular complications in patience with adult-onset diabetes. Diabetes 25:1129–1153, 1976.
31. Cahill GF, Etzwiler DD, Freinkel N. Diabetes 25 (editorial), 1976.
32. Shabo AL, Maxwell DS. Insulin-induced immunogenic retinopathy resembling the retinitis proliferans of diabetes. Trans Am Acad Ophthalmol Otolaryngol 81:497–508, 1976.
33. Engerman RL. Animal models of diabetic retinopathy. Trans Am Acad Ophthalmol Otolaryngol 81:710–715, 1976.
34. Engerman R, Bloodworth JMB, Nelson S. Relationship of microvascular disease in diabetes to metabolic control. Diabetes 26:760–769, 1977.
35. British Multicentre Randomized Controlled Trial. Prolif erative diabetic retinopathy: treatment with xenon-arch photocoagulation. Brit Med J 1:739–741, 1977.
36. The Diabetic Retinopathy Study Research Group. Preliminary report of the effects of photocoagulation therapy. Amer J Ophthalmol 81:383–402, 1976.
37. L'Esperance FA Jr. Diabetic retinopathy. In: Symposium on Diabetes Mellitus. Medical Clinics of North America 62(4): 767–785, 1978.
38. Meyer-Schwickerath G. Light-Coagulation. St. Louis: C.V. Mosby Co., 1960.
39. L'Esperance FA Jr. An ophthalmic argon laser photocoagulation system: design, construction, and laboratory investigations. Trans Amer Ophthal Soc 66:827–904, 1968.
40. L'Esperance FA Jr. Clinical photocoagulation with the krypton laser. Arch Ophthal 87:693–700, 1972.
41. L'Esperance FA Jr. Clinical photocoagulation with the frequency-doubled neodymium yttrium-aluminum-garnet laser. Am J Ophthal 71:631–638, 1971.
42. L'Esperance FA Jr. Ophthalmic lasers: photocoagulation, photoradiation and surgery. St. Louis: C.V. Mosby Co., 1983.
43. L'Esperance FA Jr., James WA Jr. Diabetic retinopathy: clinical evaluation and management. St. Louis: C.V. Mosby Co., 1981.
44. James WA Jr., L'Esperance FA Jr. Treatment of diabetic optic nerve neovascularization by extensive retinal photocoagulation. Am J Ophthalmol 78:939–947, 1974.
45. L'Esperance FA Jr. Ocular photocoagulation. St. Louis: C.V. Mosby Co., 1975.
46. Little HP. In: Diabetic Retinopathy, Lynn JR, Snyder WB, Vaiser A (eds). New York: Grune and Stratton, 1974, pp. 133–144.
47. L'Esperance FA Jr. (ed). Current diagnosis and management of chorioretinal diseases. St. Louis: C.V. Mosby Co., 1977.
48. L'Esperance FA Jr, Freidman EA, Mondschein LG. Long term retention of vision following panretinal photocoagulation in diabetics. In: Diabetic Renal-Retinal Syndrome 2 Prevention and Management, L'Esperance FA Jr., Friedman EA (eds). New York: Grune and Stratton, 1982, pp. 285–300.
49. Diabetic Retinopathy Study Research Group. Preliminary report of the effects of photocoagulation therapy. Am J Ophthalmol 81:383–402, 1976.
50. Diabetic Retinopathy Study Research Group. Four risk factors for severe visual loss in diabetic retinopathy. Arch Ophthalmol 97:654–655, 1979.
51. Davis MD. Discussion of presentation by Dr. George W. Blankenship. Ophthalmology 86(1):76–78, 1979.
52. Mandelcorn MS, Blankenship G, Machemer R. Pars plana vitrectomy for the management of severe diabetic retinopathy. Am J Ophthalmol 81:561–570, 1976.
53. L'Esperance FA Jr. In: New and Controversial Aspects of Vitreoretinal Surgery, McPherson A (ed). St. Louis: C.V. Mosby Co., 1977.
54. Okun E. In: New and Controversial Aspects of Vitreoretinal Surgery, McPherson A. (ed). St. Louis: C.V. Mosby Co., 1977.
55. Douvas NG. In: New and Controversial Aspects of Vitreoretinal Surgery, McPherson A. (ed). St. Louis: C.V. Mosby Co., 1977.

56. Kloti R. In: New and Controversial Aspects of Vitreoretinal Surgery, McPherson A. (ed). St. Louis: C.V. Mosby Co., 1977.
57. Ryan SJ, Michels RG. In: New and Controversial Aspects of Vitreoretinal Surgery, McPherson A (ed). St. Louis: C.V. Mosby Co., 1977.
58. Shea M, Young PW. In: New and Controversial Aspects of Vitreoretinal Surgery, McPherson A (ed). St. Louis: C.V. Mosby Co., 1977.
59. Machemer R. Vitrectomy for proliferative diabetic retinopathy associated with vitreous hemorrhage. Ophthalmology 88(7):643–646, 1981.
60. Aaberg TM. Pars plana vitrectomy for diabetic traction retinal detachment. Ophthalmology 88(7):639–642, 1981.
61. L'Esperance FA Jr, et al. Long term retention of vision following vitrectomy in diabetics. In: Diabetic Renal-Retinal Syndrome 2 Prevention and Management, Friedman EA, L'Esperance EA Jr. (eds). New York: Grune and Stratton, 1982, pp. 277–283.
62. Luft R, Olivecrona H, Ikkos D, Kornerup I, Ljundgren H. Hypophysectomy in man—further experiences in severe diabetes mellitus. Br Med J 2:752–756, 1955.
63. Poulsen JE. Recovery from retinopathy in a case of diabetes with Simmonds' Disease. Diabetes 2:7–12, 1953.
64. Bradley RF, Rees SB, Fager CA. Pituitary ablation in the treatment of diabetic retinopathy. Med Clin North Am 49:1105–1124, 1965.
65. Kohner EM. Diabetic retinopathy: cause, treatment and prognosis. Unpublished M.D. thesis, University of London, 1969.
66. Kohner EM. In: Diabetic Retinopathy, Lynn JR, Snyder WB, Vaiser A (eds). New York: Grune and Stratton, 1974, pp. 205–214.
67. Kohner E, Hamilton A, Joplin G, Fraser TR. Florid diabetic retinopathy and its response to treatment by photocoagulation. Diabetes 25:104–110, 1976.
68. Marble A. Late complications of diabetes. A continuing challenge. Diabetologia 12:193–199, 1976.
69. Kohner EM. A controlled trial of pituitary ablation. In: Diabetic Retinopathy, Lynn JR, Snyder WB, Vaiser A (eds). New York: Grune and Stratton, 1974, pp. 205–214.
70. Kohner E, Hamilton A, Joplin G, et al. Florid diabetic retinopathy and its response to treatment by photocoagulation or pituitary ablation. Diabetes 25:104–110, 1976.
71. Bloodworth JMB, Engerman RL. Diabetic microangiopathy in the experimentally diabetic dog and its prevention by careful control with insulin. Diabetes 22 (suppl. 1):290, 1973.
72. Didier Jr, Eschwege E, Guyot-Argenton C, et al. Effect of multiple daily injections on the course of diabetic retinopathy. Diabetes 25:463–469, 1976.
73. Cahill CF Jr, Etzwiler DD, Freinkel N. Blood glucose control in diabetes. Diabetes 25:237–239, 1976.

5. NATURAL HISTORY OF DIABETIC NEPHROPATHY

ELI A. FRIEDMAN

Pathophysiologic and clinical manifestations of kidney damage are duration related in the type I diabetic. They appear according to a well-described sequence beginning with glomerular hyperfiltration and reversible proteinuria, progressing through fixed massive proteinuria (nephrotic syndrome), and ending in renal insufficiency. Uremia, the end result of relentless nephropathy, is usually associated with severe visual loss or blindness (renal-retinal syndrome). A similar sequence may take place in the type II diabetic. Lack of precision in establishing the onset of type II diabetes, however, prevents construction of a timed natural history. Furthermore, the type II diabetic is older and may have systemic atherosclerosis, with consequent strokes and heart attacks, obscuring the course of kidney damage. Over the past decade, in the United States and Western Europe, uremia complicating diabetic nephropathy has emerged as the most prevalent (12.2% of Medicare funded uremic patients), accurately diagnosed cause of renal failure treated by maintenance hemodialysis or renal transplantation [1]. While "glomerulonephritis" (28.4%) and "hypertension" (17.4%) are reported more frequently, these diagnoses are usually employed as synonyms for unexplained kidney failure associated with small kidneys in the majority of patients so labeled. Diabetic nephropathy is the diagnosis applied to a minimum of 20% and as many as 45% of new dialysis patients, depending on the region of the country reporting. What makes the high prevalence of diabetic nephropathy so important is that despite expenditure of extra resources in the diabetic's care, the outcome of uremia therapy is generally unsatisfactory as measured by survival rate or proportion of patients attaining rehabilitation. As described elsewhere in this book, coincident vasculopathy—especially retinopathy, peripheral arterial insufficiency, and coronary artery disease—limit rehabilitation in many diabetics being treated for renal insufficiency.

EARLY RENAL CHANGES

The course of renal malfunction in type I diabetics has been well defined. At its onset, type I diabetes alters renal morphology and function [2]. Kidney size, glomerular diameter, tubular size and glomerular capillary filtration surface area are all increased by about one-third in type I diabetics. Renal and glomerular hypertrophy has also been noted in the streptozotocin-induced diabetic rat [3]. Vital to unravelling the pathogenesis of diabetic glomerulopathy was the demonstration that correction of hyperglycemia by insulin treatment or islet of Langerhans transplantation prevents renal and glomerular enlargement in rats made diabetic with streptozotocin, a beta cell toxin. Compelling evidence supports the contention that morphologic changes in diabetic nephropathy are mainly the consequence of protein denaturation by high ambient glucose levels. It is consequently inferred, though by no means proven, that a therapeutic regimen which sustains euglycemia will preempt the development of diabetic nephropathy (and other vascular complications of hyperglycemia).

As summarized by Viberti, major changes in function of the diabetic kidney are detectable years before any clinical manifestations of nephropathy appear [4]. Mogensen proposes the term "incipient diabetic nephropathy" for the early functional stage in which increased urinary albumin excretion without clinically demonstrable proteinuria—microalbuminuria—is present [2]. Parving and associates reported that microalbuminuria, if noted in the initial years of type I diabetes, signals a high probability of near-term progression to renal insufficiency more rapidly than in diabetics whose urine remains totally albumin free [5]. Confirmation of this observation in type I diabetics [6] and extension to type II diabetics [7] underscore the importance of testing for microalbuminuria.

In newly diagnosed type I diabetics, albumin excretion is a functional abnormality which usually reverts to normal upon establishment of good glycemic control. Positively charged particles penetrate the glomerular capillary wall more easily and anionic particles less easily than neutral particles of equivalent size [8]. Human albumin has a molecular size smaller than the limiting pore size of the glomerular capillary wall, but is repelled because of its negative charge by electrostatic interaction against the negative charge of the glomerular basement membrane [9]. Protein leakage through the glomerular basement membrane in the diabetic may reflect reduction in or loss of membrane electronegativity (early) and superimposed physical damage (later). At least one kidney disorder, the congenital nephrotic syndrome, may be the consequence, solely, of a loss of electronegativity on the glomerular basement membrane [10].

Measurements of apparent glomerular pore radius by fractional clearances of dextran polymers of molecular radii of 20 to 40° indicate a pore size of 54 to 55° in short-duration type I diabetics, which is similar to the pore size in nondiabetics [25]. Albuminuria in diabetes is now viewed as resulting from a reduction of electronegativity on the glomerular basement membrane on which is superimposed the effect of glomerular structural damage.

Whatever the exact mechanism for increased permeability of glomerular capillaries to large molecules in the diabetic kidney, there follows an accumulation of large macromolecules, immune globulins, and nonimmune circulating aggregates within the glomerular wall and mesangium [11]. It is these plasma constituents which are thought to stimulate mesangial matrix production, leading to diffuse and nodular intercapillary glomerulosclerosis.

Understanding of the glomerular mesangium was clarified by Mauer and Shvil [12] who investigated the function of this active part of the glomerulus. Within the mesangium, nerve endings, smooth muscle, and angiotensin II receptors have been identified. In diabetic nephropathy, the mesangium enlarges and contains a marked increase in smooth muscle. Mauer and associates speculate that some of the functional and hemodynamic abberations of the diabetic kidney may be attributable to altered mesangial contractibility, which in turn, affects angiotensin and prostaglandin secretion and metabolism [13]. The mesangium clears macromolecles, which pass through intercellular channels from the periphery of the mesangium to the juxtaglomerular apparatus, and then the distal tubular cells. Diabetic rats have impaired clearance of macromolecules [14] including products of normal glomerular basement membrane turnover, a defect which could accelerate glomerular injury.

In the type I diabetic, Osterby demonstrated correlation between the rate of glomerular basement membrane thickening and increased mesangial size after three and one-half to five years of insulin use [15]. Beginning diabetic microangiopathy, according to Osterby, is associated with increased synthesis of glomerular basement membrane [16]. Most investigators do not discern ultrastructural thickening of the glomerular basement membrane at onset of insulin dependence [17], a key point tying genesis of microangiopathy to hyperglycemia rather than genetic predisposition.

PATHOLOGY OF GLOMERULOSCLEROSIS

After years of functional renal abnormalities, the type I diabetic develops distinct morphologic glomerular alterations beginning in the mesangium (figures 5–1–5–3). In 10 type I adolescents subjected to percutaneous renal biopsy one to seven years after the onset of diabetes, Castells and associates observed diffuse glomerulosclerosis in one patient, afferent or efferent arteriosclerosis in seven patients, and diffuse mesangial matrix increase in three patients [18]. Only two of these adolescent diabetics had normal renal morphology, while three subjects excreted > 50 mg albumin/24 hr. Of extreme import to the clinician attempting to prognosticate the course of a young type I diabetic, was the finding that the patient with the most advanced glomerular damage had a creatinine clearance of 141 ml/min. Dissociation between assessment of renal function and the extent of glomerular destruction evident by light microscopy is characteristic of diabetic nephropathy.

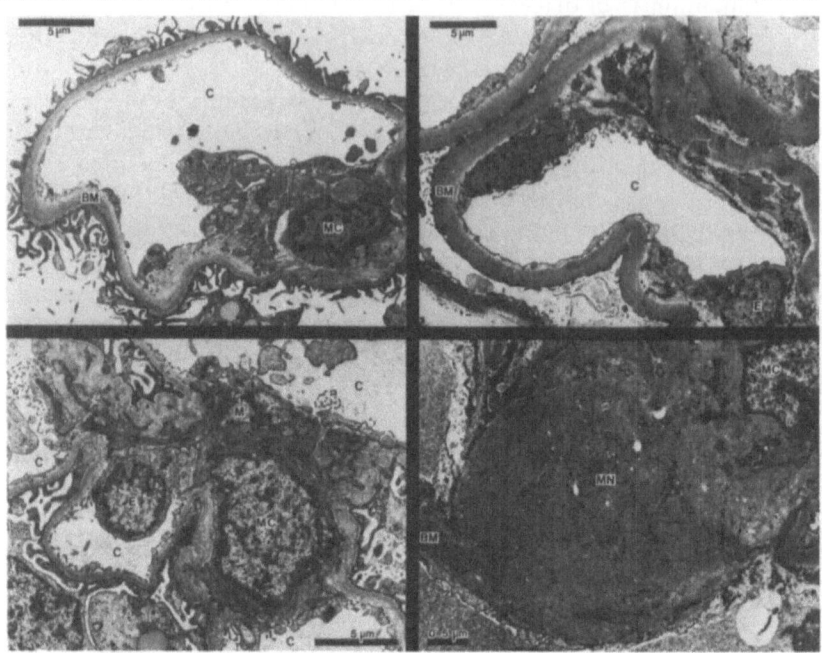

Figure 5–1. Mesangial and basement membrane changes of diabetic glomerulosclerosis. Composite electron photomicrograph contrasting normal glomerular anatomy on the left with early diabetic changes. Upper left, a biopsy from a nondiabetic, shows normal glomerular basement membrane (BM) with finger like projections of epithelial foot processes, surrounding the capillary lumen (C), adjacent to a mesangial cell (MC). Upper right, from a type I diabetic with normal renal function after 11 years, illustrates the thickened, dense glomerular basement membrane and an epithelial cell (E). Lower left, normal mesangium in a nondiabetic adult including a monocyte (M). Lower right, the mesangium from a type I diabetic with normal renal function has a large mesangial nodule (MN) composed of mesangial matrix with mesangial cell debris. See figure 5–2 for the appearance of mesangial on light microscopy.

Brenner's group relates the eventual development of glomerular pathological injury in diabetics and other pathophysiologic chronic kidney disorders to the nephron–damaging effect of glomerular hyperfiltration [19]. Based on studies of reduced nephron mass in the rat, they suggest that following an 80% nephrectomy, compensatory changes occur in remaining nephrons subjected to hyperfiltration and increase in single nephron glomerular flow and pressure [20]. These increases act —by an undefined mechanism, it is thought—to alter glomerular permselectivity, inducing proteinuria. In diabetic rats, increases in mesangial volume and capillary basement membrane thickness reduce glomerular filtering surface and precede the development of segmental glomerular sclerosis, a lesion not typical of human glomerulosclerosis. The relevence of the hyperfiltration hypothesis to progression in diabetic nephropathy has yet to be established [21].

Nodular intercapillary glomerulosclerosis is a specific lesion present in about half of diabetic kidneys examined at autopsy [22, 23]. Nodules first appear as an increase

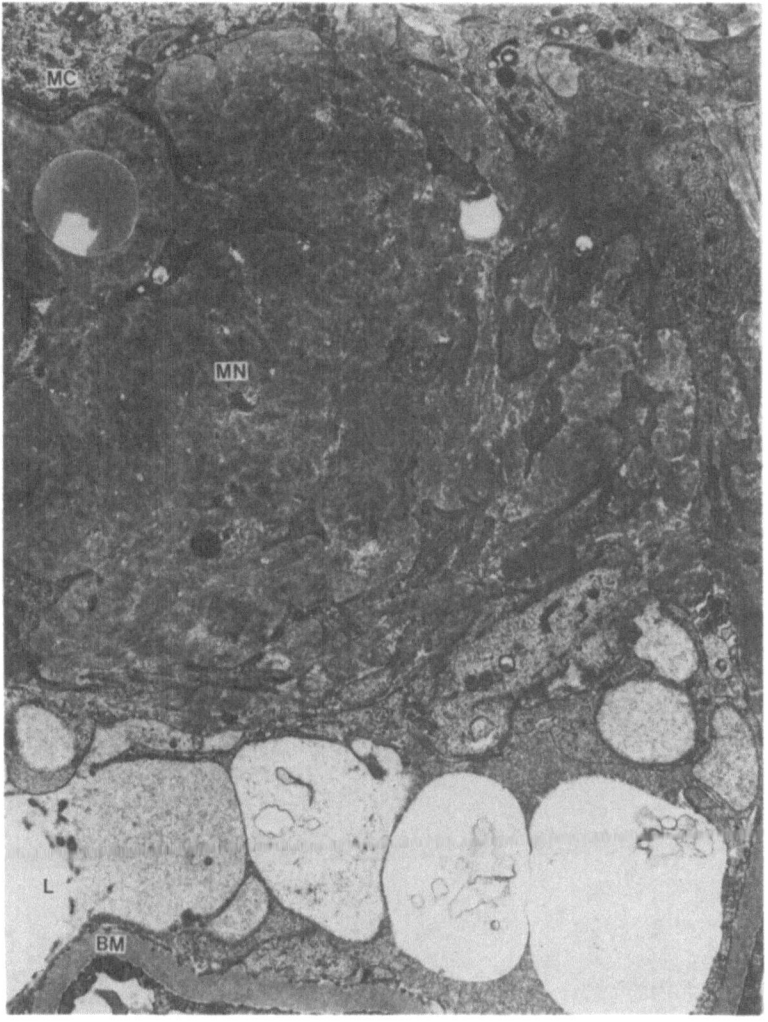

Figure 5–2. Expanded view of mesangial nodule (MN) in glomerulosclerosis (X11598). MC: nucleas of mesangial cell, BM: capillary basement membrane, L: capillary lumen.

in glomerular mesangial matrix growing into single or multiple spherical lesions which encroach on patent capillary loops (figures 5–4 to 5–6). A more prevalent abnormality in the diabetic glomerulus is diffuse intercapillary glomerulosclerosis, which begins as a thickened glomerular basement membrane, associated with an enlarging mesangium filled with amorphous material that stains with periodic acid-Schiff (PAS) (figure 5–7).

Study of renal biopsies by immunofluorescence techniques, has detected plasma proteins, particularly albumin, deposited in a ribbon-like pattern along the tubular

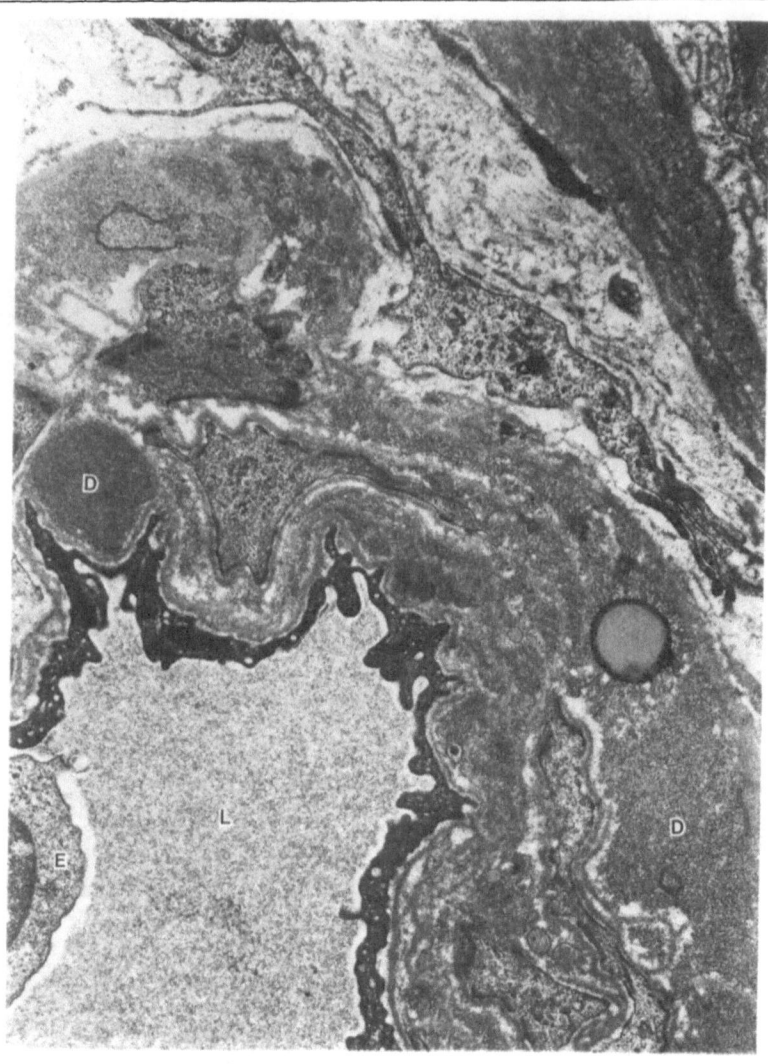

Figure 5–3. Afferent glomerular arteriole demonstrating arteriolosclerosis (X21411). L: arteriolar lumen, D: electron dense deposit in the arteriolar wall lying in a fold of basement membrane which surrounds smooth muscle cells.

basement membrane and Bowman's capsule [24]. The significance of this abnormality, which also occurs in muscle and skin, is obscure.

TYPICAL COURSE OF DIABETIC NEPHROPATHY

In type I diabetes, proteinuria by dipstick testing—which fails to detect microalbuminuria—is first noted in routine urine samples after 10 to 15 years of insulin dependence. By the 20th year of insulin treatment, about one-half of patients

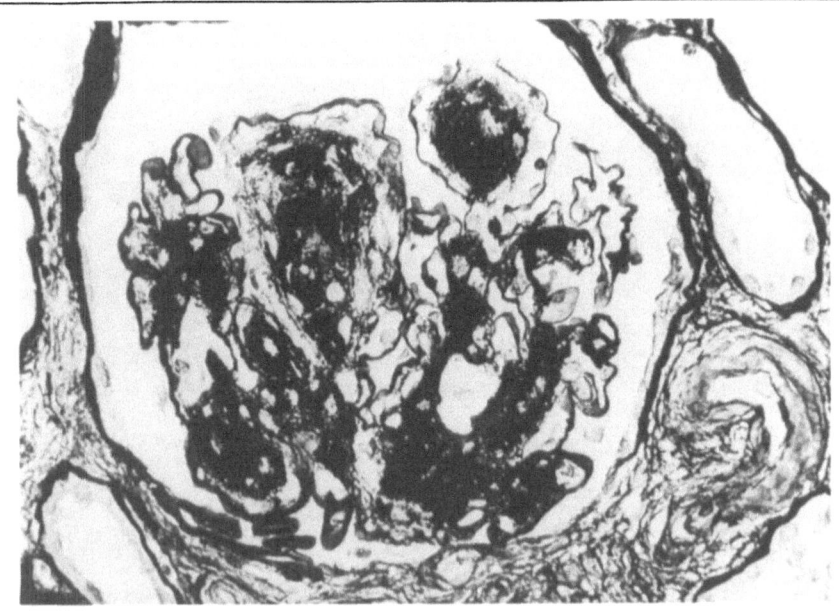

Figure 5–4. Silver-stained glomerulus in kidney biopsy of type I diabetic with 2+ proteinuria (<2g/day) showing mesangial prominence, a fully formed nodule at top right, and arteriolosclerosis in the vessel at the lower right.

have continuous proteinuria [11]. So-called fixed proteinuria is an ominous sign, heralding impending azotemia. Discovery of fixed proteinuria in a type II diabetic is less clearly interpretable, because the older type II patient may have nephrosclerosis (a cause of proteinuria on its own) in addition to intercapillary glomerulosclerosis.

Proteinuria in excess of 500 mg daily, mainly consisting of unmodified albumin, is a constant correlate of advanced glomerulosclerosis. Differences in the technique employed for protein measurement probably account for the varying proportion of diabetics found to be proteinuric. Proteinuria has been noted in all diabetics after six months to 39 years [25], or only after 10 or more years of insulin dependence [26]. Jerums and associates have recently observed in six type I diabetics aged 31 to 59 years, whose duration of diabetes ranged from 0 to 33 years, that "remission and progression of proteinuria may occur frequently in the same individual" [27]. Serial measurements of urinary B_2-microglobulin excretion may provide a reliable prospective means of estimating decline in glomerular filtration rate in type I diabetics [28].

NEPHROTIC SYNDROME

The true significance of finding fixed nephrotic range proteinuria in a type I diabetic becomes evident from examination of their subsequent course. Survival curves in a 1961 study indicated that only 28% of diabetics would live for 10 years

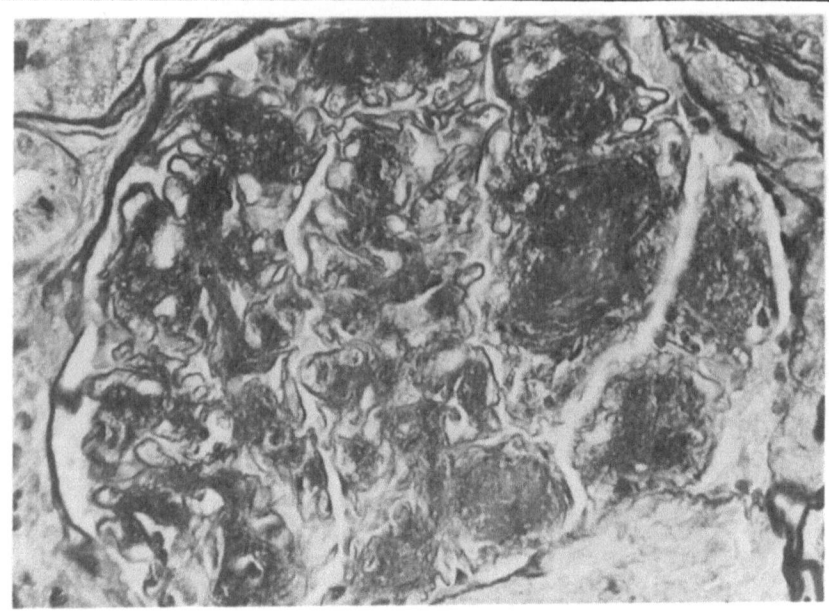

Figure 5–5. More advanced nodular intercapillary glomerulosclerosis in a nephrotic type II diabetic of 16 years' duration. PAS stain.

beyond the onset of "clinical" proteinuria [29]. Before the importance of blood pressure regulation was appreciated, vide infra, Mogensen calculated that diabetics who had a normal glomerular filtration rate (GFR) at the onset of proteinuria, would lose GFR at the rate of 11 ml/min per year. Elevation of serum creatinine concentration usually follows fixed proteinuria within about one year, though there is wide variability; some patients evince proteinuria without azotemia for five or more years [30]. There are few clinical consequences of the early stages of nephrotic syndrome due to glomerulosclerosis despite urinary protein losses of 10 to 30 g/day.

Typically, nephrosis has an insidious onset, with the patient unsure of its presence until a weight gain of 15 or more pounds forces a change in belt or shoe size. Corroboration of the presumption that massive (greater than 4 g/day) proteinuria in a diabetic is due to glomerulosclerosis is afforded by documented transition from microalbuminuria, through fixed proteinuria, and finally a nephrotic syndrome. More than 90% of nephrotic type I diabetics who have intercapillary glomerulosclerosis also have easily diagnosable retinopathy. It follows that the absence of retinopathy in a nephrotic diabetic is reason to suspect some cause for the kidney disorder other than diabetes. Should the funduscopic examination in a nephrotic diabetic be benign or the urinalysis unusual (red cell casts, for example), a percutaneous renal biopsy should be performed to clarify the renal diagnosis.

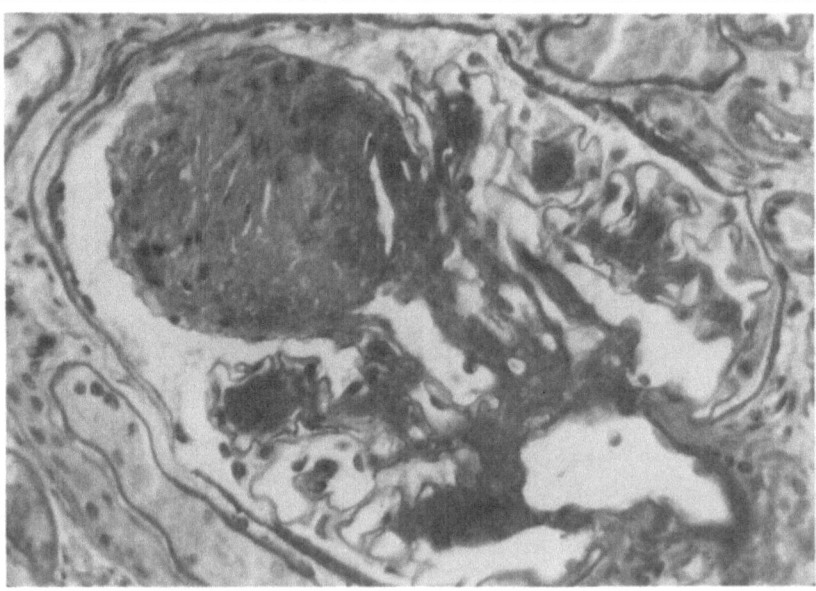

Figure 5–6. Enormous nodule, mesangial proliferation, and arteriolosclerosis in a nephrotic type II diabetic of 14 years duration with advanced glomerulosclerosis.

RENAL INSUFFICIENCY

The penultimate phase in a diabetic's march toward kidney failure is the transition after a decade or longer of normal or supernormal function to a diminished glomerular filtration rate. Correlation of serum creatinine or blood urea nitrogen (BUN) levels with creatinine clearances indicates that a rise above normal (azotemia), in these nitrogenous waste products indicates a residual clearance below 25 to 30 ml/min. Azotemia, which occurred after a mean of 17.3 years of type I diabetes, in the study by Rutherford and associates [31], is a marker, therefore, for the loss of at least 75% of kidney reserve. Subsequent loss of remaining renal function follows an exponential course over a mean of three years [32].

The rate of deterioration in renal function, however, varies considerably from one diabetic to another, but its rate is constant in individuals. Jones and associates [32] observed a linear relation between the months that elapse from the time at which serum creatinine reaches 2.3 mg/dl and the inverse (reciprocal) of the serum creatinine. Of nine patients whose course was plotted starting at a serum creatinine of 2.3 mg/dl, seven reached end stage uremia in 5 to 43 months, but two others had only minimal decline after 35 and 47 months, respectively. As a clinical generalization, the duration of azotemia in a type I diabetic only rarely exceeds three years. Modification of the preceding conclusion may be required because of the salutory effect of better control of hypertension and hyperglycemia which is now the rule rather than the exception. Figure 5–8 shows the composite clinical

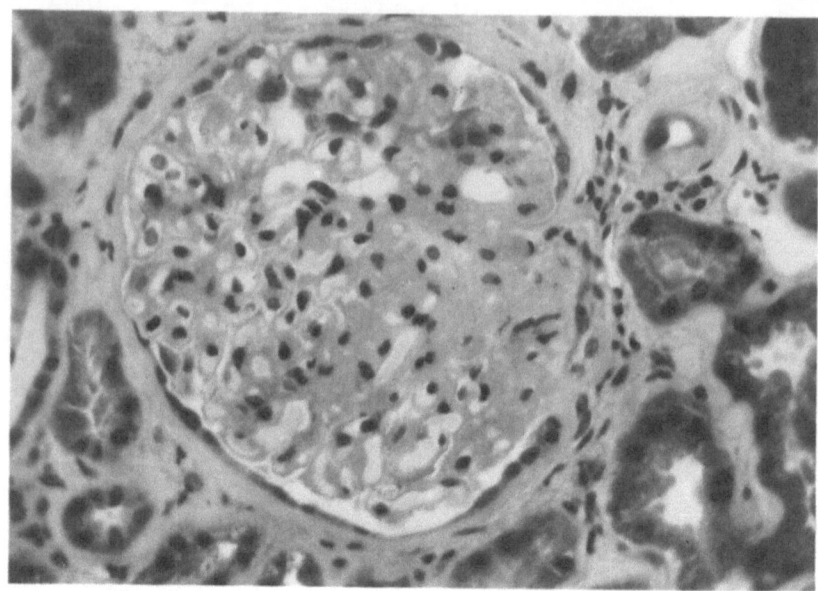

Figure 5–7. Diffuse intercapillary glomerulosclerosis in a nephrotic type I diabetic of 19 years' duration. This appearance in a kidney biopsy stained with hematoxylin and eosin and eosin is similar to that seen in idiopathic membranous glomerulonephritis, or lupus nephritis. Distinguishing diabetic glomerulosclerosis from other glomerulopathies may require multiple stains of light microscopic sections plus examination by flourescence and electron microscopy.

course of renal function in type I diabetics with and without strict regulation of blood pressure.

SPECIFICITY OF GLOMERULOSCLEROSIS FOR DIABETES

Occasional reports describe the finding of nodular and/or diffuse so-called diabetic glomerulosclerosis in nondiabetics. We believe these are in error. Complete examination of biopsy or autopsy kidney specimens requires light, fluorescence, and electron microscopic study. Partial evaluation may confuse membranoproliferative (lobular) glomerulonephritis, myeloma kidney, or idiopathic membranous glomerulonephritis for diabetic glomerulosclerosis. Prior literature descriptions of severe diabetic glomerulosclerosis in autopsy and biopsy kidney specimens, in the absence of proteinuria [33], or carbohydrate intolerance were based on outdated criteria.

CLINICAL MANIFESTATIONS

For most of the course of progressive kidney and other target organ damage, diabetes is, unfortunately, clinically silent. There are no clinical manifestations of glomerular hyperfiltration, microalbuminuria, or mesangial matrix increase (see table 5–1). In the majority of type I diabetics, the first 13 to 18 or more years of glomerulosclerosiss take place while attention is directed to hyperglycemia, ketosis,

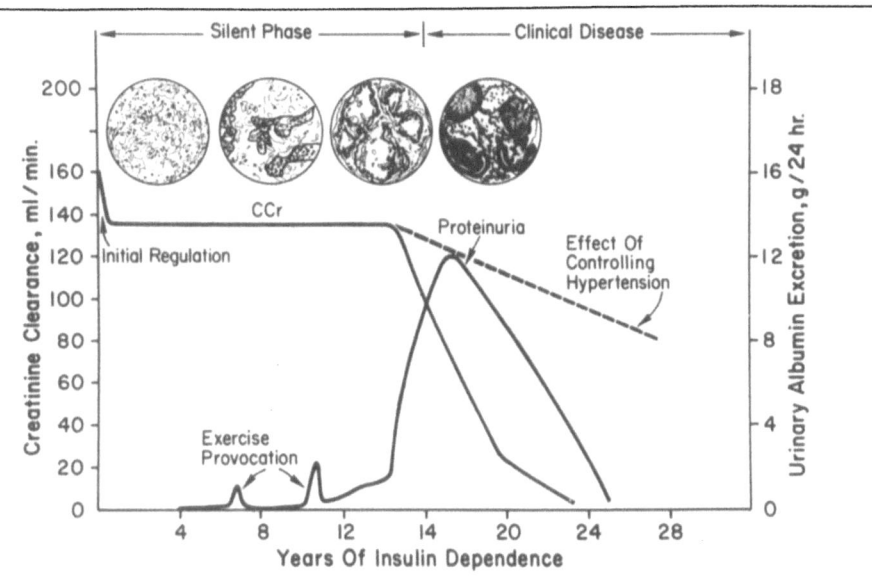

Figure 5–8. Composite course of glomerulopathy in type I diabetes. Early microalbuminuria is not shown. Proteinuria upon exercise provocation precedes fixed proteinuria. Note that severity of glomerular histopathology does not correlate with assessment of renal functional integrity. Advanced glomerulosclersis may be present while measurements of glomerular filtration are normal (or supernormal). The dashed line shows that strict regulation of blood pressure slows the rate of decline in renal function.

candidiasis, or gestational complications, which are thought to be the only manifestation of diabetes. From kidney biopsies obtained in diabetic children and adolescents, however, it is starkly apparent that very advanced intercapillary glomerulosclerosis has developed in kidneys which by function have been incorrectly designated as normal or even supernormal. The onset of proteinuria is not the start of diabetic nephropathy but rather the first clinical sign that renal damage is present.

Once the type I diabetic becomes nephrotic, it is evident that he is sicker at every point in his illness than a nondiabetic with an equivalent degree of renal insufficiency. The cumulative stresses of marginal cardiac compensation and alternating hypoglycemia and hyperglycemia, in a fluid-overloaded diabetic, can make each day an enervating experience. Sequential complications, such as infection in an ischemic foot ulcer, or a vision-impeding vitreous hemorrhage, block the harassed diabetic's effort to continue work, home, or school responsibilities.

Diabetics experience uremic signs and symptoms at a higher level of residual renal function than do nondiabetics. Adult nondiabetics in renal failure due to polycystic kidney disease, chronic glomerulonephritis, or nephrosclerosis can nearly always be managed without need for dialytic therapy as long as their creatinine clearance is greater than 7 to 10 ml/min (serum creatinine concentration > 8 mg/dl). By contrast, the type I diabetic whose creatinine clearance has fallen below 10 ml/min (serum creatinine concentration > 5 mg/dl) is usually too sick to sustain

Table 5–1. Genitourinary complications
of diabetes mellitus

Exacerbation of bacteruria to severe infections
  Pyelonephritis
  Renal carbuncle
  Septicemia
Enhanced susceptibility to renal toxins
  Contrast media-induced nephropathy
  Interstitial nephritis (diuretic induced)
Neuropathy of bladder-simulating obstruction
  Bladder atony (hydronephrosis)
Large artery degenerative syndromes
  Nephrosclerosis
  Atheromatous embolic disease
Microvasculopathy afflicting glomerulus and retina
  Diffuse intracapillary glomerulosclerosis
  Nodular intracapillary glomerulosclerosis

---

work, home, or school responsibilities. Coincident microvasculopathy and macrovasculopathy in vital organ systems (particularly the eye, heart, and central nervous system), and peripheral vascular system account in large part for the significantly higher morbidity and mortality. Management of the azotemic diabetic thus demands attention to extrarenal complications of diabetes as well as formulation of a strategy that anticipates the onset of uremia (figure 5–9).

As glomerulosclerosis progresses and renal catabolism of exogenous insulin (normally about one-third of insulin is metabolized by the kidney) diminishes, episodic profound hypoglycemia may result from formerly safely tolerated doses of insulin. With reduction in GFR to below 10 ml/min, anemia, acidosis, lethargy, nausea, and uncontrollable hypertension dictate the end of conservative care and signal the need for dialysis or renal transplantation. Table 5–2 suggests appropriate interventive actions for each stage of renal disease as a correlate of residual GFR. Lacking an overall plan, the azotemic diabetic faces fragmented, often contradictory approaches to correcting organ or system disease. Medical supervision of a diabetic with progressing nephropathy requires a team approach in which a single physician, identifiable as the patient's doctor, follows through in intergrating the needed services of ophthalmologist and nephrologist. Patients tolerate full disclosure of available options, including the statistical chances of success for each.

ADVERSE EFFECT OF HYPERTENSION
At every stage of diabetic nephropathy, careful attention must be devoted to blood pressure regulation. Normalization of hypertensive blood pressures unquestionably slows the rate of decline of glomerular filtration in the type I diabetic [5]. Because of its intensified adverse effects in diabetics, hypertension should be reduced to a standing blood pressure of about 120/80 mm Hg employing diuretic and vasodila-

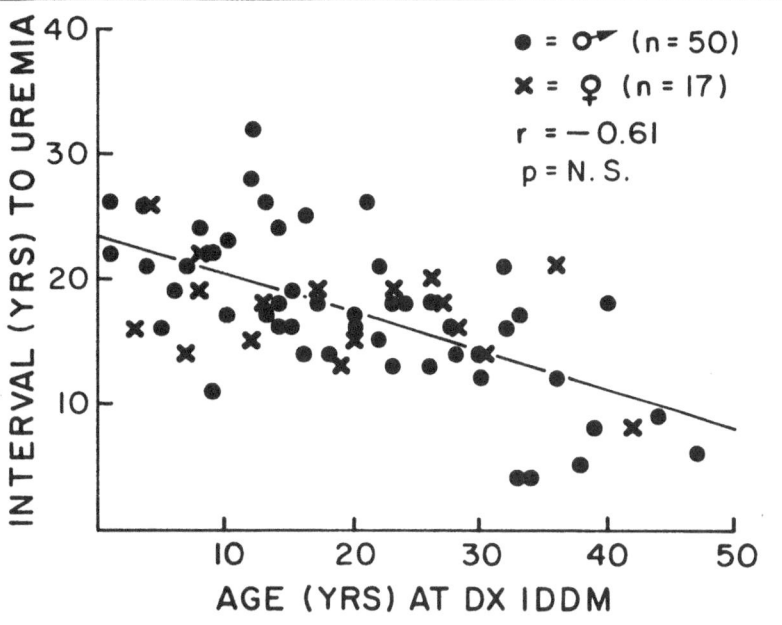

Figure 5–9. Interval between onset of insulin dependence and treatment for uremia in type I diabetics. While the small number of older patients appears to have an accelerated course, the mean duration of diabetes in this whole group of transplant recipients is typical for the 40% to 50% of type I diabetics who develop renal insufficiency is about 20 years.

tor drugs. For diastolic pressures above 120 mm Hg, the addition of captopril, nifedipine, or minoxidil is nearly always effective.

Effective hypertensive management in azotemic diabetics demands sufficient dosage of diuretics. As renal reserve declines to about 25% of normal, chlorthiazide and hydrochlorthiazide become ineffective and must be replaced by a loop diuretic such as furosemide. To effect diuresis at creatinine clearances as low as 10 to 20 ml/min may require total doses as high as 480 mg of furosemide daily. Adding metolazone, a long-acting thiazide-retaining activity in renal insufficiency, in daily doses of 5 to 20 mg, often promotes diuresis in resistant cases. Binephrectomy for control of intractable hypertension has not been required in our program in over 10 years. Diabetics may develop unusual or particularly severe complications of antihypertensive drugs including worsened hyperglycemia from diuretics, muted or altered signs and symptoms of hypoglycemia from beta blockers, and intensified fluid retention from sympathetic inhibitors and vasodilators. Lipson, in reviewing the management of hypertension in diabetes, suggests a logical "stepwise progression . . . with the use of drugs that interfere least with the diabetic state and its complications" [34].

The limit of conservative management may be signaled by persistent hypertension, no longer responsive to antihypertensive drugs. Of 67 diabetics undergoing

Table 5–2. Progression of diabetic nephropathy

Stage	Creatinine clearance	Strategy
Silent	Normal to super normal	Maintain euglycemia Control hypertension Consult ophthalmologist Document microalbuminuria
Early proteinuric	30 ml/min to normal	As in silent stage ? other renal diseases Educate patient
Late proteinuric (nephrotic)	20 to 80 ml/min	Plot 1/creatinine versus time Consider dialysis access Inventory kidney donors Review eye status Antihypertensive regimen Assess cardiac status
Azotemic	5 to 25 ml/min	Review uremia therapies Review eye status Create dialysis access Treatment if symptomatic (early dialysis) Emphasize transplant
Renal death	5 ml/min	Uremia therapy

kidney transplantation in our program, 60 (90%) were hypertensive pretransplant, a finding that underscores the correlation of elevated blood pressure and renal failure in diabetes. Reduction of elevated blood pressure will reduce proteinuria [35] and slow the rate of declining GFR [36] in nephropathic diabetics. Christlieb reviewed the mechanism(s) for an increased rate of hypertension in diabetics without evidence of nephropathy and suggested that hyperglycemia-induced expanded blood volume might be responsible [37]. Most hypertensive diabetics without renal disease have normal plasma renin activity (PRA). In nephropathic diabetics with proteinuria of 2g or more daily, both plasma renin activity and plasma aldosterone concentration are significantly reduced, characterizing a "low-renin hypertension" [38].

Low-renin hypertensive diabetics evince: decreased sympathetic activity altering stimulation of renin release [39]; defective synthesis of prorenin [40]; hyalinization of afferent arterioles inhibiting passage of renin from juxtaglomerular cells into the lumen [41]; and expanded intravascular volume. Arteriolar hyalinization is a component of diabetic vasculopathy, and also contributes to hypertension by raising peripheral vascular resistance. An additional factor responsible for hypertension is an increased cardiac output as a compensation (tachycardia) to the anemia of renal insufficiency. In this light, hypoaldosteronism (promoting natriuresis and plasma volume fall) and low-renin activity (decreased circulating angiotensin II and lowered peripheral vascular resistance) can be viewed as compensatory mechanisms to counteract hypertension.

LIMIT OF CONSERVATIVE THERAPY

Neither patient nor physician should be surprised by the ultimate need for dialysis or kidney transplantation in a diabetic who has undergone years of declining renal reserve. Timing of initiation of uremia therapy has been advocated early (creatinine clearance of 10 to 25 ml/min) or later, though all would agree that a creatinine clearance of less than 5 ml/min is an absolute indication for switching from conservative to more aggressive treatment. Dialytic treatment or a kidney transplant is urgently required by diabetics found to have a serum creatinine concentration above 8 mg/dl and bleeding due to gastritis or colitis, pericarditis, or convulsions.

Rather than a specific complication precipitating uremia therapy, the diabetic in renal insufficiency more typically ends conservative management due to a nonspecific deterioration characterized by weight loss, worsening hypertension, and lethargy. Lacking either prospective or retrospective studies of the ideal time to start dialysis, it is reasonable to select that point in a patient's course at which further deterioration, especially of visual acuity and the cardiovascular system, appears inevitable. Proper anticipatory planning should prepare for smooth initiation of uremia therapy, in which an informed patient has selected the most appropriate course. This is the time for young type I diabetics to consider the feasibility of a kidney transplant, reflecting on potential intrafamilial donors.

URINARY INFECTIONS

Diabetics develop kidney disorders other than or in addition to glomerulosclerosis. Of these, urinary tract infection is the most common. Few data detailing the incidence, prevalence, and therapy of urinary infections in diabetics distinguish between type I and type II diabetics. Hospitalization and bladder catheterization impose extra risks of bacteriuria to diabetics who are more often hospitalized than nondiabetics. Bacteriuria has been found in increased incidence in diabetics in some but not all surveys [42]. Kass detected bacteriuria in 18% of 54 asymptomatic diabetic women and 5% of 37 diabetic men [42]. Other surveys, however, have not confirmed an increased incidence of bacteriuria in either diabetic school girls or pregnant diabetics [43]. Our own study of bacteriuria in diabetic renal transplant recipients revealed a prevalence rate of 4%, no greater than in nondiabetics. Urinary infection, once established, is many times more likely to become seriously complicated in diabetics than in nondiabiabetics. Treatment of urinary infection in diabetics requires (1) precise identification of the organism(s) and a search for urease-positive organisms; (2) normalization of blood glucose concentration; (3) relief of mechanical obstruction due to ureteric or bladder calculi, tumor, or an enlarged prostate; (4) removal wherever possible of a bladder catheter; and (5) adjustment, according to renal function, of the doses of antimicrobial drugs mainly excreted by the kidney.

TOXIC NEPHROPATHY

Azotemic diabetics, especially those whose serum creatinine concentration exceeds 3 mg/dl, should avoid radiocontrast media studies in any circumstance in which

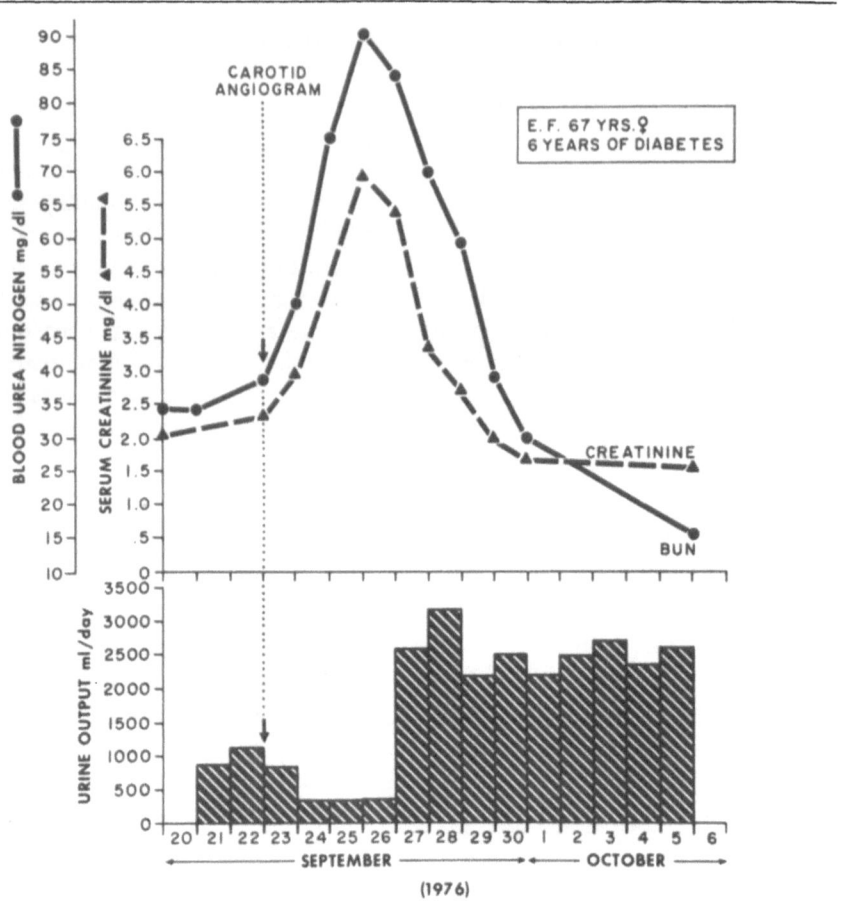

Figure 5–10. Toxic nephropathy in a type II diabetic. Administration of contrast media to a diabetic with azotemia (in this instance evidenced by a serum creatinine of 2.0 mg/dl) risks acute renal failure which in the majority of instances is reversible.

the information needed can be developed by other diagnostic means. Both type I and type II diabetics may respond to intravenous urography or intravenous or intraarterial angiographic procedures with the acute onset (hours to two days) of oliguria and renal insufficiency [10]. Renal failure has been reported after meglumine iothalamate, meglumine diatrizoate, and sodium diatrazoate given in doses of 36 to 300g. Contrast-agent-induced nephropathy has been attributed to the osmotic burden of injected contrast media (about 2,000 mOsm/kg H20), added to hyperviscous diabetic plasma, which in a patient dehydrated by a preparatory cathartic predisposes to reduced renal perfusion and ischemic injury. If angiography is unavoidable in an azotemic diabetic—for evaluation of a transient ischemic attack, for example—normal hydration should be maintained and 25g of mannitol administered intravenously one hour prior to the study to maintain urine flow.

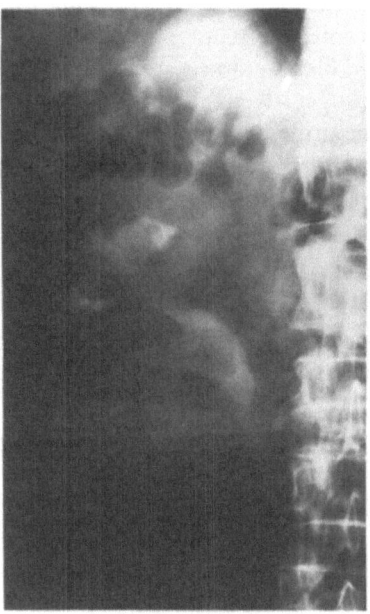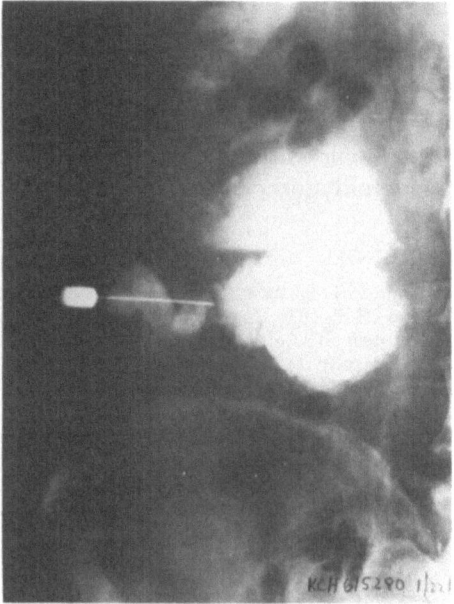

Figure 5–11. Diabetics are more likely than nondiabetics to develop a renal carbuncle as the result of an intrarenal infection. The findings in a type II diabetic woman who had fever, flank pain, and pyuria are shown. Distorted renal calyces in an excretory urogram are evident in the left panel. The right panel illustrates the abscess cavity injected percutaneously with contrast media.

Our own experience suggests that in the absence of azotemia or proteinuria, intravenous urography is safe in type II diabetics. In patients with creatinine clearances below 25 ml/min, however, postcontrast-agent acute renal failure occurs with increasing frequency, afflicting the majority of patients with a clearance of less than 10 ml/min [44].

Although the duration of acute renal failure is variable, most patients recover renal function after 3 to 10 days of oliguria. Acute renal failure due to drug toxicity, renal ischemia, or ingestion of or exposure to noxious chemicals may afflict the diabetic at any stage of his illness. Because moderately advanced renal insufficiency (creatinine clearance less than 40 ml/min), though common, may be unrecognized, potentially toxic drugs excreted by the kidneys, such as aminoglyco-side antibiotics, must be monitored and administered in reduced dosage. Reference to published tables relating serum levels of drugs to renal reserve [45] minimizes the complexity of prescribing essential yet hazardous drugs.

INTRARENAL INFECTION

Intrarenal infection leading to ischemic infarction of the renal medulla and papilla may occur in a single papilla without clinical consequence as in sickle cell trait, or may involve multiple papillae leading to destruction of the kidney and obstruction of the ureter by sloughed papillae in analgesic abuse, alcoholism, and diabetes. Fever, flank pain, and dysuria, which may progress to septicemia and shock, are the presenting findings (figure 5–11). Urine and blood cultures are usually positive for a bacterial or fungal (sometimes both) pathogen. Renal fragments, sometimes as large as 1 cm in length, may be passed in the urine. Papillary necrosis is treated by cystoscopic extraction of any renal tissue fragments causing obstruction and by the administration of antibiotics or antifungal drugs.

REFERENCES

1. Sugimoto T, Rosansky SJ. The incidence of treated end stage renal disease in the Eastern United States: 1973–1979. Amer J Public Health 74:14–17, 1984.
2. Mogensen CE. Editorial review: microalbuminuria and incipient diabetic nephropathy. Diabetic Nephropathy 3:75–78, 1984.
3. Rasch R. Prevention of diabetic glomerulopathy in streptozotocin diabetic rats by insulin treatment. Kidney size and glomerular volume. Diabetologia 16:125–128, 1979.
4. Viberti GC. Early functional and morphological changes in diabetic nephropathy. Clin Nephrol 12:47–53, 1979.
5. Parving HH, Osenboll B, Svendsen PA, Christiansen JS, Andersen AR. Early detection of patients at risk of developing diabetic nephropathy: a longitudinal study of urinary albumin excretion. Acta endocrinol 100:550–555, 1982.
6. Mogensen CE, Christensen CK. Predicting diabetic nephropathy in insulin-dependent patients. N Engl J Med 311:89–93, 1984.
7. Mogensen CE. Microalbuminuria predicts clinical proteinuria and early mortality in maturity-onset diabetes. N Engl J Med 310:356–360, 1984.
8. Brenner BM, Hostetter TH, Humes HD. Molecular basis of proteinuria in glomerular origin. N Engl J Med 298:826–833, 1978.
9. Editorial. Charge and the kidney. Lancet 3:732, 1984.
10. Vernier RL, Klein DJ, Sisson SP, Mahan JD, Oegema TR, Brown DM. Heparin sulfate rich anionic sites in the human glomerular basement membrane. Decreased concentration in congenital nephrotic syndrome. N Engl J Med 309:1001–1009, 1983.
11. Mauer SM, Fish AJ, Day NK, Michael AF. The glomerular mesangium. II. Quantitative studies of mesangial function in nephrotoxic nephritis in rats. J Clin Invest 53:431–439, 1974.
12. Mauer SM, Shvil Y. The glomerular mesangium. In: Renal Disease, Black Sir D, Jones NF (eds). Oxford: Blackwell Sci Publ 93:106, 1979.
13. Mauer SM, Steffes MW, Brown DM. The kidney in diabetes. Am J Med 70:603–612, 1981.
14. Mauer SM, Steffes MW, Chern M, Brown DM. Mesangial uptake and processing of mac-romoleculles in rats with diabetes mellitus. Lab Invest 41:401–406, 1979.
15. Osterby R. Early phases in the development of diabetic glomerulopathy. Acta Med Scand (Suppl) 574:1–82, 1975.
16. Foglia VG, Manccini RE, CarCardeza AF. Glomerular lesions in the diabetic rat. Arch Pathol Lab Med 50: 75–83, 1950.
17. Ireland JT. Diagnostic criteria in the assessment of glomerular capillary basement membrane lesions in newly diagnosed juvenile diabetics. In: Early Diabetes, Camerini-Davalos RA, Cole HS (eds). New York: Academic Press, 1970, p. 273.
18. Castells S, Tejani A, Nicastri AD, Chen CK, Fusi M-A, Sen D. Diabetic nephropathy: early renal changes in adolescent insulin-dependent diabetics. Diabetic Nephropathy 3:15–18, 1984.
19. Hostetter TH, Olson JL, Rennke HG, Venkatachalam MA, Brenner BM. Hyperfiltration in remnant nephrons: a potentially adverse response to renal ablation. Am J. Physiol 24:F85–93, 1981.
20. Olson JL, Hostetter TH, Rennke HG, Brenner BM, Venkatachalam MA. Altered glomerular permselectivity and progressive sclerosis. Kidney Internat 22:112–116, 1982.
21. Deckert T, Bo F-R, Mathiesen ER, Baker L. Pathogenesis of incipient nephropathy: a hypothesis. Diabetic Nephropathy 3:83–88, 1984.
22. Kimmelstiel P, Wilson C. Intercapillary lesions in glomeruli of kidney. Am J Pathol 12:83–98, 1936.

23. Gellman DD, Pirani CC, Soothill JF, Muehreke RC, Kark RM. Diabetic nephropathy; a clinical and pathologic study based on renal biopsies. Medicine 38:321–368, 1959.
24. Burkholder PM. Renal disease associated with diabetes mellitus. In: Atlas of Human Glomerular Pathology, Burkholder PM (ed). Hagerstown, Md.: Harper and Row, 1974, p. 325.
25. Mogensen CE. Renal function changes in diabetes. Diabetes 25:872–879, 1976.
26. Parving H-H, Oxenboll B, Svendsen PA, Christiansen JS, Andersen An AR. Early detection of patients at risk of developing diabetic nephropathy. A longitudinal study of urinary albumin excretion. Acta Endo 100:550–555, 1982.
27. Jerums G, Seeman E, Murray RML, Edgley S, Markwick K, Goodall I, Young VH. Remission and progression of trace proteinuria in type I diabetes. Diabetic Nephropathy 3:104–111, 1984.
28. Viberti GC. Effect of control of blood glucose on urinary excretion of albumin and B2-microglobulin in insulin-dependent diabetes. New Eng J. Med 300:638–641, 1979.
29. Caird RI. Survival of diabetics with proteinuria. Diabetes 10:178–181, 1961.
30. Mogensen CE. Renal function changes in diabetes. Diabetes 25:872–879, 1976.
31. Rutherford WE, Blondin J, Miller JP, Greenwalt AS, Vavra JD. Chronic progressive renal disease: rate of change of serum creatinine concentration. Kid Int 11:62–70, 1977.
32. Jones RH, Mackay JD, Hayakawa H, Parsons V. Progression of diabetic nephropathy. Lancet I:1105–1106, 1979.
33. Hatch FE, Watt MF, Kramer NC, Parrish AE, Howe JS. Diabetic glomerulosclerosis: a long-term follow-up study based on renal biopsies. Am J Med 31:216–230, 1961.
34. Lipson LG. Special problems in treatment of hypertension in the patient with diabetes mellitus. Arch Int Med 144:1829–1831, 1984.
35. Morgensen CE, Christensen CK, Christensen NJ, Gundersen HJG, Jacobssen FK, Pedersen EB, Vittinghus E. Renal protein handling in normal hypertensive and diabetic man. Contr Nephrol 24:139–152, 1981.
36. Morgensen CE. Antihypertensive treatment inhibiting the progression of diabetic nephropathy. Acta endocr, Copenh 94:(suppl 238) 103–108, 1980.
37. Christlieb AP. Diabetes and hypertensive vascular disease. Am J Cardiol 32:592–606, 1973.
38. Christlieb AR, Kaldany A, D'Elia JA. Plasma renin activity and hypertension in diabetes mellitus. Diabetes 25:969–974, 1976.
39. Christensen NJ. Plasma catecholamines in long-term diabetics with and without neuropathy and in hypophysectomized subjects. J Clin Invest 51:779–787, 1972.
40. Day RP, Leutscher JA, Gonzales CM. Occurrence of big renin in human plasma, amniotic fluid, and kidney extracts. J Clin Endocrinol Metab 40:1078–1084, 1975.
41. Schindler AM, Sommers SC. Diabetic sclerosis of the renal juxtaglomerular apparatus. Lab Invest 15:877–884, 1966.
42. Kass EII. Asymptomatic infections of the urinary tract. Trans Assoc Am Physicians 69:56–64, 1956.
43. Kunin CM, Southall I, Paguin AJ. Epidemiology of urinary tract infection: pilot study of 3057 school children. N Engl J Med 263:817–823, 1960.
44. Harkonen S, Kjellstrand CM. Exacerbation of diabetic renal failure following intravenous pyelography. Am J. Med 63:939–946, 1977.
45. Bennett WM, Muther RS, Parker RA, Feig P, Morrison G, Golper TA, Singer I. Drug therapy in renal failure: dosing guidelines for adults. Part I: Antimicrobial agents, analgesics. Ann Int Med 93:62–89, 1980.

6. HEMODIALYSIS FOR THE UREMIC DIABETIC

KATHLEEN Y. WHITLEY
FRED L. SHAPIRO

RENAL REPLACEMENT THERAPY IN DIABETICS: HEMODIALYSIS

It has been estimated that approximately 3,200 patients with diabetes mellitus will develop end-stage renal disease per year in the United States. The uremic diabetic must utilize at least one of several modalities of renal replacement therapy in order to survive. These options include hemodialysis, intermittent automated peritoneal dialysis, chronic ambulatory peritoneal dialysis, and renal transplantation from a living related or cadaver donor. A randomized, prospective trial comparing the efficacy of these treatments for the diabetic in renal failure is not feasible. Therefore, the selection of one of these therapies for each individual patient must be made by matching the specific needs of the patient to available clinical data demonstrating the advantages and indications for each of the different end-stage renal replacement therapies.

Hemodialysis has been the renal replacement therapy used most widely both in the United States and Europe for patients with end-stage diabetic nephropathy. Because of dismal survival and progressive handicaps (e.g., blindness) in diabetic patients treated by hemodialysis early in the development of this therapy, and because of limited availability of this resource for patients with complications of multisystemic disease, diabetic patients initially composed only 1–5% of all chronic hemodialysis patients. However, as resources have become more plentiful and survival in diabetic patients has improved, patients with end-stage renal disease secondary to both type I and type II diabetes mellitus have contributed increasing numbers of patients now utilizing hemodialysis. In fact, in several centers in the United States and in European countries such as Sweden and Finland, diabetic patients comprise 20–30% of all patients now initiating dialysis.

Since 1966, the Regional Kidney Disease Program (RKDP) in Minneapolis has provided regular hemodialysis care to 421 diabetic patients. The proportion of new patients entering the RKDP program who are diabetic has also increased in recent years. During the past few years, approximately 30% of our new patients have endstage diabetic nephropathy (figure 6–1). As has been observed throughout the United States, our chronic dialysis patient population of both diabetic and nondiabetic patients has also been increasing in age. Selected aspects and results of the RKDP experience treating diabetic patients with hemodialysis will be discussed in this review of hemodialysis for patients with diabetic nephropathy.

TIMING OF ACCESS AND DIALYSIS

The clinical progression of diabetic nephropathy is remarkably predictable and particularly well characterized in the type I (insulin-dependent, ketosis-prone) diabetic patient of whom 30–50% develop renal failure. The earliest clinical manifestation of diabetic nephropathy is intermittent proteinuria which is invariably followed by persistent proteinuria, the latter occurring predictably 15–20 years after onset of disease. This phenomenon is often accompanied by hypertension. Approximately four years after onset of proteinuria, diabetic nephropathy progresses to end-stage renal failure.

Less well characterized is the clinical course of the type II (non-insulin depen-

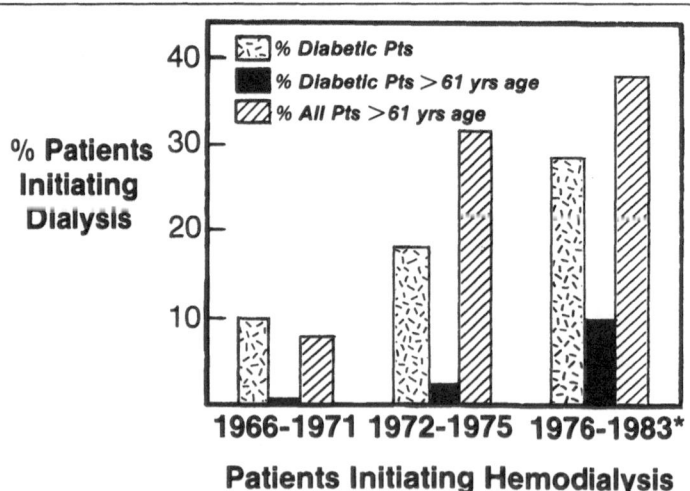

Figure 6–1. Patients with type I and type II diabetes mellitus contribute an increasing percentage of patients now initiating dialysis in the Regional Kidney Disease Program in Minneapolis. The average age of both diabetic patients and nondiabetic patients also continues to increase. Includes patients through June 30, 1983.

dent, non-ketosis prone, maturity onset, often obese) diabetic patient. Although this is the more common type of diabetes, a much smaller percentage of patients with type II diabetes mellitus will develop renal failure, particularly as age of onset increases. However, Goldstein and Massry have previously described, and Avram has more recently noted, that clinical evidence of diabetic nephropathy occurs earlier in these patients, approximately 12–13 years after diagnosis with subsequent rapid deterioration in renal function. In the RKDP experience, the time course from onset of diabetes to end-stage renal disease in type I and type II diabetic patients follows patterns similar to those noted above (table 6–1).

Other multisystemic manifestations of diabetes mellitus cascade in parallel with renal dysfunction. In the two years prior to development of end-stage renal failure, the diabetic patient often experiences an accelerated progression of diabetic retinopathy, diabetic neuropathy, and hypertension. The patient often has a very rapid deterioration in renal function when serum creatinine reaches 5–8 mg/dl.

It is during this time period when significant handicaps such as blindness and preventable causes of accelerated decline in renal function can be avoided by close medical supervision of patients with diabetes mellitus. This is also a time when the desired effects of antihypertensive therapy and insulin therapy regimens may be complicated by autonomic insufficiency and uremic symptomatology. For example, orthostatic hypotension is a common manifestation of autonomic neuropathy which limits the types of medications that can be utilized for blood pressure control. Gastrointestinal dysmotility disorders (gastroparesis) may be incapacitating and are worsened by uremia. Anorexia, nausea, and vomiting often result in decreased and variable caloric intake, and detrimentally affect glycemic regulation and secondarily exacerbate diabetic visceral and peripheral neuropathies. Hyperglycemia also stimulates thirst, and as a result, extracellular fluid volume overload is common and in turn worsens hypertension. The development of a neurogenic

Table 6–1. Clinical presentation of type I and type II diabetic patients with end-stage renal disease initiating dialysis in the Regional Kidney Disease Program 1966–83[1]

	Type I	Type II
Number of patients	266	187
Males	154 (58%)	71 (38%)
Females	112 (42%)	116 (62%)
Mean age (yrs)	41.9	62.9
Age range (yrs)	21–77	25–84
Duration of diabetes (yrs)	22.5	13.1
Range (yrs)	2–48	0–48
Number 15 + yrs	237 (89%)	62 (33%)
Retinopathy	257 (97%)	126 (67%)
Blind	89 (33%)	24 (13%)

1. 421 patients began hemodialysis and 32 patients initiated peritoneal dialysis during this time period.

bladder may cause accelerated deterioration of renal function by predisposing the patient with diabetic renal insufficiency to urinary tract infection and obstructive uropathy. In contrast to patients with advanced renal failure of other etiologies, the patient with diabetic nephropathy exhibits symptoms of uremia at a higher measured creatinine clearance. Thus, patients with diabetic nephropathy should begin dialysis when serum creatinine reaches 8–9 mg/dl.

Planning for hemodialysis as renal replacement therapy must, therefore, begin early in the patient with diabetic nephropathy for several reasons. Since the patient with diabetes often has extensive underlying vascular disease, the creation of a simple fistula as vascular access is often difficult and the success rate is very low. Therefore, an attempt at formation of a simple fistula should be made when the patient's creatinine is between 4–5 mg/dl to allow ample time for fistula maturation. An end artery anastomosis should be created to avoid a steal syndrome which can complicate a side-to-side radial artery anastomosis and result in ischemia distal to the fistula, digital gangrene, and necessitate amputation. If, at the time of surgery, the cephalic vein or radial artery is not suitable for fistula formation, a bovine carotid artery or Gortex graft should be placed as the primary internal vessel access. These grafts, once successfully established, compare favorably in diabetic patients with results in nondiabetic patients and avoid loss of valuable time awaiting the maturation of a fistula which will never occur because of poor arterial flow or a sclerotic vein which will not dilate. Only rarely, in the patient with diabetes, these grafts must be banded to diminish flow rates which otherwise would result in ischemic contractures.

Complications of external devices for hemodialysis access such as the Scribner cannula or the subclavian catheter are more common in diabetic patients, and therefore they are utilized only for temporary use until internal access has been firmly established. Alternatively, peritoneal dialysis may also be employed as a temporizing measure.

Tables 6–1 and 6–2 summarize the clinical presentation of RKDP patients

Table 6–2. Mean serum creatinine and creatinine clearance of diabetic patients initiating dialysis during 1966–71, 1972–75, 1976–83

	Serum creatinine (mg/dl)	Creatinine clearance (ml/min)
Type I		
1966–71	11.2	5.6
1972–75	12.7	4.8
1976–83	9.0	5.9
Type II		
1972–75	12.0	3.2
1976–83	9.6	5.5

Note: Although renal function at the time of initiation of dialysis for the average patient is slightly better than before, survival has markedly improved during these periods.

initiating hemodialysis between January 1966 and June 1983. Of note, the mean duration of diabetes in type I diabetic patients before initiation of dialysis was 22.5 years. In type II diabetic patients the mean duration of disease was 13.1 years. Almost universally, the type I diabetic patients demonstrated at least background retinopathy, with 33% of patients being legally blind. Although diabetic retinopathy in type II diabetic patients was not quite as pervasive, 13% of these patients were blind at the time hemodialysis was initiated. Mean serum creatinine at the time of initiation in both type I and type II diabetics has been 9.0 and 9.6 mg/dl, respectively, during the last seven years.

STABILIZATION OF NEWLY INITIATED HEMODIALYSIS PATIENTS

Hemodialysis in patients with end-stage renal disease secondary to diabetic nephropathy presents some unique problems in patient management. During the initial stabilization period, which often lasts four to six weeks, several clinical and metabolic changes occur in the diabetic patient. Patients may initially note increasing weakness and malaise after starting dialysis. Vomiting without associated nausea also occurs commonly secondary to delayed gastric emptying. Both of these problems usually improve during the first month of dialysis. Managing changes in insulin therapy, changes in diet, control of hypertension and hypotension during dialysis and between dialysis therapies, and control of fluid gains between dialysis runs are some of the therapeutic challenges presented by the newly initiated diabetic hemodialysis patient.

Diet

The onset of uremia and dialysis therapy requires further dietary restriction of the diabetic patient which makes planning a palatable diet difficult and requires some ingenuity. There are three goals in regulating the diet in the diabetic dialysis patient: (1) maintenance of nitrogen balance; (2) minimization of the sensation of thirst and excess fluid intake secondary to hyperglycemia or excess dietary sodium intake; and (3) minimization of hyperkalemia induced by hyperglycemia or excess dietary potassium intake. Caloric requirements are similar to those of nondiabetic patients: 35 kcal/kg/day, divided into three meals and two snacks. Calories should be supplied as 50% carbohydrate, particularly complex carbohydrate to provide better glucose and lipid control. Protein requirements include 1.5 grams protein/kg/day with two-thirds provided as high biological protein. Polyunsaturated fats should supply 30–35% of calories and have an added role in inducing satiety and adding interest to the diet. Fiber may also be important in minimizing postprandial hyperglycemia. Daily sodium chloride intake is limited to 4 grams, and daily potassium intake should not exceed 70 mEq.

Insulin

During the time when end-stage renal failure is reached and dialysis is initiated, insulin requirements may again increase, although this is quite variable and is also dependent on the patient's appetite, frequency of vomiting, other associated medical complications, and physical activity. Variations in insulin requirements needed to maintain euglycemia also result from the balance between several pathophysiologic effects of end-stage renal disease in diabetic patients. Increased sensitivity to insulin occurs because of diminished excretion and degradation of insulin by the kidney. Glycogen stores in the uremic diabetic patient are also decreased, and as a result, hypoglycemic episodes may be profound. On the other hand, increased insulin resistance occurs in both peripheral tissues such as adipose and muscle, and also in the liver. In peripheral tissues, this resistance appears to be an abnormality in tissue binding of insulin to its receptor or a postreceptor defect. Also peripheral tissues may have an increased sensitivity to the insulin antagonistic effects of the hormone glucagon which is present in higher quantities in renal failure. Finally, in the liver, the usual modulation of glucose production from gluconeogenesis and glycogenolysis appears to be impaired. Elevated parathyroid hormone (PTH) may have a role in this latter effect. At least peripheral insulin resistance is reversible by chronic hemodialysis. As a result of these cumulative effects, and often by the end of the stabilization period, patients usually require the same total dosage of insulin that they previously needed prior to the development of renal insufficiency. Acceptable glucose regulation is usually achieved by twice-daily insulin injections containing regular and NPH insulin in a mixture of 3–5:1. Self-monitoring of blood glucose by reagent strips and/or reflectance meters is necessary in patients with diabetic nephropathy and also in patients with end-stage diabetic renal disease since urine testing is inaccurate or impossible in both of these groups.

Insulin regulation of serum glucose is extremely important in the dialysis patient to insure nutrition, prevent life-threatening hyperkalemia, prevent hyperlipidemia, and control extracellular fluid volume. In fact, at one extreme, pulmonary edema has been reported in diabetic dialysis patients secondary to rapid intracellular to extracellular fluid shifts caused by increase in extracellular fluid osmolality from hyperglycemia.

Hypotension/hypertension
Episodes of hypertension and hypotension during hemodialysis are much more common and problematic in patients with end-stage diabetic nephropathy. Hypotension during dialysis is usually precipitated by autonomic insufficiency manifested by orthostatic hypotension and a fixed heart rate. This complicates the process of establishing the patient's optimum dry weight by ultrafiltration. Orthostatic hypotension is also a problem between dialysis runs and can be incapacitating. This circumstance can be improved by the use of elastic support stockings during the day and elevation of the head of the bed by 8 to 10-inch blocks during the night.

Hypertension in the diabetic patient initiating dialysis is overwhelmingly volume-dependent and does respond to ultrafiltration during dialysis and fluid restriction between dialysis runs. It has previously been reported that interdialytic weight gains are much greater in diabetic patients than in nondiabetic patients. Because of difficulty with autonomic insufficiency during dialysis, hypotension may prevent effective ultrafiltration and rapid establishment of ideal dry weight.

In the RKDP experience, normalization of blood pressure and acceptable levels of orthostasis have, however, been achieved in the great majority of patients without resorting to antihypertensive agents by gradually reducing the patient's weight over several weeks with ultrafiltration. This process has the additional benefit of improvement in visual acuity in patients because of decreasing macular edema as optimal dry weight is achieved.

Technical aspects of dialysis
Two specific details of hemodialysis technique in the diabetic patient deserve special emphasis. The first of these is that dialysate without glucose may complicate long-term hemodialysis by stimulating glycogenolysis and gluconeogenesis and, as a result, can cause negative nitrogen balance. Glucose should therefore be included in dialysate in the concentration of 150–200 mg/dl.

Second, it was previously thought that much of the blindness in diabetic hemodialysis patients was caused by intermittent heparinization. Over the last 15 years, despite little change in heparinization regimens during dialysis, the incidence of new blindness in diabetic patients has progressively and impressively declined in our dialysis population as well as in other centers. Therefore, regular heparinization schedules may be used routinely in diabetic dialysis patients. However, long-term anticoagulation with coumarin may pose considerable increased risk of intraocular hemorrhage. Therefore, oral anticoagulation should be avoided if its sole or major purpose is to preserve function in a tenuous hemoaccess, and alternatively definitive surgical access repair should be accomplished.

SURVIVAL
Prolongation of life by the technique of hemodialysis in patients with end-stage renal disease secondary to diabetic nephropathy can be evaluated by comparison with survival in patients with end-stage renal disease of other etiologies maintained by hemodialysis or by comparison with diabetic patients whose lives are prolonged by other renal replacement therapies. As previously mentioned, hemodialysis has been the replacement therapy for end-stage renal disease used most often in diabetic patients. In more limited numbers, diabetic patients have also been treated by renal transplantation. Long-term survival is significantly better in younger diabetic patients treated with living related donor renal transplantation, and to a lesser degree cadaver donor renal transplantation, than is survival with chronic hemodialysis. In more recent times, there has also been a special interest in continuous ambulatory peritoneal dialysis (CAPD) in diabetic patients. The survival results of CAPD are encouraging but still very preliminary. The technique, however, has some advantages for the patient with diabetes which include obviating the need for vascular access, intraperitoneal insulin administration, and narrowing the swings in fluid balance by very gentle continuous ultrafiltration.

During the past year, Krakauer and associates have reported survival data on end-stage renal disease therapy collected through the Medical Information System of the Health Care Financing Administration of the U.S. Department of Health

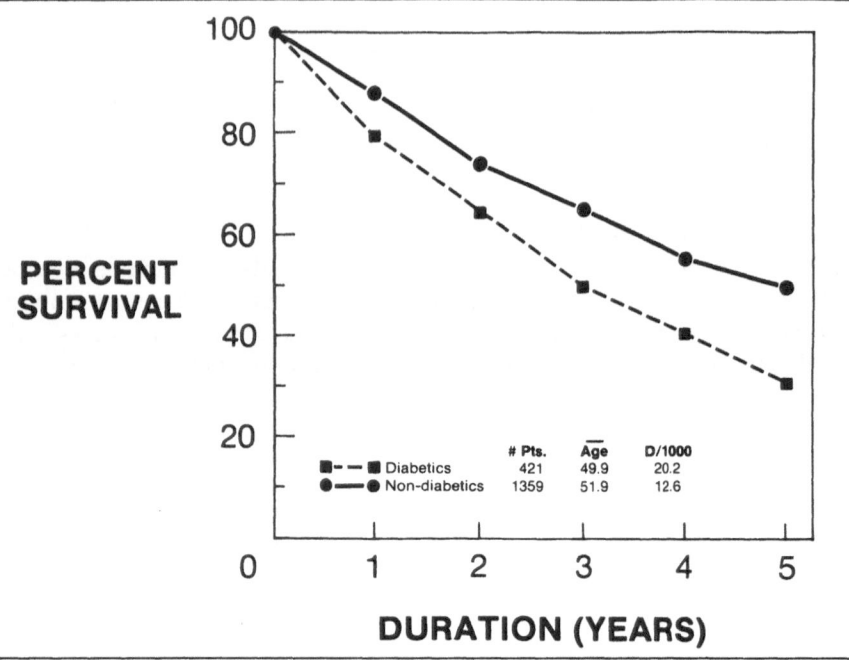

Figure 6–2. Cumulative survival of patients with end-stage renal disease secondary to diabetes mellitus is compared to patients with end-stage renal disease of other etiologies during 1966–83. Diabetic patients have consistently lower five-year survival rates compared to patients with end-stage renal disease of other etiologies.

and Human Services. Between 1977 and 1980, 65,000 patients were treated by hemodialysis, and 7,500 were treated by transplantation. This study demonstrated that survival in the patient with end-stage renal disease secondary to diabetic nephropathy is worse than other etiologies of renal failure. Survival of diabetic patients was 75% at one year and 39% at three years, data very comparable to those at the University of Washington, Seattle, experience [23]. Cumulative survival of all hemodialysis patients in this study demonstrated first-year survival of 81% and third-year survival of 56%, representing a substantial difference compared to diabetic patients. This study also confirmed the observation that irrespective of etiology of end-stage renal disease, survival decreased with increasing age at initiation of dialysis [15].

Of special note, survival rates of diabetic patients treated with hemodialysis was comparable during the first year to those treated with cadaveric renal transplantation. However, long-term survival in these two groups was strikingly different. Three-year survival in transplant patients was 65% in contrast to 39% survival in hemodialysis patients. The difference between survival in diabetic patients receiving dialysis as renal replacement therapy versus patients who received living related donor transplants was even more significant.

Cumulative survival in patients with diabetes mellitus compared to nondiabetic

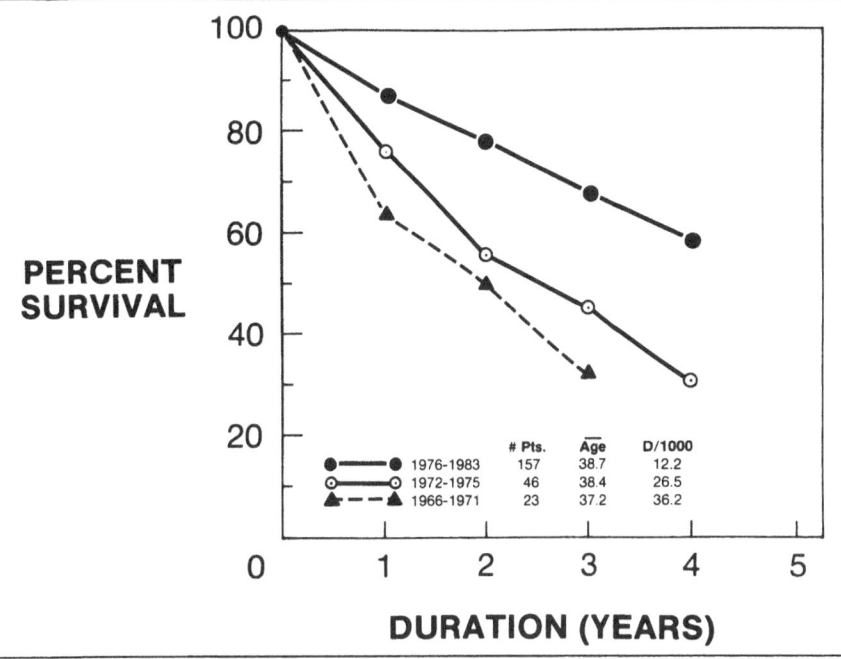

Figure 6–3. Improving actuarial survival curves in patients with type I diabetes mellitus for the last 17 years are depicted in this figure. Although mean age has remained relatively constant in patients less than 61 years of age, survival has dramatically improved in these patients. Death rate has fallen from 36.2 and 26.5 deaths per 1,000 treatment months to 12.2 deaths per 1,000 treatment months. Patients with endstage renal disease secondary to type I diabetes mellitus initiating dialysis after age 61 years still have extremely poor survival.

patients in the RKDP program from 1966 to December 31, 1983, is illustrated in figure 6–2. One-year and three-year cumulative survival in nondiabetic patients was 86.4% and 64.7%, respectively. In diabetic patients, first-year and third-year cumulative survival was 79.5% and 48.6%, with long-term survival comparing less favorably with that of patients with ESRD of other etiologies. Unlike the study above, RKDP cumulative survival in type I diabetic patients less than 61 years of age has steadily improved from 1966 to 1983 (figure 6–3). Similarly, the cumulative survival in all type II diabetic patients has improved in comparison of patients initiating dialysis from 1972–1975 versus 1976–1983 (figure 6–4).

The possible reasons for our sizable and sustained improvement in survival over time are multiple. Two technical aspects of hemodialysis may help explain these improving survival rates. First, higher sodium levels in dialysate baths (140 mEq/L) permit better tolerance of ultrafiltration and therefore more effective continuous blood pressure control in the majority of diabetic patients without the added risk of antihypertensive agents. The duration of dialysis has also been reduced to between four and five hours by utilizing more efficient dialyzers. Finally, special emphasis has been placed on achieving and maintaining adequate nutritional status

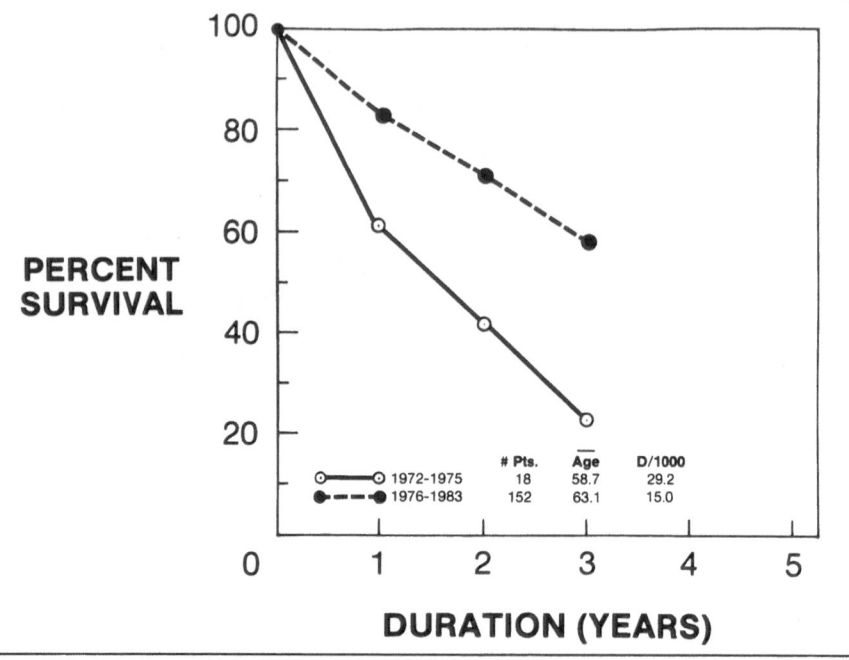

Figure 6–4. Improving actuarial survival curves over time are demonstrated in patients with end-stage renal disease secondary to type II diabetes mellitus. Despite a small rise in patient mean age, type II diabetic patient survival has improved since 1976. Death rate has fallen from 29.2 deaths per 1,000 treatment months to 15.0 deaths per 1,000 treatment months.

of the individual patient which may have contributed to improved survival. Since 1976, serum creatinine at the time of initiation of dialysis has been slightly lower in both type I and type II diabetic patients (table 6–2). However, this small difference in renal function cannot fully explain this yearly improvement in patient survival.

Death rates and cumulative survival in type I and type II diabetic patients and nondiabetic patients vary with patient age in the RKDP experience and the previously mentioned studies. Type I diabetic patients over age 60 have essentially no patient survival beyond three years of dialysis (figures 6–5 and 6–6). In general, cumulative survival in type I diabetic patients is identical to survival curves in nondiabetic patients 30 years older than type I diabetic patients. Cumulative survival in type II diabetic patients over 60 years of age at initiation of dialysis is very similar to nondiabetic patients in this same age group (figures 6–6 and 6–7). Death rates and cumulative survival in type II diabetic patients are also fairly similar to nondiabetics between ages 31 and 60.

The causes of death in diabetic patients treated with hemodialysis are depicted schematically in figure 6–8. During the first two years after initiation of hemodialysis, the majority of deaths are secondary to cardiovascular or cerebrovascular events (i.e., cardiac arrest, arrhythmia, myocardial infarction, congestive heart

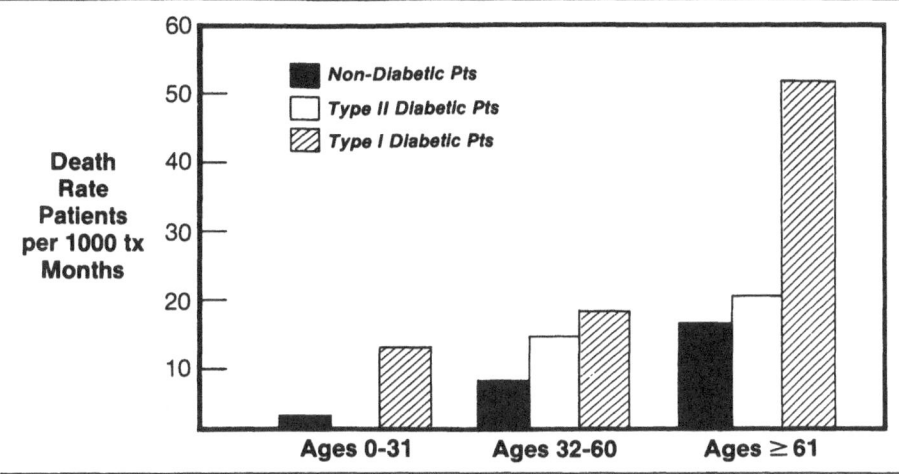

Figure 6–5. Death rate per 1,000 treatment months for type I and type II diabetic patients as well as nondiabetic patients are depicted by age of initiation. Death rates in type I diabetic patients in particular are two to three times greater than nondiabetic patients at each age interval. Death rates in type II diabetic patients greater than age 61 is similar to nondiabetic patients greater than 61 years of age. 1976–1983

failure, cerebrovascular accident). A smaller but important cause of death during this time includes uremia (patients with overwhelming medical complications or failure to thrive that discontinue dialysis). After two years of dialysis, infectious complications or septicemia become an increasingly important cause of death (45%), although cardiovascular causes of death remain high (30%)

Few clinical criteria help define prognosis for survival of the diabetic patient on hemodialysis. Age greater than 61 years in type I diabetic patients predicts very poor survival. Early studies among RKDP patients had demonstrated that those patients with angina, congestive heart failure, or electrocardiogram (ECG) abnormalities appeared to have a poorer prognosis among RKDP patients. Over time, these observations have not remained prognostically helpful. Recently, coronary arteriography in small series of diabetic patients with end-stage renal disease have demonstrated some predictive survival data. Although patients studied in these series were asymptomatic and had no ECG abnormalities, several of the subjects had significant macrovascular coronary artery disease. These studies demonstrated markedly increased cardiovascular mortality in patients with 50–70% stenosis of at least one coronary artery vessel when compared to patients with no angiographic evidence of coronary artery disease [3,25].

MEDICAL COMPLICATIONS OF DIABETIC HEMODIALYSIS PATIENTS

Hospitalizations

Table 6–3 depicts the number of hospital days per patient-treatment month in diabetic and nondiabetic patients receiving chronic hemodialysis within the RKDP

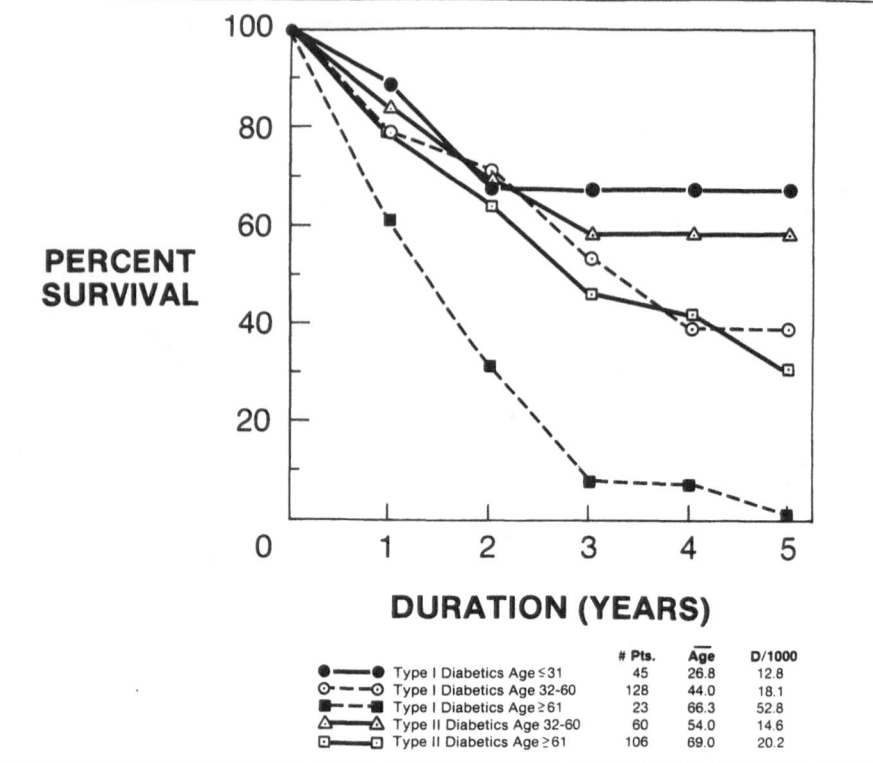

	# Pts.	Age	D/1000
Type I Diabetics Age ≤31	45	26.8	12.8
Type I Diabetics Age 32-60	128	44.0	18.1
Type I Diabetics Age ≥61	23	66.3	52.8
Type II Diabetics Age 32-60	60	54.0	14.6
Type II Diabetics Age ≥61	106	69.0	20.2

Figure 6–6. Cumulative survival of type I and type II diabetic patients with end-stage diabetic nephropathy treated by hemodialysis are shown by age of onset. As is also true for nondiabetic patients, survival decreases as age of onset increases. Survival in type I diabetic patients is similar to nondiabetic patients 30 years older. 1976–1983.

program. Of note, the in-hospital complication rate for diabetic patients is very similar to the rate for nondiabetic patients. As might be expected, there is a trend for older diabetic patients to spend more time in hospital than younger patients. The most common reasons for hospitalization of RKDP chronic diabetic hemodialysis patients, in order of decreasing frequency, include: infectious complications (most commonly hemo-access related and pneumonia), cardiovascular complications, hemo-access problems, and gastrointestinal complaints (nausea, vomiting, diarrhea, and gastrointestinal blood loss). Also, particularly in the type I diabetic patient, admission for metabolic regulation of recurrent episodes of hyperglycemia or hypoglycemia is common. Admission for complications of peripheral vascular disease were more frequent in the type II diabetic patient than in the type I diabetic patient.

Several complications of diabetic patients receiving hemodialysis renal replacement therapy deserve further discussion. Two of these complications, retinopathy

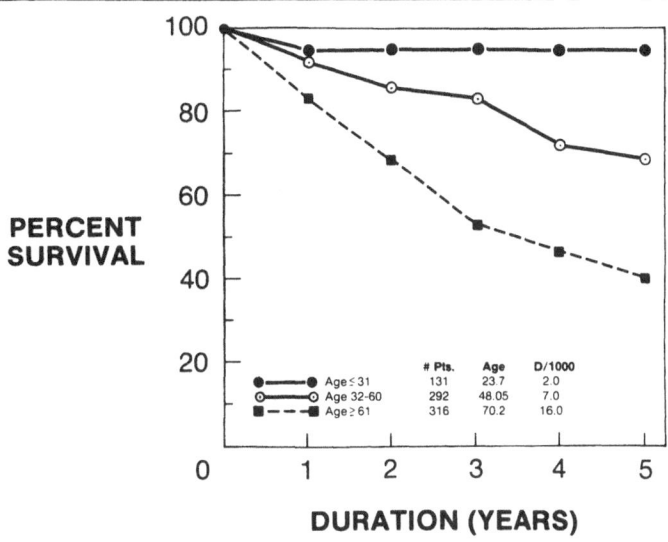

Figure 6–7. Cumulative survival of nondiabetic patients initiating dialysis between 1976–83 is compared by age at initiation of dialysis. Survival markedly decreases as age at onset of dialysis increases.

and amputation, have contrasted sharply in clinical outcome among patients treated by hemodialysis compared to those treated with transplantation.

Retinopathy

One of the most debilitating complications of the diabetic dialysis patient, particularly in the early years of chronic hemodialysis as renal replacement therapy, was the extremely high incidence of new blindness after initiating hemodialysis. This was in striking contrast to the very low incidence of development of blindness in renal transplant recipients. However, the number of patients in whom blindness has ensued after initiating dialysis has more recently fallen from 44% in the group of type I dialysis patients initiating dialysis in 1966–71 to 3% in type I patients initiated since 1976. Although not quite as dramatic, the development of blindness in type II diabetic patients treated by hemodialysis has also significantly declined over this same time period (figure 6–9). Presumed explanations for this marked improvement in visual status in patients treated with dialysis are: more intensive ophthalmologic care, including panretinal photocoagulation; more stringent control of blood pressure; and, although somewhat controversial, better control of blood glucose. Of note, the percentage of patients who are blind at the time of initiation of dialysis has not changed to any considerable degree. Diabetes is still the leading cause of new blindness in the United States. In fact, approximately 5,000 people become blind each year as the result of diabetes. Since effective therapy now exists for proliferative retinopathy, macular degeneration, and glaucoma, it appears

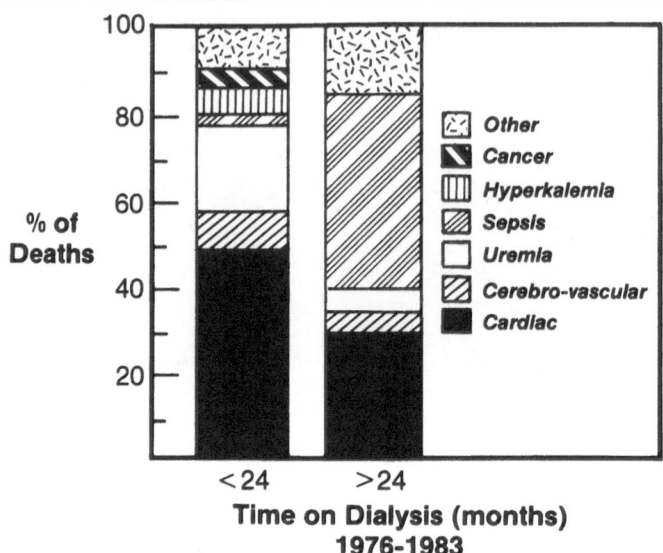

Figure 6–8. Cause of death in diabetic dialysis patients (1976–1983) during the first two years of dialysis and dialysis thereafter is depicted. Early dialysis deaths are cardiovascular or cerebrovascular deaths. After two years of dialysis, infectious complications are responsible for increasing diabetic deaths, although cardiovascular deaths continue to contribute to diabetic mortality.

that special ophthalmologic surveillance should be started earlier and maintained consistently in diabetic patients long before dialysis is initiated.

Amputations

Peripheral vascular disease is present in 30–50% of patients with end-stage diabetic nephropathy when they initiate hemodialysis. Peripheral neuropathy in these patients is even more common. As a result of inadequate peripheral blood supply and insensitive feet, these diabetic patients are highly susceptible to injury, ulceration,

Table 6–3. Medical complication rates of diabetic hemodialysis patients resulting in hospitalization compared to nondiabetic patient complication rates during 1976–83

Patients	Hospital days/ TX months	Admissions	Average hospitalization (days)
Nondiabetic patients	1.54	2,067	11.5
Type I diabetic patients	1.50	361	11.4
Type II diabetic patients	1.69	481	11.6

Note: Diabetic patients utilizing hemodialysis have very similar rates of hospitalization as do nondiabetic patients in the RKDP program.

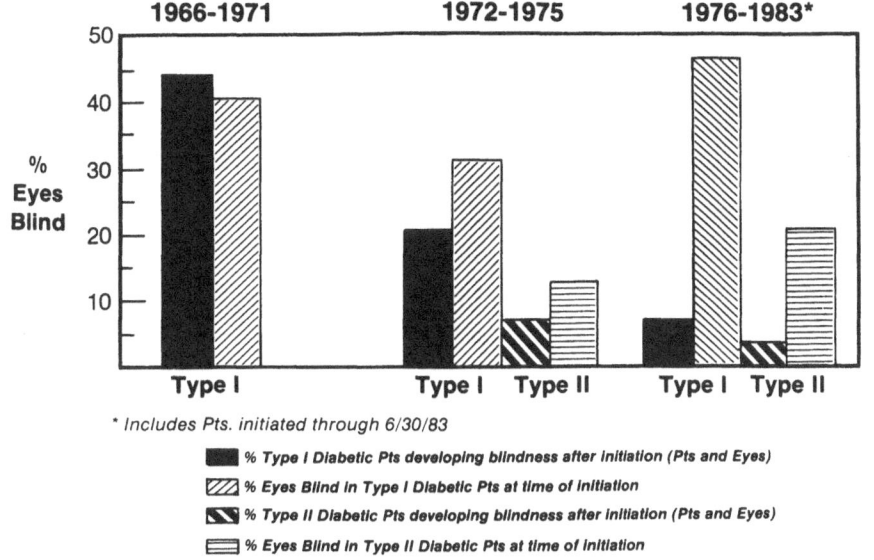

Figure 6–9. Blindness in both type I and type II hemodialysis diabetic patients both prior to onset of dialysis and after initiation of dialysis are separated by time intervals between 1966–61, 1972–75, and 1976–83. The number of patients developing blindness after initiating dialysis has markedly declined, particularly in type I patients with diabetes mellitus. Although blindness is decreasing once dialysis has been initiated, the number of patients that present to the Regional Kidney Disease Program already blind has not declined.

gangrene, infection, and ultimately amputation of a digit or extremity. As a result, patients with diabetes mellitus account for 50–70% of all nontraumatic amputations in the United States. After initiating hemodialysis, amputations in diabetic patients have been reported to occur infrequently. In the Regional Kidney Disease Program, 16 of 453 diabetic patients (4%) who subsequently received either hemodialysis or peritoneal dialysis as renal replacement therapy had experienced amputation before initiating dialysis. Of this group, 30 patients (7%) have since required 44 amputations of either a digit or limb subsequent to initiating dialysis (table 6–4). Similar numbers of type I and type II diabetic patients have undergone amputations. On the average, these patients had been receiving maintenance hemodialysis for 18 months prior to amputation. Amputations have not appeared to have any significant prognostic value for survival in dialysis patients. In contrast, amputations in diabetic renal transplant recipients are much more frequent and, when they occur, portend both poor graft and patient survival. In a study reviewing 373 type I diabetic renal transplant recipients at the University of Minnesota, 65 patients (17%) had 151 amputations posttransplant [20]. Amputation in the transplant recipient may be a marker of other medical complications that alter both graft and patient survival. Therefore, diabetic patients with severe peripheral

Table 6–4. Amputations required after initiating dialysis
in diabetic patients with end-stage renal disease between 1966–83

Patients	Type I diabetes	Type II diabetes
Total # dialysis patients requiring amputation[1]	15(22)	15(22)
Total # hemodialysis patients requiring amputation	8(13)	11(13)
Total # peritoneal dialysis patients requiring amputation	7 (9)	4 (9)
Site of amputation		
Upper extremity	3	3
AK	3	4
BK	11	9
Toes/foot	5	6

1. Total amputations are shown in parentheses.
Note: Comparable numbers of amputations have been done in both type I and type II diabetic patients. Only 16 patients in a total of 453 patients initiating dialysis in the 1966–83 period had undergone amputation prior to dialysis.

vascular disease may possibly be a unique group in which dialysis may be superior to transplantation as renal replacement therapy judged by both survival and rehabilitation.

Cardiovascular disease

Cardiovascular complications in diabetic patients account for a large percentage of hospital admissions in this group as well as early hemodialysis mortality, as has previously been discussed. Myocardial infarction, angina, and congestive heart failure often precipitated by extracellular fluid volume overload are common manifestations of diabetic cardiovascular disease in dialysis patients. In our experience, pericarditis may also be somewhat more common in patients with diabetes mellitus. Both microvascular and macrovascular cardiac disease exist in diabetics with end-stage renal disease. Myocardial dysfunction without coronary artery disease documented by coronary angiography has been observed in recent studies. Although difficult, both patient and physician attention to interdialytic weight gains may minimize these admissions.

Osteodystrophy

Renal osteodystrophy in patients with end-stage diabetic renal disease appears to be of a lesser degree than in other hemodialysis patients. The explanation for this fascinating observation is unclear. However, diabetic PTH levels, with serum calcium levels similar to nondiabetic patients, are decreased. This may represent a relative "hypoparathyroid" state, analogous to other endocrinologic deficiency syndromes in the diabetic patient.

Infections

Infections in hemodialysis patients with diabetes are a major source of increased morbidity. Although subtle immune deficiencies may exist in diabetic patients, particularly those with poor glucose control, most infections in hemodialysis diabetic patients result from local problems with breaks in skin barriers, such as infected foot ulcers and access site infections. The tenuous fistula which requires multiple needle punctures or the shunt which requires declotting often start infections. Bacteremias associated with access infections are more frequent among diabetic patients compared to nondiabetic patients. Pulmonary and access infections account for the majority of infection-related hospital admissions in our diabetic patients. In addition, osteomyelitis also occurs in diabetic patients with increased frequency.

Neuropathy

Although the peripheral neuropathy of diabetes is difficult to separate from uremic neuropathy, uremic neuropathy usually improves after adequate dialysis. On the other hand, although diabetic neuropathy may have remissions, it is generally progressive. The pain and paresthesias of diabetic neuropathy have been treated in a number of ways. Carbamazepine has been effective for pain relief in controlled clinical trials. More recently, fluphenazine and amitryptiline in combination have been used with some success.

Improvement in visceral autonomic neuropathy may be observed with dialysis. Gastroparesis, orthostatic hypotension, and bladder neuropathies have been noted to improve. Metoclopramide has been extremely helpful, in addition, to ameliorate diabetic gastroparesis. In dialysis patients, neurogenic bladders are usually of minor significance since urine volumes are quite small. Impotence in the diabetic male does not usually respond to dialysis. Consideration should be given in the individual patient to penile prosthesis implantation.

Rehabilitation

The success of a renal replacement therapy must be judged not only on the increased survival that it provides but also on the quality of the life it prolongs. The rehabilitation of diabetic patients treated with hemodialysis as renal replacement therapy has been uniformly poor. Few diabetic hemodialysis patients are employed after one year of dialysis. In one large multicenter study, only 23% of 289 patients with diabetes were able to carry out normal physical activities. In fact, 77% of diabetic patients were unable to accomplish any activities beyond caring for themselves. Furthermore, 51% of these patients were not even capable of independent self-care [11].

Many of the psychosocial problems that patients with end-stage diabetic nephropathy manifest are the result of multiple medical complications of diabetes and their resultant handicaps, particularly loss of vision, peripheral vascular disease with amputation, and peripheral and autonomic neuropathies. These handicaps cause increasing dependence on family members. Special psychosocial support is extremely important, therefore, not only for the patients but also for their families.

Transplantation, in contrast, has a much better rehabilitation record. Preliminary results in some studies with CAPD suggest that this therapy may also be associated with improved rehabilitation potential in the diabetic patient with end-stage renal disease.

SUMMARY

Hemodialysis has been the renal replacement therapy used most commonly in patients with end-stage diabetic nephropathy. Although actuarial survival has improved for diabetic hemodialysis patients over the last several years, survival is still inferior to patients with other types of end-stage renal disease. Improvement has recently been demonstrated in the decreasing number of patients developing blindness after initiating hemodialysis, minimizing one of the most devastating secondary handicaps of these patients. Morbidity and mortality are still most commonly associated with cardiovascular and infectious complications of diabetes mellitus. Finally, long-term survival and rehabilitation of diabetic hemodialysis patients are still inferior to transplantation results.

SELECTED BIBLIOGRAPHY

1. Amair P, Khanna R, Leibel B, Pierratos A, Vas S, Meema E, Blair G, Chisolm L, Vas M, Zingg W, Digenis G, Oreopoulous D. Continuous ambulatory peritoneal dialysis in diabetics with endstage renal disease. N Engl J Med 306:625, 1982.
2. Avram, MM. Diabetic renal failure. Nephron 31:285–288, 1982.
3. Braun WE, Phillips D, Vidt DG, Novick AC, Nakamoto S, Popowniak KL, Magnusson MO, Pohl MA, Steinmuller D, Protiva D, Buszta C. Coronary arteriography and coronary artery disease in 99 diabetic and nondiabetic patients on chronic hemodialysis or renal transplantation programs. Transplantation Proc 13:128–135, 1981.
4. Davis JL, Lewis SB, Gerich JE, Kaplan RA, Schultz TA, Wallin JD. Peripheral diabetic neuropathy treated with amitriptyline and fluphenazine. JAMA 238:2291–2291, 1977.
5. Davis M, Comty C, Shapiro F. Dietary management of patients with diabetes treated by hemodialysis. J Am Diet Assoc 75:265–269, 1979.
6. D'Elia JA, Weinrauch LA, Healy RW, Libertino JA, Bradley RF, Leland OS. Myocardial dysfunction without coronary artery disease in diabetic renal failure. Am J Cardiol 43:193, 1979.
7. Ellenberg M. Diabetic neuropathy; clinical aspects. Metabolism 25:1627–1654, 1976.
8. El Shahar Y, Rottembourg J, Bellio P, Guimont MC, Rousselie F, Jacobs C. Visual function can be preserved in insulin dependent diabetic patients treated by maintenance hemodialysis. Proc Eur Dial Transplant Assoc 17:167–172, 1980.
9. Fluckiger R, Harmon W, Meier W, Loo S, Gabbay KH. Hemoglobin carbamylation in uremia. N Engl J Med 304:823–827, 1981.
10. Goldstein DA, Massry SG. Diabetic nephropathy. Clinical course and effect of hemodialysis. Nephron 20:286–296, 1978.
11. Gutman RA, Stead WW, Robinson RR. Physical activity and employment status of patients on maintenance dialysis. N Eng J Med 304:309–313, 1981.
12. Keane WF, Shapiro FL, Raij L. Incidence and type of infections occurring in 445 chronic hemodialysis patients. Trans Am Soc Artif Inter Organs 23:4, 1977.
13. Kjellstrand C, Comty C, Shapiro FL. A comparison of dialysis and transplantation in insulin dependent diabetic patients. In: Diabetic Renal-Retinal Syndrome, Friedman EA, L'Esperance FA (eds). New York: Grune & Stratton, 1983.

14. Knowles HC. Magnitude of the renal failure problem in diabetic patients. Kidney Int 6(Suppl 1):S2–S7, 1974.
15. Krakauer H, Grauman JS, McMullan MR, Creede CC. The recent U.S. experience in the treatment of endstage renal disease by dialysis and transplantation. N Engl J Med 308:1558–1563, 1983.
16. Kussman MJ, Goldstein HH, Gleason RE. The clinical course of diabetic nephropathy. JAMA 236:1861–1863, 1976.
17. Mauer SM, Steffes MW, Brown DM. The kidney in diabetes. Am J Med 70:603–612, 1981.
18. Page MM, Watkinsn PJ. The heart in diabetes: autonomic neuropathy and cardiomyopathy. Clin Endocrinol Metab 6:377–385, 1977.
19. Parving HH, Andersen AR, Smidt U, Friisberg B, Bonnevie-Nielsen V, Svendsen PA. The natural course of glomerular filtration rate and arterial blood pressure in diabetic nephropathy and the effect of anti-hypertensive treatment. Acta Endocrinol 97(Suppl 242):39–40, 1981.
20. Peters C, Sutherland DER, Simmons RL, Fryd DS, Najarian JS. Patient and graft survival in amputated versus nonamputated diabetic primary renal allograft recipients. Transplantation 32:498–503, 1981.
21. Snape WJ, Battle WM, Schwartz SS, Braunstein SN, Goldstein HA, Alavi A. Metoclopramide to treat gastroparesis due to diabetes mellitus. Ann Intern Med 96:444–446, 1982.
22. Vincenti F, Hattner R, Amend WJ, Feduska NJ, Duca RM, Salvatierra O. Decreased secondary hyperparathyroidism in diabetic patients receiving hemodialysis. JAMA 245:930–933, 1981.
23. Vollmer WM, Wahl PW, Blagg CR. Survival with dialysis and transplantation in patients with endstage renal disease. N Engl J Med 308:1553–1558, 1983.
24. Wathen RL, Keshaviah P, Honmeyer P, Cadwell K, Comty CM. The metabolic effects of hemodialysis with and without glucose in the dialysate. Am J Clin Nutr 31:1870, 1978.
25. Weinrauch LA, D'Elia JA, Healy RW, Gleason RE, Takacs FJ, Libertino JA, Leland OS. Asymptomatic coronary artery disease: angiography in diabetic patients before renal transplantation. Relation of findings to postoperative survival. Ann Intern Med 88:346–348, 1978.
26. West KM, Erdreich LJ, Stober JA. A detailed study of the risk factors for retinopathy and nephropathy in diabetes. Diabetes 29:501–508, 1980.

7. CONTINUOUS AMBULATORY PERITONEAL DIALYSIS IN END-STAGE DIABETIC NEPHROPATHY

RAMESH KHANNA
and
DIMITRIOS G. OREOPOULOS

Centers throughout North America are experiencing a remarkable rise in the proportion of newly diagnosed diabetic uremic patients requiring kidney replacement treatment [1–3]. Approximately 30% of all insulin–dependent (type I) diabetic patients die of renal failure. In the United States each year by conservative estimate, between 2,500 and 3,200 diabetics die of kidney disease [4]. Despite this large number, a decade ago diabetics with uremia comprised only 1–7% of all patients accepted for dialysis in Europe and the United States [5, 6]. These patients were excluded from dialysis for reasons that were multiple and complex, but the most important factors were the uniformly poor outcome of dialysis and transplantation [7–16], and the progressive deterioration of visual function. By 1978, however, due to technical advances in hemodialysis and better understanding of the factors contributing to the progression of diabetic complications, survival among chronically hemodialysed diabetics improved considerably [17–20].

In assessing chronic peritoneal dialysis as an alternative to hemodialysis for renal failure of all causes, it appears that this form of dialysis is especially useful in diabetic patients in particular because, in them, vascular access (for hemodialysis) is often difficult to establish and maintain. The medical literature in the mid-1970s showed a varying response of diabetics with end-stage renal disease (ESRD) to chronic peritoneal dialysis [21,22].

Compared to hemodialysis, intermittent peritoneal dialysis (IPD) in 31 diabetic patients at the Toronto Western Hospital [23] seemed to offer the potential advantage of reduced cardiovascular stress; however, the survival of these patients was poor—only 24% survived for two years. A positive aspect was that retinopathy did not progress on IPD. After a nonrandomized comparison [24] between diabetic patients on peritoneal and hemodialysis, workers at the Mayo Clinic reported a 50% survival at one year in both groups. Despite the disappointing survival of diabetics on chronic peritoneal dialysis (PO), most centers reported slower progression of retinopathy and a level of general well-being that was significantly better in PD patients than those maintained on chronic hemodialysis [22–32].

Since its introduction, continuous ambulatory peritoneal dialysis (CAPD) has offered better management of diabetic patients with ESRD and, at the same time, provides control of blood sugar (by the intraperitoneal administration of insulin) in a way that resembles an artificial pancreas [33–35]. In a short time CAPD established itself as a viable alternative to hemodialysis in the treatment of ESRD [36–40]. After the encouraging preliminary results this method is now used extensively in diabetics who require dialysis. In many centers survival has been so encouraging that CAPD has become the preferred mode of dialysis for diabetics [41–43].

ADVANTAGES OF CAPD

In the treatment of diabetics with ESRD, CAPD offers several medical advantages: for example, a steady-state control of uremia, good control of hypertension, and stable cardiovascular status without the rapid fluid shifts. An additional advantage is good, tight control of blood sugar achieved by intraperitoneal administration of insulin, which eliminates the need for multiple subcutaneous insulin injections and promotes the patient's compliance. Eliminating the need for vascular access and heparinization removes access-related complications—a major cause of morbidity while on hemodialysis.

The social advantages include freedom from machine and electrical outlets, thereby reducing the difficulties associated with travel, especially overseas. Also, CAPD patients do not have to learn to operate complex machinery, and training time can be reduced to 10–15 days. Finally, the capital cost of home dialysis is low.

TECHNIQUE OF CAPD

Patients are dialyzed through an in-dwelling Tenckhoff or Toronto Western Hospital catheter [44], using the same technique as for nondiabetics [45]. The patients exchange four two-liter bags per day. Dialysis solutions are available in four dextrose concentrations—0.5, 1.5, 2.5, and 4.25 g/dl. The patients are taught to add insulin into the dialysis solution according to the protocol described below. The exit site is dressed daily with a gauze soaked with poviodine, or after a daily shower the patient paints the exit site with poviodine. The patients are seen weekly during the first month after the completion of training and monthly thereafter. The connection tubing is changed by the nurses every month at the time of clinic visits.

METHOD FOR BLOOD SUGAR CONTROL

The intraperitoneal administration of insulin during CAPD in diabetics has been compared to treatment with an artificial pancreas [33], and indeed there are certain similarities between physiological insulin secretion and the response to intraperitoneal insulin administration [46–51]. Thus, in the normal state, insulin is secreted into the portal vein in response to various secretagogues [46], and the peak blood insulin level is attained approximately 40 minutes after a carbohydrate load [46]. Fifty percent of the insulin secreted into the portal vein is removed as the blood flows through the liver [50].

Intraperitoneally administered insulin closely mimics these physiological events. Thus it appears that a large percentage of intraperitoneal insulin is absorbed into the portal vein [47]. The administered dose varies according to the glucose load. Peak insulin levels lag about 20–30 minutes behind the physiological peak, and the duration of peak achieved is longer [46–50,52]. From the peritoneal cavity insulin can be absorbed into the portal circulation and the lymph [53]. The studies of Zingg and associates [54] suggest that part of the insulin administered intraperitoneally is absorbed from the peritoneal cavity through the capsule and parenchyma of the liver. The reaction to insulin given as bolus injection is different from that produced when insulin is added through a dialysate [55]. The form in which insulin is absorbed from the peritoneal cavity is not known. Based on research obtained in dogs, Shapiro and associates [56] postulated that the insulin molecule is absorbed as a monomer. In contrast, Brachet and Rasio [57], while studying insulin transport across the isolated rat mesentery in vitro, reported that transport is by passive diffusion of insulin in the trimeric form. Shade and colleagues [53] concluded, as a result of their studies on anesthetized dogs, that interperitoneal insulin administration is followed by increased absorption into the portal vein and, therefore, may be more physiological than other conventional routes. However, studies of Zingg and associates [54] failed to demonstrate a preferential absorption of the insulin into the portal vein in conscious rats. Consequently, the specific value of this route of insulin administration remains uncertain. Despite the lack of clear understanding of the kinetics of insulin absorption across the peritoneum, the similarities observed between the physiological state of insulin secretion and intraperitoneal insulin administration during CAPD encourage us to believe that this method will give excellent blood sugar control and achieve more desirable long-term results in diabetic patients with ESRD.

Clinical results with CAPD and intraperitoneal (IP) insulin administration appear superior to those achieved with subcutaneous injections, although the IP route usually requires higher daily insulin doses. These high insulin requirements may be due to such factors as: substantial binding and retention of insulin in the dialysis bag and tubing [58–63]; slow absorption from the peritoneal cavity with losses in the drained dialysate; degradation of insulin by insulinases in the peritoneum or during transit to the systemic circulation; altered effectiveness of insulin absorbed via the portal system; or a combination of these. Studies in dogs of the kinetics of insulin transport across the peritoneum have shown that insulin (MW

6,000 daltons) peritoneal permeance is 3–6 ml/min [56]. Such absorption is independent of either blood or dialysate glucose concentration [64].

PROTOCOL FOR INSULIN ADMINISTRATION

This chapter outlines the protocol developed in the Toronto Western Hospital for insulin administration in diabetics on CAPD and describes two other protocols [65]. For the three centers table 7–1 shows the route of administration, initial dose, nighttime corrections, additional insulin increments for different dialysis glucose concentrations, and average insulin requirements. It also shows the number of CAPD exchanges per day and recommended daily calorie and protein intake per day.

The Toronto Western Hospital protocol is as follows: the patient is hospitalized for four to six days before training begins in order to establish the individual's insulin requirements. During the day the bags are exchanged 20 minutes before the three major meals and for a fourth time about 11 P.M. At this time a snack is provided consisting of a sandwich and a small drink. The patient is encouraged to follow a diet providing 20 to 25 kcal per kilogram of body weight per day and containing 1.2 to 1.5 g of protein per kg. B.W. During this control period, blood sugar is measured four times a day—i.e., in the morning fasting, and one hour after breakfast, lunch, and supper. Regular insulin is added to each bag just before the fluid is infused, and the bag is inverted two or three times to aid mixing. The dose is proportional to the concentration of glucose in the dialysate.

On the first day, one-quarter of the previous day's insulin is added to each bag of dialysate, with a supplemental dose determined according to the concentration of dialysate glucose (table 7–1).

On the second day, the insulin added to each bag is increased or decreased according to the previous day's blood sugar levels. The insulin dose in the 11 P.M. exchange is based on the level of fasting blood sugar six to eight hours later, the next morning. The adjustment of the insulin dose in the dialysate exchange immediately before meals is based on the blood sugar level after the corresponding meal.

Table 7–1. Amount of regular insulin (above baseline amount) added to the dialysis solution, according to the concentration of dialysate glucose

Concentration of glucose in dialysate (g/dl)	Additional insulin units/liter of solution
0.5	0
1.5	1
2.5	2
4.25	3

After the period of assessment, because of the occasional anorexia, nausea and vomiting, and inherent diabetic lability, it is necessary to monitor the blood sugar level at least weekly. As an additional precaution, patients are trained to check the blood sugar level by the "finger prick" technique. This method gives a quick result which correlates reasonably well with the true blood sugar levels [64], and helps to detect unexpected fluctuations in blood sugar. The test is performed 5 to 10 minutes before each bag exchange, and whenever necessary the insulin added to the next bag is adjusted according to a sliding scale (table 7–2). During the training period, the patient becomes familiar with the principles described in table 7–2 and practices them under observation. It should be emphasized that the finger-prick blood sugar test is for guidance only and is used only to adjust the insulin dose in the relevant bag.

Initial blood sugar control requires three or four days in hospital, with insulin requirements that may vary from 50 to 200 units per day. Nocturnal insulin requirements are 30–50% of the daytime dose.

Hyperglycemia is frequent in association with peritonitis, systemic infection, and in the period immediately following discontinuation of CAPD. During these periods a higher dose of insulin is required to control hyperglycemia than is usual during CAPD, and some patients may require intravenous infusions of insulin for 24 to 48 hours. Hyperglycemic ketoacidosis is extremely uncommon during CAPD. However, hypoglycemia does occur during intraperitoneal administration of insulin, and patients and/or family should be trained to respond by draining the dialysis fluid from the peritoneal cavity and, if necessary, providing additional oral glucose. If the situation warrants, a solution containing no insulin should be infused into the peritoneal cavity without delay.

Table 7–2. Suggested change in basal dose of insulin added to dialysate solution, according to blood sugar levels (−) indicates decrease and (+) increase

Blood sugar level[1] (mg/dl)		Change in baseline insulin dose units/2 liters of solution
Fasting	1 hr after meals	
80–140	120–180	No change
40	80	−2
< 40	40	−4
—	< 40	−6
180	240	+2
240	> 240	+4
> 400		+6 or more

1. To convert to millimoles per liter, multiply by 0.0555.

Other published protocols

Table 7–3 shows highlights of the Iowa Lutheran and Pitie-Salpetriere protocols.

The Iowa Lutheran protocol [65] aims at the same levels of blood sugar control as the Toronto Western Hospital. Additionally, it measures glycosylated hemoglobin and attempts to maintain a level equal to or less than 10%.

It recommends strict control of diet but leaves it unspecified. Exchanges are done at 0600, 1400, and 2200 hours. Initially blood sugar is measured at two hourly intervals, then one hour before each exchange. In followup, the Iowa plan does fasting blood sugars monthly with a measurement of glycosylated hemoglobin.

The initial IP dose is equal to the previous total daily requirement. The second dose is 0.8 of the first, and the third (nighttime) dose is 0.5 of the first with a 2.5% or 4.25% glucose exchange and only 0.3 of the first, with a 1.5% exchange (table 7–3).

The Pitie-Salpetriere protocol [65] monitors blood sugar by Dextrostix, four

Table 7–3. Protocols of insulin administration in diabetics on CAPD in Toronto Western Hospital (TWH) and two other centers

	TWH	Pitie-Salpetriere		Iowa Lutheran
Insulin administration	intraperitoneal	intraperitoneal		intraperitoneal
Initial dose per bag	¼ previous daily requirement	Arbitrary reflects previous requirement		total previous daily requirement
Nighttime	reduced 30–50%	Unspecified		0.3 of 1.5% dose 0.5 of 2.5% dose or 4.25% dose
			Hours	
			0600	20–100 (53)
			1400	12–90 (43)
			2200	10–70 (33)
Insulin units per glucose concentration				
0.5 g%	¼ previous +0	0		
1.5 g%	¼ previous +1	4–30 (18)		
2.5 g%	¼ previous +2	unspecified		
4.25 g%	¼ previous +3	10–45 (30)		
Subcutaneous	not used	not used		not used
Daily range	70–200 (−)	36–96 (68)		42–260 (129)
No. of CAPD exchanges/day	four	three/four		three
Diet: calories Kcal/kg B.W.	20–25	not specified		not specified
protein g/kg B.W.	1.2–1.5	not specified		not specified

times a day, immediately before each exchange. Followup sugars are done twice daily by the finger-prick method. Six Dextrostix measurements are made on one day each week. Glycosylated hemoglobin is measured every second month. Insulin, administered exclusively by the intraperitoneal route, is added directly into the administration tubing before instillation of a new bag.

Rottembourg and associates [66] investigated the advantage of different insulin injection sites in the CAPD system in order to study the insulin retention at the injection site, the amount of insulin contained in the first ml of dialysate entering the peritoneal cavity, and the amount of insulin in the last ml of the dialysis solution. Their study suggested an important adsorption of insulin entered the peritoneal cavity. However, the studies of Twardowski and colleagues showed no important loss of insulin in the bag when the insulin was injected into the dialysis bag.

RESULTS OF BLOOD SUGAR CONTROL

Many centers have reported that insulin absorbed from the peritoneal cavity, as the sole route of administration during CAPD, achieves good glucose control [67–72].

In 37 CAPD patients at the Toronto Western Hospital (TWH) the protocol described above gave tight control of blood sugar (table 7–4). Mean fasting and one-hour, postmeal blood sugar values were within the desired range. These mean values were derived by averaging all the measurements available in each patient for one month. Table 7–5 shows the results of glucose monitoring in the same patients done at home by the finger-prick technique for the month; they correspond to the laboratory values shown in table 7–4. The correlation between the two methods is good.

VALUE OF GLYCOSYLATED HEMOGLOBIN (HBA,C) IN CAPD

It might be asserted that mean blood sugar values do not provide a good indication of the clinical efficacy of any method of insulin administration, and this is supported by the large standard deviations in table 7–4. Some sensitive and/or noncompliant patients will show very high and low blood sugar values. In recent years, several investigators have tried to assess the blood sugar control in diabetics with normal renal function, by estimating the level of glycosylated hemoglobin (HbA_1C). They found a significant correlation between fasting blood glucose and HbA_1C levels,

Table 7–4. Mean blood sugar levels in 37 diabetics on CAPD[1]

	No. of observations	X blood sugar + SD (mg/dl)
Fasting	200	119.9 + 50
1 hr p.c. breakfast	180	202.2 + 61
1 hr p.c. lunch	151	180.5 + 78

1. These mean values were derived from all the available values of every patient over one month.

Table 7–5. Blood sugar levels estimated by the finger-prick technique in diabetics on CAPD

	No. of observations	$\overline{X}$ blood sugar $\pm$ SD (mg/dl)
1st exchange (fasting)	153	135.3 $\pm$ 49
2nd exchange (prelunch)	141	152.6 $\pm$ 57
3rd exchange (presupper)	147	140.2 $\pm$ 52
4th exchange (midnight)	108	121.8 $\pm$ 53

in normal subjects and untreated diabetic patients [73] in whom the level of Hb_{1C} is determined by the blood glucose level in the previous two to three weeks and the life span of the erythrocytes. Impaired glucose metabolism, which may be present in about 50% of patients with renal failure, may contribute to the formation of glycosylated hemoglobin. It is more likely, however, that some unknown uremic toxins interfere with the measurement of glycosylated hemoglobin, and hence that elevated levels do not necessarily indicate poor blood glucose control. The level of HbA_{1C} in uremic patients on intermittent hemodialysis is high—a situation similar to that seen in nondiabetics with renal failure [74]. Diabetics on CAPD always have a high HbA_{1C} level despite good blood glucose control. As table 7–6 shows, the mean HbA_{1C} level in our 31 diabetic patients on CAPD is higher than that of normal subjects. Serkes and associates [75] also showed that HbA_{1C} values for CAPD diabetic patients recruited from various centers were higher than normal controls but were significantly lower than those of diabetics on hemodialysis. The high level of HbA_{1C} in dialyzed and nondialyzed uremic patients suggests that chronic renal failure per se, rather than hyperglycemia, is responsible for this increase.

COMPLICATIONS OF CAPD

Peritonitis

In the first report of CAPD in 1976, Popovich and Moncrief [76] recognized that this treatment would not be accepted widely unless means were found to lower the high incidence of peritonitis. The TWH technique brought a significant reduction [77] in peritonitis and, as a result, CAPD—as a treatment for end-stage renal disease, has shown an exponential growth all over the world. The gradual

Table 7–6. Glycosylated hemoglobin values in 31 diabetic patients on CAPD at the Toronto Western Hospital

No.	$\overline{X} \pm$ SD level in CAPD patients	$\overline{X} \pm$ SD level in control normal persons
31	9.1 $\pm$ 1.0	6.2 $\pm$ 0.9

introduction of various innovations [78,79] will further reduce the frequency of peritonitis. However, despite these improvements, peritonitis remains the leading cause of CAPD morbidity in most centers.

In the initial phases it was feared that intraperitoneal administration of insulin to diabetics on CAPD would increase the frequency of peritonitis. In a preliminary report, however, Katirtzoglou and associates [23] reported a peritonitis incidence of one episode every 11.9 patient months in nine insulin-dependent diabetics on CAPD—an incidence slightly better than that observed in nondiabetics. Subsequently other centers have reported a similar if not lower incidence of peritonitis in diabetics compared to nondiabetics (table 7–7) [80–84]. Furthermore, over the past few years, the incidence of peritonitis in CAPD patients has been gradually decreasing. For example, at TWH the incidence of peritonitis among 37 diabetics during 1982 was one episode every 20.3 patient months—a rate similar to that for our total group of 210 patients (one episode every 18 patient months). Similarly, in a larger group of diabetics on CAPD in the area of Metropolitan Toronto (table 7–8) the incidence of peritonitis in diabetics (one episode every 10.9 patient months) did not differ significantly from that of nondiabetics (one episode every 11 patient months).

As in nondiabetics, peritonitis in diabetics is caused predominantly by skin flora bacteria; for example, about 40% of bacterial peritonitis is due to *Staphylococcus epidermidis*. While this organism is a weak pathogen, in recent years it has been recognized with increasing frequency as a cause of wound infections, endocarditis, etc. *Staph. epidermidis* does not produce toxins, and pathogenicity depends entirely on its ability to initiate a pyogenic process. The clinical illness usually is mild, and the disease responds well to antibiotic treatment. Other organisms isolated during

Table 7–7. Incidence of peritonitis in diabetics compared to the nondiabetics on CAPD reported in the literature during 1982–83

Authors	Year	No. of patients in the study D/ND[1]	Incidence of peritonitis one episode/patient months	
			Diabetic	Nondiabetic
Khanna et al. [68]	1983	37/173	20.3	18
Toronto Collaborative Group [80]	1983	89/419	10.9	11.2
Nolph et al. [97]	1983	31/105	7.0	8.1
Rottembourg et al. [72]	1983	31/	12.2	
Flynn et al. [81]	1983	26[2]/37	10.6	9.7
		12[3]	7.4	—
Grefberg et al. [83]	1983	26/24	6	6
Madden et al. [84]	1982	14/27	3.7	3.2
Slingeneyer et al. [82]	1981	22/57	13	18.7

1. D = diabetic; ND = nondiabetic
2. Blind diabetics on CAPD
3. Sighted diabetics on CAPD

Table 7–8. Incidence of peritonitis (expressed as one episode per patient month) in diabetic and nondiabetics in the Toronto area hospitals

	Nondiabetic (N=419)	Type I (N=60)	Type II (N=29)
No. of patients with peritonitis	263 (62.8%)	27 (45%)	21 (72%)
No. of episodes	666	65	47
Total followup (patient months)	7453	747	448
Incidence (one episode per patient months)	11.2	11.5	9.5

episodes of peritonitis include *Staph. aureus, Strep. viridans,* gram-negative enteric organisms, and very rarely, anaerobic organisms. A very small fraction of peritonitis is caused by fungi. The pathogenesis and clinical presentation, and the spectrum of peritonitis in diabetics on CAPD, does not differ from that seen in the nondiabetics.

Treatment for peritonitis during CAPD is the same for both groups. Due to the enhanced and rapid absorption of glucose during peritonitis, hyperglycemia is observed frequently in diabetics, and insulin requirements increase. Some may need intravenous infusion of insulin for the control of blood glucose. The rapid glucose absorption may provoke fluid retention, and these patients may require additional dialysis. Due to increased protein losses during peritonitis, the patient's nutrition must be watched closely during the acute phase and, in some, parenteral nutrition should be considered.

Generally the outcome of peritonitis treatment is good. Most patients continue on CAPD after the peritonitis is cured. A small percentage (2–5%) will drop out of the CAPD program for a variety of reasons. Some fail only after one or two episodes of peritonitis, while others fail because of the severity of peritonitis.

Complications other than peritonitis during CAPD
Complications which are a direct result of increased intraabdominal pressure such as dialysate leaks, hernia, hemorrhoids, and cardiopulmonary compromise occur with the same frequency in diabetics and nondiabetics. In diabetics, because of the delayed wound healing, dialysate leakage is more frequent during the initial dialysis after catheter insertion [85]. To minimize this risk we recommend that when a new catheter is implanted in diabetics, it be placed through a lateral approach rather than in the midline and that dialysis be postponed for 24–48 hours [85].

Some diabetics have complications which are due to loss of proteins, amino acids, polypeptides, and vitamins in the dialysate; these contribute to morbidity and slow rehabilitation. Such losses pose a special problem in diabetics who may be wasted and malnourished because of poor food intake, vomiting, catabolic stresses, and intercurrent illness.

Twenty-four hour amino acid losses in the dialysate average 2.25 g/day with about 8 g/day of protein [86]. These losses are small in comparison to the intake of 1.1–1.3 g protein per kg BW per day. Protein losses correlate with serum protein concentration and body surface area. During peritonitis the protein losses are excessive and, associated with inadequate food intake due to poor appetite or inability to eat, may produce severe hypoproteinemia, hypoalbuminemia, and hypoimmunoglobulinemia. Therefore, early in the course of a peritonitis episode which appears to be responding poorly, the physician should consider parenteral nutrition. Various studies have shown that plasma levels of the essential amino acids are low in CAPD patients [86–88]. Of the nonessential amino acids, tyrosine and serine are low, whereas half-cystine, citrulline, and 3-methylhistidine are high [86]. However, in comparison with the nondiabetic patients, diabetics on CAPD tend to show fewer abnormalities perhaps because intraperitoneal administration of insulin does much to correct the metabolic abnormalities [86]. On the other hand, in diabetics, plasma amino acid uptake by tissues may be reduced and release increased, which may tend to balance the effect of uremia. Therefore, the more normal pattern resulting from the combination of these two factors may not necessarily indicate that diabetics have a better nitrogen economy. This view is supported by the presence, in diabetics on CAPD, of abnormal levels of nonessential amino acids.

Continuous absorption of glucose during CAPD may aggravate the hypertriglyceridemia, which is common in both dialyzed and nondialyzed uremics. Many patients develop hyperlipidemia and obesity after commencing CAPD. As a group, diabetics on CAPD have less hypertriglyceridemia than nondiabetics [41]. This improvement is attributed to the effect of intraperitoneal insulin, and some centers now advocate the administration of [89] intraperitoneal insulin to nondiabetics with hypertriglyceridemia, although others do not believe this is effective [90]. Uremics have concentrations of high-density lipoproteins (HDL) significantly lower than normals: CAPD appears to reverse this trend but does not return the HDL-C concentration to normal [91].

Retinopathy

One of the most dreaded complications of diabetes is progression of retinopathy. Most insulin-dependent diabetics have irreversible visual lesions before they start dialysis, especially during the terminal phase of renal failure when hypertension tends to be severe. In the great majority by the time they reach the stage of dialysis, ocular lesions are far too advanced to expect any useful recovery. Therefore, better preservation of ocular function depends on a more aggressive approach to blood pressure regulation and glucose control during the predialysis phase.

Factors that accelerate the progression of retinopathy during dialysis include retinal ischemia made worse by the rapid fluctuations in the intravascular volumes during intermittent therapy, severe hypertension, hyperglycemia, and systemic heparinization. CAPD avoids many of the problems inherent in the intermittent forms of dialysis: by its design, CAPD does not involve volume fluctuations; blood pressure control during CAPD is much easier; no heparinization is required; and intraperitoneal insulin gives tight blood sugar control. Therefore, many have reported stabilization or even improvement of ocular function in diabetic patients maintained on CAPD. In the experience of Toronto Western Hospital [68], diabetic patients starting CAPD with normal visual function tend to preserve their visual acuity during CAPD (figure 7–1). Those in whom vision deteriorates already have far-advanced proliferative retinopathy or other ophthalmological diseases.

Peripheral and autonomic neuropathy

Clinically obvious peripheral neuropathy is extremely rare in nondiabetic CAPD patients; however, abnormal motor-nerve conduction velocities are noted frequently. These abnormalities tend to stabilize during CAPD. Similarly, diabetic peripheral and autonomic neuropathy seem to persist despite adequate dialysis. Autonomic nerve dysfunction with severe orthostatic hypotension and hypertension in the supine position and bladder and bowel dysfunction constitute a real challenge to persons treating diabetics. Gastroparesis and the associated obstacles to nutrition that this implies are most frustrating complications. None of these problems is reversed by CAPD. With respect to orthostatic hypotension, it may be blunted by a combination of slight fluid excess with minimal leg edema; potent vasodilators, flurohydrocortisone, and beta blockers may lower blood pressure in the supine position. Metoclopropamide 10–30 mg/day facilitates gastric emptying and may minimize gastric symptoms.

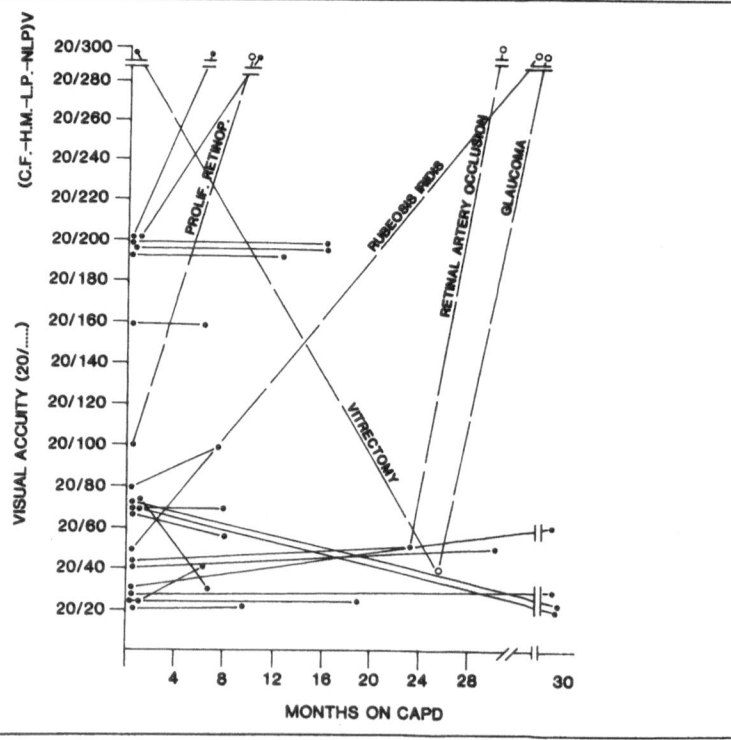

Figure 7–1. Changes in visual acuity in 22 eyes of diabetics on CAPD.

Peripheral vascular disease

Small-vessel disease leading to ischemic gangrene of the extremities is a common complication of type I diabetes. Initial short-term experience with CAPD does not suggest that this complication is more frequent in diabetics than in nondiabetics. Since CAPD is not believed to prevent macrovascular disease, one might expect to encounter this complication in long-term CAPD patients. Preexisting vascular disease might accelerate during CAPD in the presence of persistent hypertension. In such patients, it is wise to accept a lower standard of blood pressure control.

Foot care is of paramount importance in the prevention of vascular complications (tables 7–9 and 7–10).

LONG-TERM ABDOMINAL COMPLICATIONS

Loss of ultrafiltration capacity in diabetics on CAPD has been observed with or without the past history of recurrent peritonitis [72,92,93]. However, Nolph [37] observed an increased ability to ultrafiltrate very early on during the course of

Table 7–9. List of things CAPD diabetic patients should do to prevent foot complications such as an ulcer, necrosis, gangrene, etc.

WHAT YOU SHOULD DO
1. Wash feet daily with mild soap and luke warm water. Dry thoroughly especially between toes. Use blotting pressure—no rubbing.
2. When feet are dry, apply emollient to be prescribed by doctor to keep the skin soft and smooth.
3. Cut nails straight across, not shorter than flesh; this should be done by a podiatrist.
4. Socks or stockings should be of unmercerized cotton or wool about ½″ lower than longest toe and should be unwrinkled.
5. If feet are cold, use woolen bed socks or stockings when going to bed.
6. Keep feet warm and dry. Wear warm socks in winter, two pairs if necessary.

Table 7–10. List of things that should not be done by diabetic patients in order to avoid foot complications

WHAT YOU SHOULD NOT DO
Do not use any sharp or dull instrument on feet.
Do not cut corns or callouses.
Do not use corn cures or any medication to remove corns or callouses.
Do not pick or tear toenails.
Do not scratch, rub, or tear skin.
Do not use any medication that is not prescribed by doctor.
Do not use hot water, hot water bottles or bags, baking lamps, heating lamps, pads, electrical heaters, or massaging devices.
Do not walk barefoot.
Do not expose feet to cold weather.
Do not wear shoes that hurt or rub, cut, or blister.
Do not get feet wet or walk when shoes are wet.

CAPD treatment in diabetics as compared to nondiabetic normotensive patients. When loss of ultrafiltration occurs, patients are exposed to a risk of chronic overhydration and may end up discontinuing CAPD treatment. Recovery of ultrafiltration capability has been observed after a temporary cessation of peritoneal dialysis treatment [93].

Changes in residual kidney function during CAPD

During the predialysis phase of chronic renal failure in diabetics, the important factors in the steady decline of kidney function are hypertension and hyperglycemia. In view of its ability to control blood pressure and blood glucose, one would anticipate that after starting CAPD the decline in residual kidney function would stop or be slowed. However only Rottembourg and associates [94] have demonstrated preservation of residual kidney function in a diabetic population on CAPD; most centers report a steady decline in residual kidney function over the first year on CAPD [45]. Rottembourg and associates [94] attributed their results to the concomitant use of high doses of furosemide. This possibility should be studied further especially by serial measurements of inulin clearance because, at high serum creatinine values, the 24-hour creatinine clearance is not a good index of kidney function.

Adequacy of dialysis

Most patients treated by CAPD appear to have a good clinical status and enjoy a sense of general well-being. They have a higher hemoglobin concentration than nondiabetics [68, 37], and this may contribute to their feeling of well-being. As in nondiabetics on CAPD, levels of blood urea and creatinine are maintained at a steady state. Serum phosphorus is held at normal levels with only small doses of phosphate binders.

During the first year, body weight returns more or less to the preillness level; if they had lost significant weight, they have a rapid weight gain if they had significant fluid accumulation. After these initial changes, body weight generally stabilizes unless the patient has a complicating intercurrent illness. Day-to-day fluid balance is maintained by hypertonic solutions. We recommend no more than one hypertonic exchange per day to minimize the ill effects of excessive glucose absorption. Many centers now use diuretics to enhance the urine output.

In most patients blood pressure control is easy unless there is associated orthostatic hypotension due to autonomic neuropathy. In 37 diabetics on CAPD, we encountered only 2 who required antihypertensive medication for control of elevated blood pressure; of this group, almost 80% were hypertensive and required several drugs before starting CAPD. Persistent hypertension in diabetics on CAPD usually is part of a complex disorder in which supine hypertension is associated with severe orthostatic hypotension.

BACKUP HOSPITALIZATION

As would be expected, the various complications seen in this population increase the number of days they spend in the hospital for treatment. At the Toronto Western Hospital diabetics on CAPD spent 33 days/patient year in hospital— almost twice as long as nondiabetic CAPD patients (16 days per patient year). For types I and II diabetics, the rate of hospitalization appears to be similar. Fifty percent of these hospitalization days is due to peritonitis and related complications. However, improvement in CAPD techniques and the introduction of new devices for reduction of peritonitis should decrease further the rate of hospitalization in diabetics.

This high rate of hospitalization reflects the morbidity which compounds the management of diabetics on dialysis. Diabetics on hemodialysis [95] have similar high hospitalization rates (table 7–11).

CAUSES OF DEATH AMONG DIABETICS ON CAPD

In most centers, the most common causes of death among diabetics on CAPD are cardio- or cerebrovascular events and infection. Table 7–12 shows the causes of death in 21 CAPD diabetic patients treated in the Toronto area. Contrary to expectation and unlike the experience in nondiabetics, infection does not seem to be a major cause of death in this group of diabetics. Cardiovascular events were the single most important cause of death.

Table 7–11. Rate of hospitalization for diabetics on CAPD at the Toronto Western Hospital (TWH) compared with diabetics managed by hemodialysis at the University of Minnesota (UM) by Shapiro and Comty

	Days/patient months	
	TWH	UM
Insulin-dependent diabetics	2.86 (29)[1]	2.37 (129)
Non-insulin dependent diabetics	2.86 (8)	1.87 (81)
Nondiabetics	1.33 (210)	1.56 (552)

1. The numbers in the parentheses indicate the number of patients in each group.

Table 7–12. Causes of death in diabetics and nondiabetics maintained on CAPD in the Toronto area hospitals

	Nondiabetic	Type I diabetic	Type II diabetic
Cardiovascular	28 (52%)	11 (73%)	5 (83%)
Peritonitis	17 (31%)	1 (7%)	1 (17%)
Other	9 (17%)	3 (20%)	0

TECHNIQUE SURVIVAL OF DIABETICS ON CAPD

Despite the impressive improvement in survival among diabetics, these patients leave CAPD programs at a high rate for causes that include deaths and transfers to other forms of treatment. Figures 7–2, 7–3, and 7–4 show the cumulative technique survival rate for 60 type I and 29 type II patients in the Toronto area. Table 7–13 shows the causes of CAPD failure. The drop in rate for diabetics does not differ from that in nondiabetics. In both groups the main reason for transfer to other forms of treatment is peritonitis. Membrane failure, an entity that has been recognized only in the past year or so [93], has not been observed among diabetics.

OUTCOME OF DIABETICS ON CAPD

The two-year cumulative survival rate of diabetics treated by CAPD has shown remarkable improvement compared to that achieved by IPD. This may be because diabetics, who tend to have significant cardiovascular disease, seem to tolerate CAPD better. Furthermore, during the past four to five years, significant improvement made in peritoneal dialysis undoubtedly have influenced survival rates. Thus our ability to handle complications has improved considerably; CAPD gives better control of blood pressure than IPD and has clearly reduced morbidity.

On the average CAPD patients with diabetes are 10 years younger, but they tend to have significantly more cardiovascular disease than nondiabetics; this may explain the lower survival of diabetics than of nondiabetics of the same age [80].

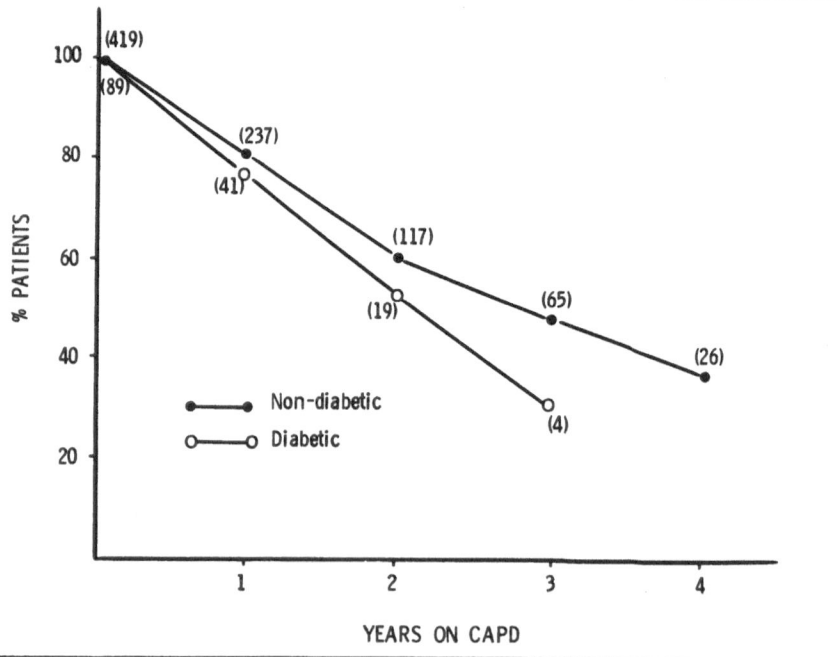

Figure 7–2. Technique survival for Type I and II diabetics on CAPD in Toronto area.

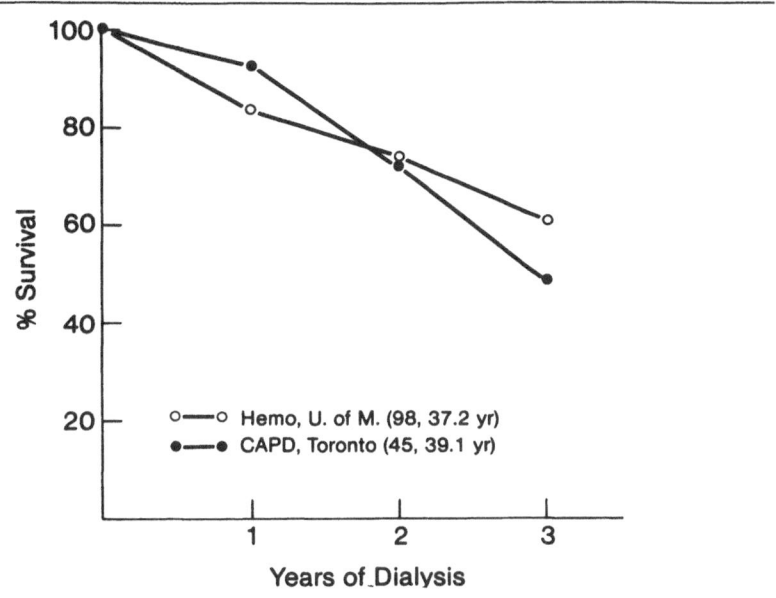

Figure 7–3. Patient survival. Type I diabetics under 61 years of age in Toronto compared to diabetics on hemodialysis in Minnesota.

Tables 7–14 and 7–15 show the characteristic of 60 type I and 29 type II diabetics treated by CAPD in the Toronto area under the University of Toronto Collaborative Dialysis Group. These patients have been compared with 202 type I and 101 type II diabetics treated by hemodialysis at the University of Minnesota [95]. The latter group led by Shapiro and Comty have one of the largest experiences in the use of hemodialysis in diabetic ESRD patients. The Toronto CAPD and the University of Minnesota populations are similar with respect to mean age and duration of diabetes. Figures 7–2, 7–3, and 7–4 show the cumulative survival of these patients. For Type I diabetics on CAPD, one- and two-year cumulative survivals were 92% and 75%, respectively. Type II diabetics had almost similar cumulative survival rates—90% and 75% at one and two years, respectively. In the two centers there appears to be no difference between the CAPD and hemodialysis populations in the cumulative survival up to three years. This comparison suggests that in the Toronto area, diabetics maintained on CAPD have a survival rate similar to that achieved by one of the most experienced hemodialysis centers. Table 7–16 shows similarly encouraging one-year cumulative survivals for CAPD diabetics, as reported by several centers in North America and Europe [68,-72,80,81,84,96–98].

A most recent update of combined report on regular dialysis and transplantation in Europe [98] showed that after starting CAPD in 1981 or 1982 in patients with diabetic nephropathy, survival at one year was equal or better than any other form of renal replacement therapy, particularly in the young diabetics aged 15–34 years.

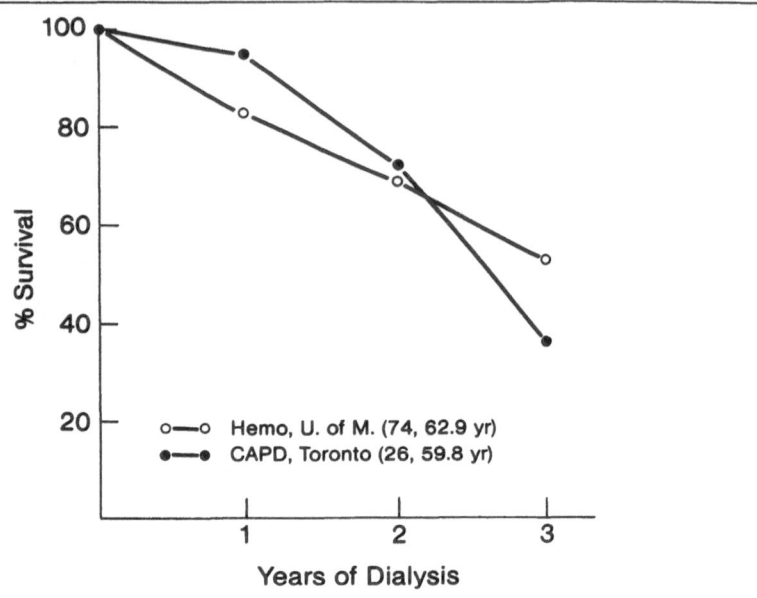

Figure 7–4. Patient survival. Type II diabetics in Toronto compared to diabetics on hemodialysis in Minnesota.

This report concluded, "Despite the limitations and in contrast to previous years, it would appear that Europe has learned how to apply CAPD and make adequate use of its potential to achieve better treatment, particularly in young diabetics."

Chiefly because of the small number of patients in each group, most centers report an overall combined cumulative survival rather than analyzing the survival data of type I and type II diabetics. The few centers that report separately the cumulative survival of type II diabetics show a comparatively poor outcome for them. This is not surprising because, as a group, type II diabetics are older, usually have severe atherosclerotic heart disease, and generally have other medical problems.

Table 7–13. Reasons for transfer to other forms of dialysis in diabetic and nondiabetic on CAPD in Toronto area

	Nondiabetics (N=419)	Type I (N=60)	Type II (N=29)
Peritonitis	45 (44.1%)	2 (25%)	2 (40%)
Membrane failure	12 (11.8%)	0	1 (20%)
Preference	9 (8.8%)	3 (37.5%)	0
Unable to cope	9 (8.8%)	0	0
Back pain	7 (6.9%)	0	1 (20%)
Technical failure	6 (5.9%)	1 (12.5%)	0
Other	14 (13.7%)	2 (25%)	1 (20%)

Table 7–14. Characteristics of type I diabetics on CAPD managed by the University of Toronto collaborative group, compared with type I diabetics on hemodialysis at the University of Minnesota managed by Shapiro and Comty [79]

	CAPD Toronto	Hemodialysis Univ. of Minnesota
Number	60	202
Sex		
Male	46 (77.1%)	121 (60%)
Female	14 (23%)	81 (40%)
Age		
Mean	39.1	41.7
(Years) Range	21–69	21–77
Duration of diabetics	24.6	22.2
Retinopathy	58 (97%)	181 (95%)

Table 7–15. Characteristics of type II diabetics on CAPD managed by the University of Toronto collaborative group compared with type II diabetics on hemodialysis at the University of Minnesota [79]

	CAPD Toronto	Hemodialysis Univ. of Minnesota
Number	29	101
Sex		
Male	20 (69%)	37 (36%)
Female	9 (31%)	64 (64%)
Age		
Mean	59.4	62.3
(Years) Range	49–68	2503
Duration of diabetes	13.4	13.0
Retinopathy	20 (69%)	62 (61%)

Although the literature shows no great difference in short-term (one to three years) survival between diabetic and nondiabetic ESRD patients, it remains to be established whether there is any difference in long-term survival. Not many diabetic patients have been on CAPD for long periods because CAPD is only five to six years old. However, on other forms of kidney replacement treatment (hemodialysis and kidney transplant) nondiabetics show a significantly longer survival mainly because of the steady progression of the underlying cardiovascular disease in the diabetic population. In the future, when large number of diabetic patients have been carried on this treatment for a longer period, we may find a similar trend with CAPD.

CAPD IN BLIND DIABETICS

Despite its simplicity, blind diabetics with ESRD found CAPD difficult to perform. However, Flynn and his colleagues have proved that when both patients and

Table 7–16. One-year cumulative survival of diabetics on CAPD

Author	Year	No. of patients treated	Cumulative one-year survival (Percent)
Madden et al. [84]	1982	14	70
Rottembourg et al. [72]	1983	24	84
Kurtz et al. [96]	1983	29	78
Flynn et al. [81]			
Blind diabetics	1983	26	92
Sighted diabetics	1983	12	64
Grefberg et al. [83]	1983	24	80
Nolph et al. [97]	1983	24	92
Khanna et al. [68]			
(Type I)	1983	29	87
(Type II)	1983	8	82
Univ. of Toronto Collaborative Group [80]			
(Type I)	1983	60	92
(Type II)	1983	29	90
Combined report of EDTA = ERA [98]			
Age 15–34 years	1983	33	92
Age 35–44 years	1983	39	77
Age 45–54 years	1983	49	80
Age 55–64 years	1983	64	71
National CAPD Registry[1]	1984	1,276	82

1. Report of the "National CAPD Registry of the National Institute of Health" January 1984

staff have enthusiasm, blind diabetics can be trained to perform CAPD safely [99]. Their long-term experience showed that the incidence of peritonitis among blind CAPD patients was, if anything, a little lower than that seen in sighted patients. Encouraged by the work of Flynn and associates [99], several other centers have started blind diabetics on CAPD with considerable success [100–102]. Despite this encouraging report we could not train our blind CAPD patients to perform CAPD until a special adaptor was introduced which makes the whole procedure simpler and safer [79]. Figure 7–5 shows the various steps in this procedure.

Despite the use of an "Injecta aid" similar to that described by Flynn [99], our patients had difficulty in injecting the insulin (prepared before hand) by a sighted person into the bag without contaminating the needle. We solved this problem by having a sighted person add the insulin in all the bags to be used for a 24- to 48–hour period; according to our findings, insulin seems to be biologically active if it is left in the peritoneal dialysis solution for this period.

Between May 1982 and December 1983 three blind diabetics have been performing their own CAPD with this system. Their characteristics, episodes of peritonitis, and rate of hospitalization are shown in table 7–17. So far we observed no peritonitis. Table 7–18 shows blood sugar control (average values of blood chemistry and that obtained by the finger-prick technique at home). Only one of these

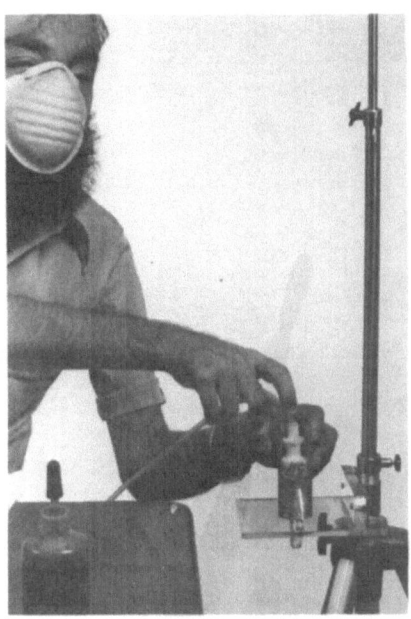

a) Insert spike coupler in the hole of the special tray with guide.

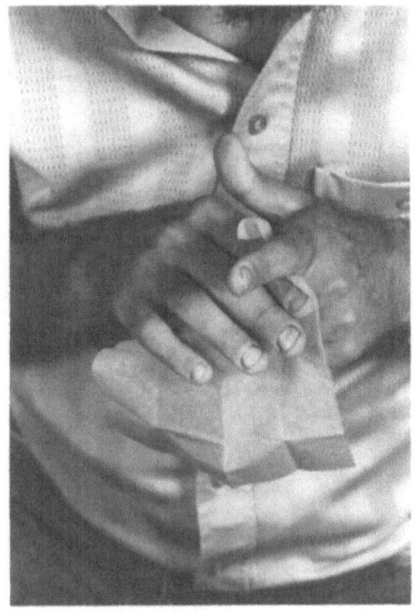

b) Wash hands with an antiseptic towelette.

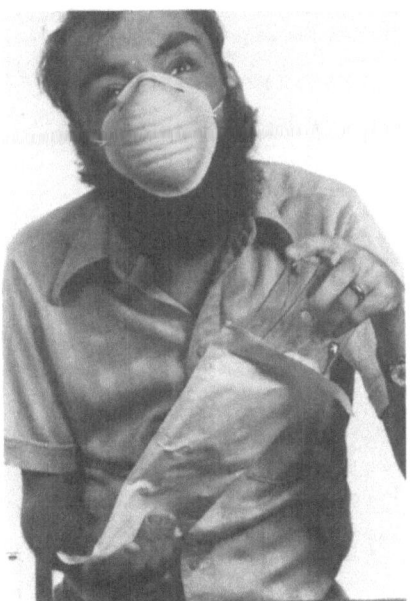

c) Open the container and remove sterile drainage bag.

Figure 7–5. Technique for the use of the Oreopoulos-Zellerman connector by blind CAPD patients.

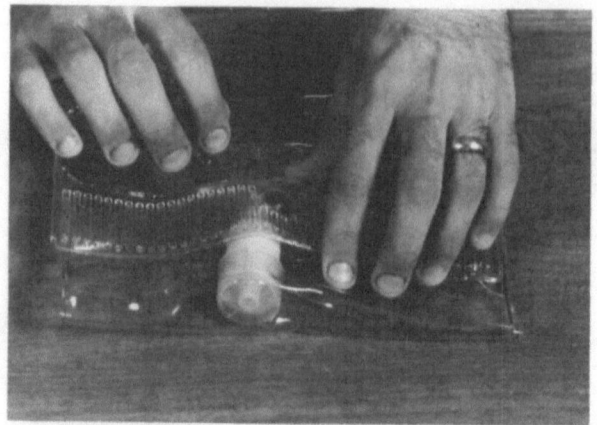

d) Feel for the rough flap of the bag and identify the female connector with the protective cap.

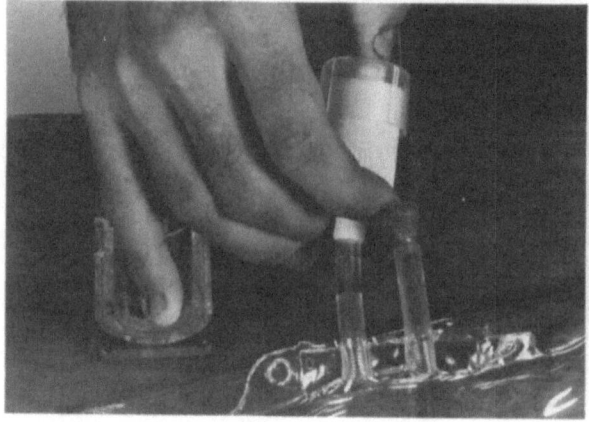

e) While holding the protective cap, feel with the little finger of the same hand the ridge of the guide on the special board.

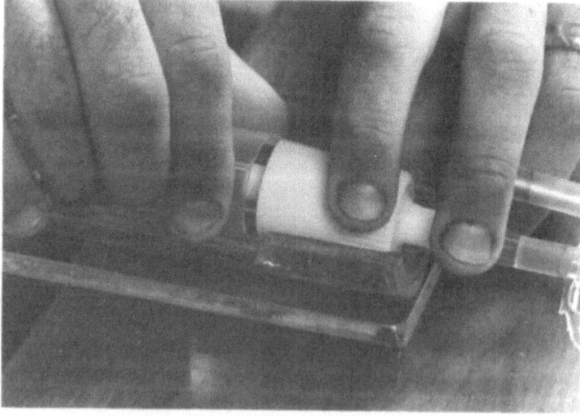

f) Place female connector in guide and remove cap. Place cap on tray with the open end upside.

Figure 7–5 (continued)

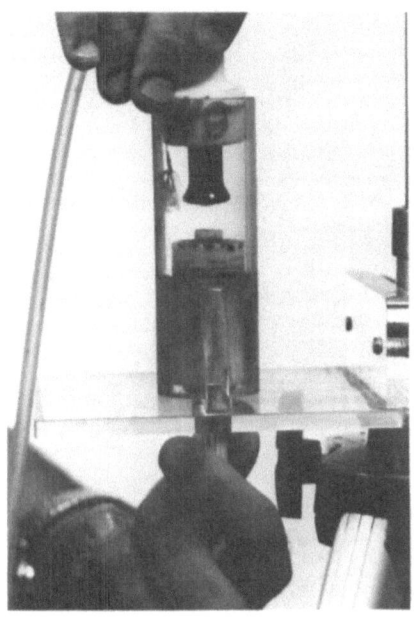 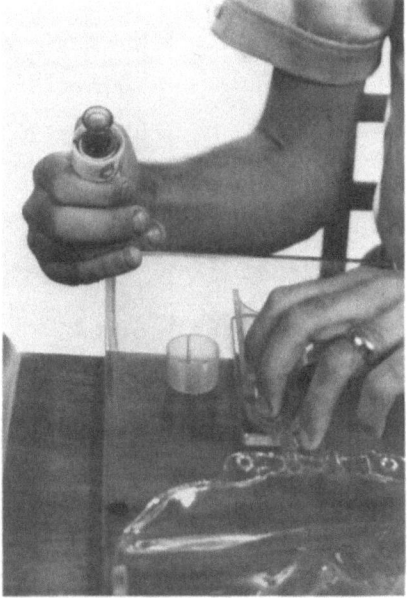

g) Unscrew and remove spike coupler from disinfectant cap.

h) With left hand, feel for the corner of the guide and with the ring and small finger of right hand feel for the center of the guide.

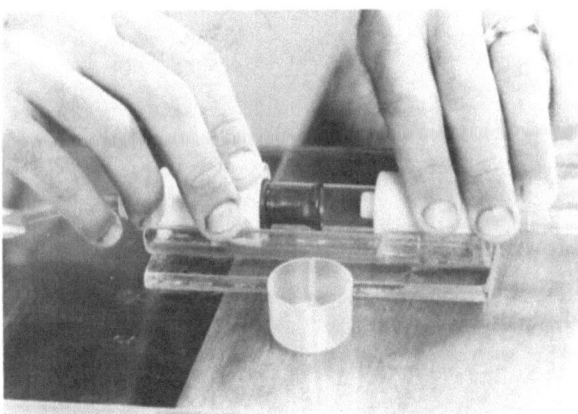

i) After placing spike coupler into guide and while holding down both parts, slide spike into female connector and screw together.

Figure 7–5 (continued)

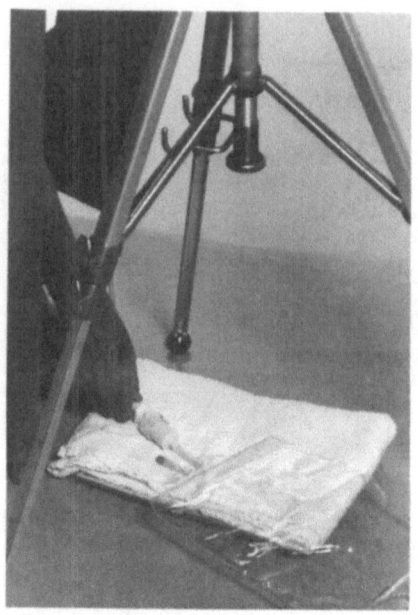

j) Place drain bag on top of a clean towel on the floor, open clamp on connection tubing and drain.

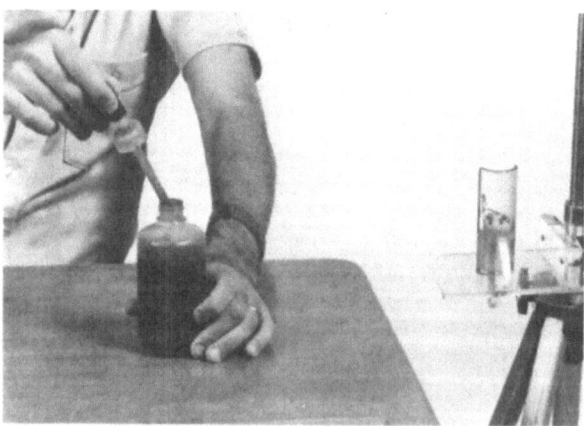

k) While draining, draw-up proviodine.

Figure 7–5 (continued)

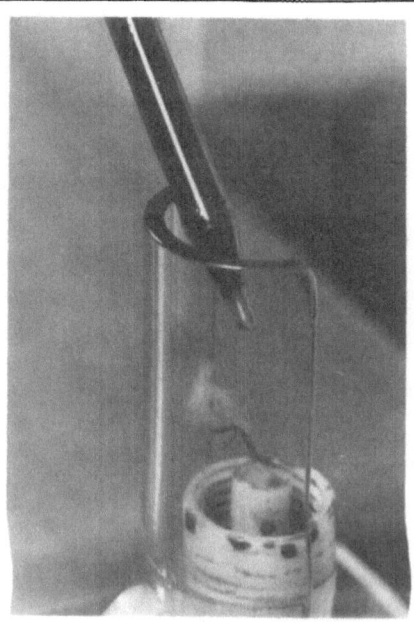

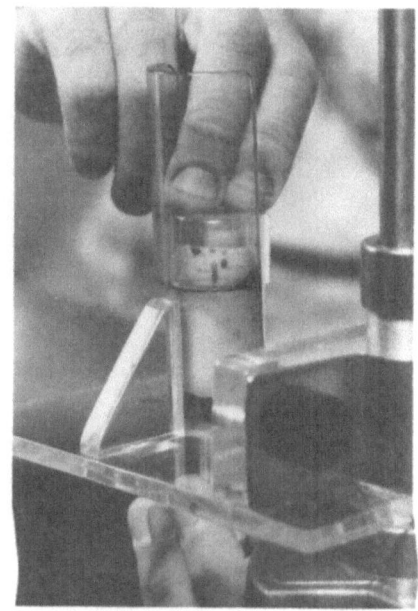

l) Drop proviodine into the disinfectant cap.

m) Place protective cap on disinfectant cap.

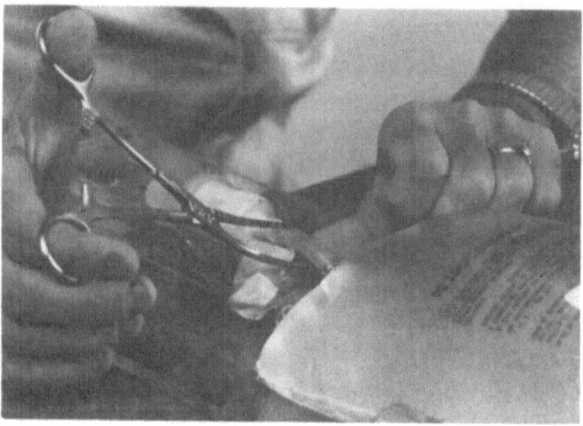

n) Place the female connector of a new bag in the guide.

Figure 7–5 (continued)

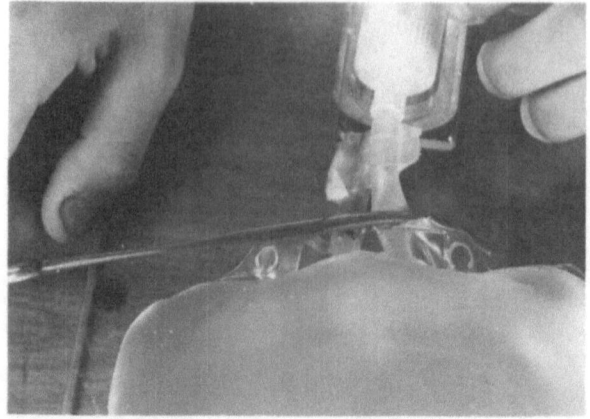

o) Clamp the port of the bag.

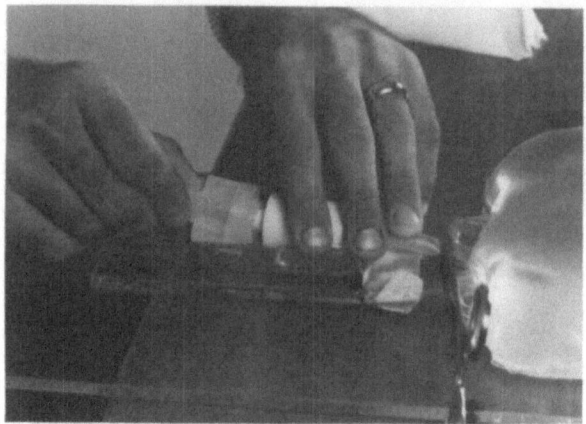

p) Remove protective cap.

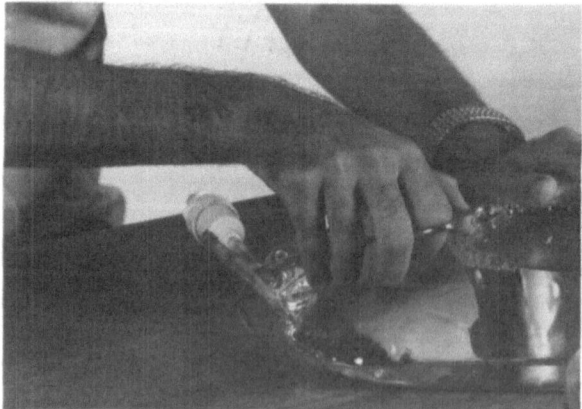

q) Place filled drain bag on the table and clamp the port of the bag.

Figure 7–5 (continued)

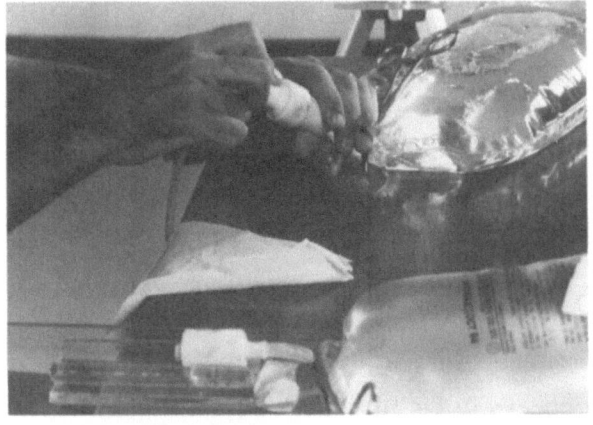

r) Unscrew and remove spike from the drainage bag.

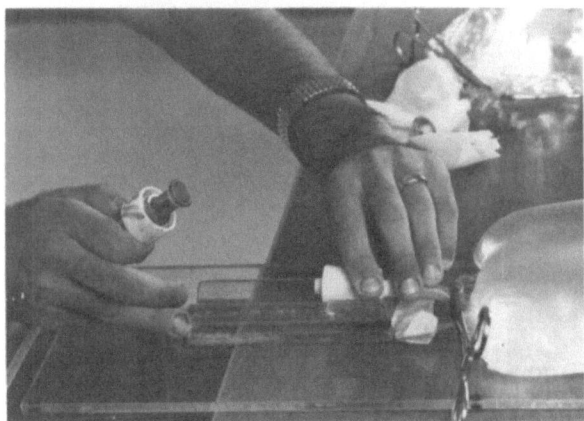

s) Approach guide with the right hand holding the spike, while with the left hand, hold down the female connector on the guide.

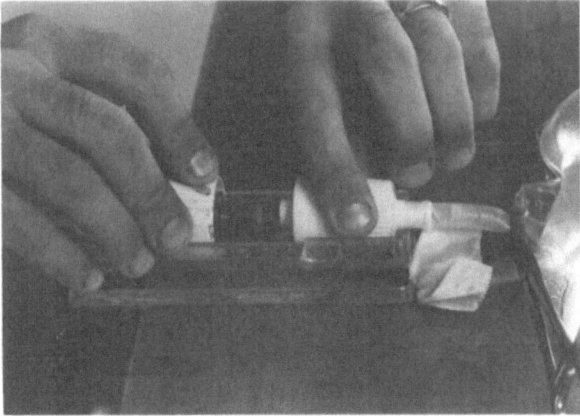

t) Connect the spike coupler with the female connector by sliding the former in the guide.

Figure 7–5 (continued)

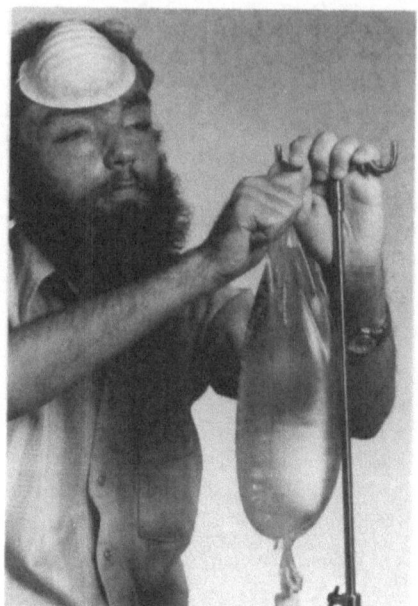

u) Hang bag on the pole and start infusion of the solution.

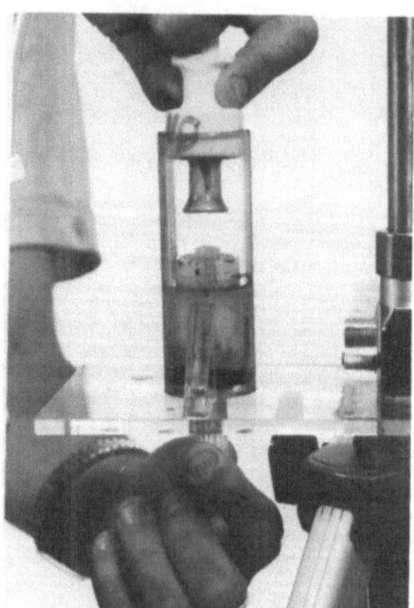

v) At the end of the infusion, remove spike coupler from the bag and insert into the disinfectant cap, with the help of the special guide.

Figure 7–5 (continued)

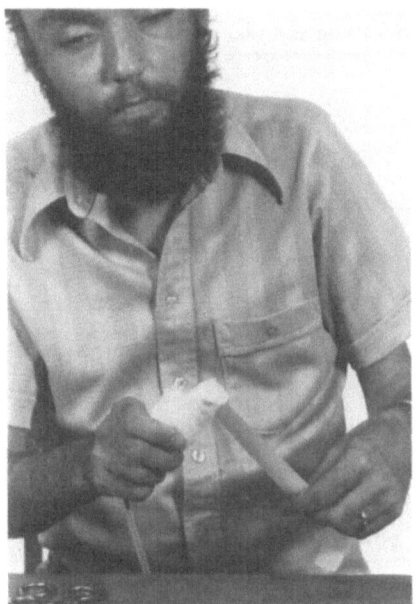

w) Wrap the O-Z connector with a 4 × 4 gauze and tape.

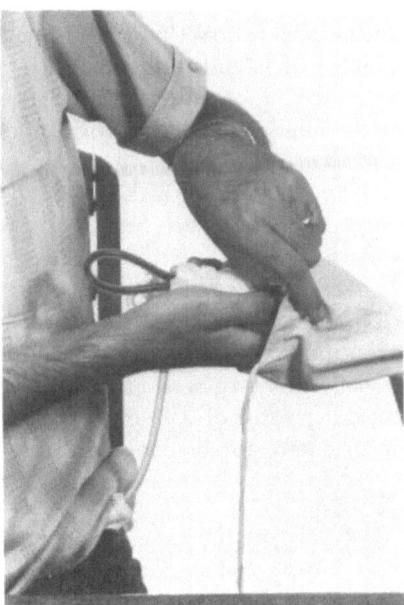

x) Place wrapped connector into the pouch.

Figure 7–5 (continued)

Table 7–17. Characteristics, episodes of peritonitis, and hospitalizations among three blind diabetics using the OZ connector for CAPD

Patient	Age/sex	Ccr/urine volume	Duration of CAPD with OZ connector (days)	Peritonitis episodes	Hospitalization/day
P.C.	../M	0	211	0	0
R.D.	../M	0	226	0	0
R.M.	../M	11/700	184	?1[1]	3/44[2]

1. First sample sterile; sample of second day grew pseudomonas.
2. 18 days for neuropathic pain of legs, five days for unexplained R.U.Q. pain, and 21 for the (?) peritonitis.

Table 7–18. Blood pressure—blood sugar and biochemical control during CAPD with the OZ connector in three blind diabetics (average of last three months)

Patient	FBS	1 hr postbreakfast	B. P. Standing	BUN	Creat	Alb/T.Pr. (g/L)
P.C.	198	360	150/85	23	1236	39/66
R.D.	171	72	110/76	19.3	968	38/64
R.M.	117	193	90/75	22.4	565	34/63

patients was admitted to the hospital for overhydration and an unexplained abdominal pain. The main advantage of having blind diabetics performing their own CAPD is that it gives them a feeling of independence, which is important for all patients and especially for the blind. In addition, such independence decreases the burden on the family.

In conclusion, the cumulative survival of diabetics on CAPD continues to rise. Good control of blood sugar, blood pressure, and steady-state control of uremia may be the contributing factors. Patients with good vision at the start tend to maintain good vision. The rate of hospitalization and other medical complication is much higher than that of nondiabetic patients. Preliminary results indicate that the residual kidney function may be preserved, or decline may be slowed while on CAPD. Because of the many advantages, and the trend for better and promising rates of survival over any other form of kidney replacement treatment, CAPD seems to be the treatment of choice for diabetics requiring dialysis.

REFERENCES

1. Friedman EA. Where are the data on America's uremic diabetics: Diabetic Nephropathy 2: 3, 1983.
2. E.S.R.D. Network dialysis and transplant survival data 1981. 1982.
3. 1981 End Stage Renal Disease Annual Report to Congress. Health care financing administration, HCFA 82-02144.
4. Knowles HC. Magnitude of the renal failure problem in diabetic patients. Kidney Int 6(SI): 2–7, 1976.

5. Drukker W, Haagsma-Schouten WAG, Alberts CHR, Baarda B. Report on regular dialysis treatment in Europe VI. Proc Euro Dial Transplant Assoc 6: 133–135, 1971.
6. Kjellstrand CM. Dialysis in diabetics. In: Strategy in Renal Failure, Friedman EA (ed). New York: J. Wiley & Sons, 1977, pp. 345–391.
7. Abella R, et al. Periodic dialysis in terminal uremia. JAMA 199: 362–368, 1967.
8. Chazan BI, Rees SB, Balodimos MC, Younger D, Ferguson BD. Dialysis in diabetics: a review of 44 patients. JAMA 209: 2026–2030, 1969.
9. Blagg CR, Eschback JW, Sawyer TK, Casaretto AA. Dialysis for endstage diabetic nephropathy. Proc Eur Dial Transplant Forum 1: 133–135, 1971.
10. Comty CM, Shapiro FL. Management and prognosis of diabetic patients treated by chronic hemodialysis. Am Soc Nephrol 5:15, 1971.
11. Ghavamian M, Gutch CF, Kopp KF, Kolff WJ. The sad truth about hemodialysis in diabetic nephropathy. JAMA 222: 1386–1389, 1972.
12. White N, Snowden SA, Parsons V, Sheldon J, Bewick M. The management of terminal renal failure in diabetic patients by regular dialysis therapy. Nephron 11: 261–275, 1973.
13. Leonard A, Comty C, Raij L, Rattazzi T, Wathen RS, Shapiro F. The natural history of regularly dialyzed diabetics. Trans Am Soc Artif Intern Organs 19: 282–286, 1973.
14. Ma KW, Masler DS, Brown DC. Hemodialysis in diabetic patients with chronic renal failure. Ann Int Med 83: 215–217, 1975.
15. Shideman JR, Buselmeier TJ, Kjellstrand CM. Hemodialysis complications in insulin dependent diabetic patient accepted for transplantation. Arch Intern Med 136: 1126–1130, 1976.
16. Avram MM, Slater PA, Fein PA, Altman E. Comparative survival of 673 patients with chronic uremia treated with renal transplantation (RT) and maintenance hemodialysis (MD). Trans Am Soc Artif Intern Organs 25: 391–393, 1979.
17. Comty C, Kuellsen D, Shapiro F. A reassessment of the prognosis of the diabetic patients treated by chronic hemodialysis. Trans Am Soc Artif Intern Organs 20: 286–296, 1978.
18. Ma K, Masler D, Brown D. Hemodialysis in diabetic patients with chronic renal failure. Ann Intern Med 83: 215–217, 1975.
19. Totten M, Izenstein B, Gleason R, et al. Chronic renal failure in diabetics. Survival with hemodialysis vs. transplantation. J Dial 2: 17–32, 1978.
20. Jacobs C, Rottembourg J, Frantz P, et al. Le traitment de l'insufficiance renale terminale du diabetique insulinodependent. In: Acutalitees Nephrologiques de L'Hopital Necker, Hamburger J, Grosnier J, Funk-Brentano J. (eds). Paris: Flammarion, 1978, p. 77.
21. Blumenkrantz M, Shapiro D, Mimura N, Oreopoulos DG, et al. Maintenance peritoneal dialysis as an alternative in the patients with diabetes mellitus and end stage uremia. Kidney Int (Suppl 1)6: 108–114, 1974.
22. Rubin J, Oreopoulos DG, Blair RG, et al. Chronic peritoneal dialysis in the management of diabetics with terminal renal failure. Nephron 19: 265–270, 1977.
23. Katirtzoglou A, Izatt S, Oreopoulos DG, et al. Chronic peritoneal dialysis in diabetics with end stage renal failure. In: Diabetic Renal-Retinal Syndrome, Friedman EA, et al. (eds). New York: Grune & Stratton, 19??, pp. 317–332.
24. Mitchell J, Fronhert P, Kurtz S, Anderson C. Chronic peritoneal dialysis in juvenile onset diabetes mellitus. A comparison with hemodialysis. Mayo Clinic Proc 53: 775–781, 1978.
25. Mion C. A peritoneal dialysis programme. Proc Eur Dial Transpl Assoc 12: 140, 1975.
26. Rubin J, Oreopoulos DG, Blair G, et al. Chronic peritoneal dialysis in the management of diabetics with terminal renal failure. Nephron 19: 265, 1977.
27. Blumenkrantz MJ, Kamdar AK, Coburn JW Peritoneal dialysis for diabetic patients with end stage nephropathy. Dial & Transpl 6: 47, 1977.
28. Blumenkrantz MJ, Shapiro DJ, Mimura, N, et al. Maintenance peritoneal dialysis as an alternative in the patient with diabetes mellitus and end-stage uremia. Kidney Int 1: S108, 1974.
29. Warden GS, Maxwell JG, Stephen RL. The use of reciprocating peritoneal dialysis with subcutaneous peritoneal catheter in end-stage renal failure in diabetes mellitus. J Surg Res 24: 495, 1978.
30. Mion C, Slingeneyer A, Selam JL, et al. Home peritoneal dialysis (HPD) in end-stage diabetic nephropathy (ESDN) (Abstr.). J Dial 2: 426, 1978.
31. Quellhorst E, Schuenemann B, Mutzsch G, Jacob I. Hemo and peritoneal dialysis treatment of patients with diabetic nephropathy. A comparison study. Proc Eur Dial Transpl Assoc 15: 205, 1978.

32. Ghantous WN, Adelson BH, Salkin MS, et al. A comparison of peritoneal and hemodialysis in the treatment of diabetic and end-stage renal failure (Abstr.). J Dial 2: 436, 1978.
33. Flynn CT, Nanson JA. Intraperitoneal insulin in diabetes. Lancet Sept. 15: 591, 1969.
34. Flynn CT, Nanson JA. Intraperitoneal insulin with CAPD—an artificial pancreas. Trans Am Soc Artif Intern Organs 25: 114–117, 1979.
35. Schade DS, Eaton RP. 1980. The peritoneum—a potential insulin delivery route for a mechanical pancreas. Diabetes Care 3: 229, 1980.
36. Oreopoulos DG, Khanna R, Williams P, Vas SI. Continuous ambulatory peritoneal—1981. Nephron 30: 293–303, 1982.
37. Nolph KD. Continuous ambulatory peritoneal dialysis. Am J Nephrol 1: 1–10, 1981.
38. Mion C, Slingeneyer A, Canaud B, Elie M. A review of seven years home peritoneal dialysis. Proc EDTA 18: 91–110, 1981.
39. Flynn T. Continuous ambulatory peritoneal dialysis in diabetic patients. Proceedings of the 1st International Symposium on CAPD. Excerpta Medica, Amsterdam 187, 1980.
40. Kuhlmann H, Thomae U. CAPD—an alternative in the dialysis treatment of diabetics suffering from kidney failure? Med Welt 31: 1140, 1980.
41. Amair P, Khanna R, Leibel B, et al. Continuous ambulatory peritoneal dialysis in diabetics with end-stage renal disease. N Engl J Med 306: 625, 1982.
42. Flynn CT. Diabetes and CAPD. Int J Artif Organs 5, 332–333, 1982.
43. Legrain M, Rottembough J, Bentchikou A, et al. Dialysis treatment of insulin dependent diabetic patients: ten years experience. Clin Nephrology 21:72–81, 1984.
44. Khanna R, Oreopoulos DG. Peritoneal access using the Toronto Western Hospital permanent catheter. Perspect Perit Dial 1; 4–7, 1983.
45. Khanna R Oreopoulos DG, Dombros N, et al. Continuous ambulatory peritoneal dialysis after three years: still a promising treatment. Perit Dial Bull 1: 24, 1981.
46. Porte D Jr, Bagdade JD. Human insulin secretion: an integrated approach. Annu Rev Med 21: 219–240, 1970.
47. Flynn CT Hibbard J, Dohrman B. Advantages of continuous ambulatory peritoneal dialysis to the diabetic with renal failure. Proc EDTA 16: 184–193, 1979.
48. Editorial. New insulin delivery system for diabetics. Lancet 1 (June): 1275–1277, 1979.
49. Greenwood RH, Davies CJ, Senator GB, et al. Intraperitoneal insulin in diabetics. Lancet 2: 312, 1979.
50. Flynn CT, Nanson JA. Intraperitoneal insulin in diabetics. Lancet 2: 591, 1979.
51. Graber AL. Chronic peritoneal dialysis in insulin dependent diabetes mellitus—diabetic clinical care conference. J Tenn Med Assoc 2: 74, 1981.
52. Schade DS, Eaton RP, et al. Five day programmed intraperitoneal insulin infusion in diabetic man. Abstract Am Diabetic Assoc, p. 71, 1980.
53. Schade DS, Eaton RP, Spencer W. The advantages of the peritoneal route of insulin delivery. In: Irsigler K., Kunz D., Owens, D., Regal, H. (Eds) New Approaches to Insulin Therapy. MTP Press, Lancaster 1981.
54. Zingg W, Shirriff JM, Liebel. Experimental routes of insulin administration. Perit Dial Bull 2: S24–27, 1982.
55. Balducci A, Slama G, Rottembourg J, Baumelou A, Delage A. Intraperitoneal insulin in uraemic diabetics undergoing continuous ambulatory peritoneal dialysis. Br Med J 283: 1021–1023, 1981.
56. Shapiro DJ, Blumenkrantz MJ, Levin SR, Coburn JW. Absorption and action of insulin added to peritoneal dialysate in dogs. Nephron 23: 174–180, 1979.
57. Brachet E, Rasio E. The passage of (125I) insulin across isolated mensentery. Effect of anti-insulin serum, Biochim Biophys Acta., 183: 162–168, 1969.
58. Twardowski ZJ, et al. Insulin binding to plastic bags: a methodologic study. Am J Hosp Pharm 40: 575–579, 1983.
59. Twardowski ZJ, et al. Nature of insulin binding to plastic bags. Am J Hosp Pharm 40: 579–582, 1983.
60. Twardowski ZJ, et al. Influence of temperature and time on insulin adsorption to plastic bags. Am J Hosp Pharm 40: 583–586, 1983.
61. Twardowski ZJ Insulin adsorption to peritoneal dialysis bags. Perit Dial Bull 3: 113–115, 1983.
62. Johnson CA, et al. Adsorption of insulin to the surface of peritoneal dialysis solution containers. Am J Kidney Disease 3: 224–228, 1983.

63. Silver MR, Sorkin MI. Insulin delivery from continuous ambulatory peritoneal dialysis bags used with peridex filters. Perit Dial Bull 4:23–27, 1984.
64. Blumenkrantz MJ, Salehmghaddan S, Salusky I. Treatment of patients with end-stage diabetic nephropathy. In: Peritoneal Dialysis, LaGreca G, et al. (eds). Milano, Italy: Wichtig, Editor, 1983, pp. 289–306.
65. Khanna R, Liebel B. The Toronto Western Hospital protocol. What is the protocol for control of blood sugar in diabetics on CAPD? Perit Dial Bul 1: 100–101, 1981.
66. Rottembourg J, Caryon A, Benoliel D, Pelluzo F, Ozzanne P. Critical evaluation of the injection site for insulin in CAPD diabetic patient. Perit Dial Bull 4: S55, 1984.
67. Reeves ML, Forhan SE, Skyler JS, Peterson CM. Comparison of methods for blood glucose monitoring. Diabetes Care 4: 404–406, 1980.
68. Khanna R, Wu G, Chisholm L, Oreopoulos DG. Further experience with CAPD in diabetics with end-stage renal disease. In: Prevention and Treatment of Diabetic Nephropathy, Keen H, Legrain M. (eds). Boston: MTP Press Limited, 1983, pp. 279–288.
69. Lameire N, Dhaene M, Matthigs E, et al. Experience with CAPD in diabetic patients. In: Prevention and Treatment of Diabetic Nephropathy, Keen H, Legrain M. (eds). Boston: MTP Press Limited, 1983, pp. 289–297.
70. Coronel F, Naranjo P, Prats D. A year of experience of CAPD in the diabetic and non-diabetic patient. In: Prevention and Treatment of Diabetic Nephropathy, Keen H, Legrain M. (eds). Boston: MTP Press Limited, 1983, pp. 315–332.
71. Grefberg N, Danielson BG, Nilsson P. Continuous ambulatory peritoneal dialysis in the treatment of end-stage diabetic nephropathy. Acta Medica Scand 215:427–434, 1984.
72. Rottembourg J, Shahat EL, Agrafiotis A, et al. CAPD in insulin dependent diabetic patients, and a 40 month experience. Kidney Int 23: 40, 1983.
73. Graft RJ, Porte DJ. Glycosylated hemoglobin as an index of glycemia independent of plasma insulin in normal and diabetic subjects. Diabetes 27: 368, 1977.
74. Boer MJ, Miedema K, Casparie AF. Glycosylated hemoglobin in renal failure. Diabetologia 18: 437–440, 1980.
75. Serkes K. Travenol Laboratories, Deerfield, Illinois, Personal communication.
76. Popovich RP, Moncrief JW, Nolph KD, et al. Continuous ambulatory peritoneal dialysis. Ann Intern Med 88: 449, 1978.
77. Oreopoulos DG, Robson M, Izatt S, et al. A simple and safe technique for continuous ambulatory peritoneal dialysis. Trans Am Soc Artif Intern Organs, 1978, pp. 484–487.
78. Slingeneyer A, Mion C, Despaux E, et al. Use of bacteriologic filter in the prevention of peritonitis associated with peritoneal dialysis: long-term clinical results in intermittent and continuous ambulatory peritoneal dialysis. In: Peritoneal Dialysis, Atkins RC, et al. (eds). Edinburgh: Churchill Livingston, 1981, pp. 114–125.
79. Oreopoulos DG, Zellerman G, Izatt S. The Toronto Western Hospital permanent peritoneal catheter and continuous ambulatory peritoneal dialysis connector. In: Continuous Ambulatory Peritoneal Dialysis, Legrain M. (ed). Amsterdam: Excerpta Medica , 1980, pp. 73–78.
80. Williams C, and the University of Toronto Collaboratory Dialysis Group. CAPD in Toronto —an overview. Perit Dial Bull 35: 2–6, 1983.
81. Flynn CT. The diabetic patient on continuous ambulatory peritoneal dialysis. Perit Dial Bull 351: 16–20, 1983.
82. Slingeneyer A, Mion C, Selam JL. Home intermittent and CAPD as a long term treatment of end-stage renal failure in diabetics. In: Advances in Peritoneal Dialysis, Gahl GM, et al. (eds). Amsterdam: Excerpta Medica, 1981, pp. 378–388.
83. Grefberg N. Clinical aspects of continuous ambulatory peritoneal dialysis. Scand J Uro & Nephrol 72: S7–38, 1983.
84. Madden MA, Zimmerman SW, Simpson DP CAPD in diabetes mellitus. Am J Nephrol 2: 133–139, 1982.
85. Ponce SP, et al. Comparison of the survival and complications of the permanent peritoneal dialysis catheters. Perit Dial Bull 2: 82, 1982.
86. Dombros N, Oven A, Marliss EB, et al. Plasma amino acid profiles and amino acid losses in patients undergoing CAPD. Perit Dial Bull 2: 27–32, 1982.
87. Giordano C, DeSanto NG, Capodicase G, et al. Amino acid losses during CAPD. Clin Nephrol 14: 230–232, 1980.
88. Randerson D, Chapman GV, Farrel PC. Amino acid and dietary status in CAPD patients. In:

Peritoneal Dialysis, Atkins RC, et al. (eds). New York: Churchill Livingston, 1981, pp. 179–191.
89. Moncrief JW, Pyle WK, Simon P, Popovich RP. Hypertriglyceridemia, diabetes mellitus, and insulin administration in patients undergoing CAPD. In: CAPD Update, Moncrief JW, et al. (eds). New York: Mason Publishing, 1981, pp. 143–165.
90. Beardsworth SF, Goldsmith HJ, Stanbridge BR. Intraperitoneal insulin cannot correct the hyperlipidemia of CAPD. Perit Dial Bull 3: 126–128, 1983.
91. Khanna R, Breckenridge C, Roncari D, Digenis G, Oreopoulos DG. Lipid abnormalities in patients undergoing continuous ambulatory peritoneal dialysis. Perit Dial Bull 35: 13–15, 1983.
92. Faller B, Marichal JD. Loss of ultrafiltration in CAPD. Clinical data. In: Advances in Peritoneal Dialysis, Gahl G, Kessel M, Nolph KD. (eds). Amsterdam: Exerpta Medica, 1981, pp. 227–232.
93. Slingeneyer A, Canaud B, Mion C. Permanent loss of ultrafiltration capacity of the peritoneum in long-term peritoneal dialysis. Nephron 33: 133–138, 1983.
94. Rottembourg J, Issad B, Poignet JL, et al. Residual renal function and control of blood glucose levels in insulin-dependent diabetic patients treated by CAPD. In: Prevention and Treatment of Diabetic Nephropathy, Keen H, Legrain M. (eds). Boston: MTP Press Ltd, 1983, pp. 339–352.
95. Shapiro FL, Comty CM. Hemodialysis in diabetics—1981 update. In: Diabetic Renal—Retinal Syndrome, Friedman EA, et al. (eds). New York: Grune & Stratton, 1982, pp. 309–320.
96. Kurtz SB, Wong VH, Anderson CF, et al. Continuous ambulatory peritoneal dialysis. Three years experience at the Mayo Clinic. Mayo Clinic Proc 58: 633–639, 1983.
97. Nolph KD, et al. Personal communication.
98. Wing AF, Broyer M, Brunner FP, et al. Combined report on regular dialysis and transplantation in Europe 1982. Proc EDTA, ERA, 1983. 20: 1–78, 1983.
99. Flynn CT. The diabetics on CAPD. In: Diabetic Renal-Retinal Syndrome, Friedman EA, et al. (eds). New York: Grune & Stratton, 1983, pp. 321–330.
100. Doughty MC, Pierie KG. Continuous ambulatory peritoneal dialysis and the blind patient. Nephrol Nurse 3: 11, 1981.
101. Knotek B. Independence for the visually impaired continuous ambulatory peritoneal dialysis (CAPD) patient. AANNT J 9: 69–71, 1982.
102. Kelman B. Diabetes and the blind new methods. New treatments. Renal Family: 35–41, 1983.

8. OPTIONS IN UREMIA THERAPY: KIDNEY TRANSPLANTATION

ELI A. FRIEDMAN

When evaluating a diabetic with kidney disease, it must be appreciated that in highly prevalent diseases such as diabetes (America has at least 10 million diabetics), any renal disorder likely to effect nondiabetics will also be encountered independently according to its frequency. An initial step in the assessment of a nephropathic diabetic becomes the distinction between diabetes-induced and nondiabetes related kidney disease. The importance of this differentiation lies in the superior prognosis, and occasional reversibility, of nephropathy *not caused by diabetes* in a diabetic.

To illustrate the favorable impact on prognosis of the finding that a renal syndrome in a diabetic is not due to diabetic nephropathy, consider the minimal immediate risk of vitreous hemorrhage, blindness, or a stroke—all are vasculopathic complications of long-duration diabetes—in a new onset type I diabetic made uremic by aminoglycoside antibiotic toxicity, or poststreptococcal glomerulonephritis. By contrast, once uremia caused by diabetic glomerulosclerosis has developed, it is likely that coincident symptomatic, eye, cardiovascular, and neurological disease will compromise rehabilitation even though the renal insufficiency is adequately treated. The point emphasized here is that once diabetes has caused renal failure due to diabetic glomerulosclerosis, multisystem complications of diabetes limit the probability of a favorable outcome no matter how well the renal disease is managed [1].

Genetic disorders individually capable of inducing renal failure may coexist, as in our series of patients with polycystic kidney disease and type II diabetes. In this remarkable subset of uremic patients, prognosis for rehabilitation is primarily

139

contingent on the polycystic disease, the diabetes adding an interesting but relatively minor "epi" phenomenon. Indeed, the toll imposed by type II diabetes on the course of treated renal failure has not been established. As shown by Ma and coworkers, for example, survival on maintenance hemodialysis for uremia therapy in type II diabetics, ones who were male veterans, was equivalent to that of age- and sex-matched nondiabetics [2]. Furthermore, differentiation of a type I from a type II diabetic late in the course of progressive renal insufficiency may, however, prove difficult.

Characteristically, nephropathy in the type I diabetic evolves through stages of functional abnormality (hyperfiltration), proteinuria, and finally azotemia (vide infra). Atypical presentations of uremia in a type I diabetic, such as the lack, during the preuremia course, of antecedent nephrotic-range proteinuria, or the presence of normal fundi, are indicative of a cause other than diabetes for the renal syndrome. For this small proportion of patients, percutaneous kidney biopsy is appropriate to distinguish between diabetic glomerulopathy alone or the presence of some other renal disorder (membranoproliferative glomerulonephritis, for example) superimposed on diabetes [3].

Devising an individualized strategy for sustaining life in diabetics whose serum creatinine concentration has risen above 5 mg/dl requires that key demographic information be collected. Without an awareness of his patient's home and life circumstances, the nephrologist will be unable to tailor an individual specific regimen. Insistence that a blind diabetic who lives alone attempt home hemodialysis, for example, is an impractical and unworkable option in uremia therapy for that patient. Similarly, recommendation of living donor kidney transplantation is obviously contingent on a knowledge of the patient's family structure, including its willingness to participate. (See Cohen's chapter on family stress in diabetic nephropathy.)

Listed in table 8–1 are the practical choices in therapy open to a uremic diabetic patient in the United States in 1985. In parts of western Europe where modern renal care is otherwise widely practiced (Great Britain, for example) diabetics may be excluded in the belief that satisfactory rehabilitation will prove to be unattainable. Heading the list is the important, frightening (to some physicians unable to accept their own mortality) "no treatment" option elected by patients for whom the concept of further life extension is unacceptable. Court decisions in the United States hold that "termination of extraordinary treatment was not homicide but a result of the free exercise of a constitutional right to privacy [4]." A diabetic losing

Table 8–1. Options in uremia therapy

---

1. No further treatment (equivalent to acceptance of death).
2. Maintenance hemodialysis (facility or home).
3. Peritoneal dialysis—PD (intermittent, continuous ambulatory—CAPD; continuous cyclic—CCPD).
4. Kidney transplantation (living or cadaver donor).

---

sight, crippled by limb amputation, and a stroke, with unremitting gastrointestinal discomfort, may understandably be unenthusiastic about his family's plea that he undertake the labor of intensified dialysis. In the absence of strong family support, such patients may "give in and give up." Visits by rehabilitated dialysis patients or transplant recipients can renew motivation and lift moderate depression. Should this maneuver fail, the physician who is satisfied that his patient appreciates the consequences of refusing dialysis must guide the renal team in providing symptomatic relief without guilt.

Physicians must resist the intuitive belief that everyone with a potentially treatable disease wishes to be treated. Our experience suggests that coercing a diabetic (in full control of his mental faculties) to accept dialysis or kidney transplantation, when life has minimal (or even negative) value to him or her, may provoke behavior patterns equivalent to suicide (figure 8–1). Twice during the past year, type I diabetics who had been coaxed to agree to a kidney transplant by forceful family members and an enthusiastic physician subsequently evinced self-destructive responses to their treatment regimen. A 52-year-old woman depressed over the seemingly relentless erosion of her health refused to ambulate post-kidney transplant; a 44-year-old clergyman unwilling to participate in glucose self-moni-

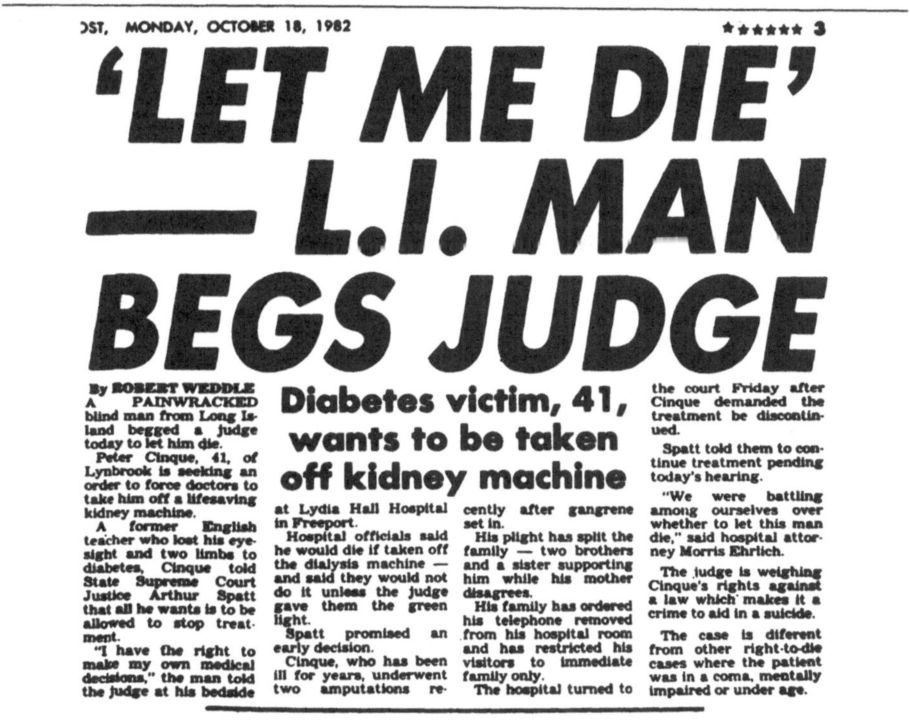

OST, MONDAY, OCTOBER 18, 1982 ★★★★★ 3

'LET ME DIE' — L.I. MAN BEGS JUDGE

By ROBERT WEDDLE

A PAINWRACKED blind man from Long Island begged a judge today to let him die.

Peter Cinque, 41, of Lynbrook is seeking an order to force doctors to take him off a lifesaving kidney machine.

A former English teacher who lost his eyesight and two limbs to diabetes, Cinque told State Supreme Court Justice Arthur Spatt that all he wants is to be allowed to stop treatment.

"I have the right to make my own medical decisions," the man told the judge at his bedside

Diabetes victim, 41, wants to be taken off kidney machine

at Lydia Hall Hospital in Freeport.

Hospital officials said he would die if taken off the dialysis machine — and said they would not do it unless the judge gave them the green light.

Spatt promised an early decision.

Cinque, who has been ill for years, underwent two amputations re-

cently after gangrene set in.

His plight has split the family — two brothers and a sister supporting him while his mother disagrees.

His family has ordered his telephone removed from his hospital room and has restricted his visitors to immediate family only.

The hospital turned to

the court Friday after Cinque demanded the treatment be discontinued.

Spatt told them to continue treatment pending today's hearing.

"We were battling among ourselves over whether to let this man die," said hospital attorney Morris Ehrlich.

The judge is weighing Cinque's rights against a law which makes it a crime to aid in a suicide.

The case is different from other right-to-die cases where the patient was in a coma, mentally impaired or under age.

Figure 8–1. News reports such as this sad example indicate the intensity of stress in complicated diabetics entered into uremia therapy programs.

toring or regulation of hypertension suffered episodic profound hypoglycemia and fluid overload. Both recipients sustained multiple, ultimately fatal complications attributable to "noncompliant" behavior.

MAINTENANCE HEMODIALYSIS

Following Avram's demonstration that hemodialysis might sustain life in diabetics with failed kidneys, maintenance hemodialysis has been progressively utilized in their care. For the majority of uremic diabetics in the United States, maintenance hemodialysis will be the main (usually sole) treatment for the duration of their post-uremia lives. Earlier problems in establishing a vascular access have been overcome by resorting to prosthetic grafts or insertion of metallic devices [5].

Type II diabetics older than 50 years, the age limit often applied for a kidney transplant, fare about as well on maintenance hemodialysis as nondiabetics of equivalent age [6]. Younger, type II, and type I diabetics of all ages have been carefully studied on hemodialysis by Shapiro and associates [7]. Over the past decade, progressive increases in survival of hemodialyzed diabetics have been effected by directing attention to blood pressure reduction and extraction of excess total body water by ultrafiltration during hemodialysis. Concern that repeated heparinization during hemodialysis would aggravate diabetic retinopathy has been assuaged by reports of equivalent retention vision in hemodialyzed and kidney-transplanted diabetics [8, 9].

HEMOFILTRATION

Extraction of solute and water from plasma by creating a pressure differential across a blood-membrane barrier, a technique called hemofiltration, is an effective means of prolonging life in uremia [10]. Segoloni and coworkers conducted a multicenter retrospective study of the "potentialities" of hemofiltration as sole therapy for uremic diabetics [11]. A total of 13 diabetics, 10 type I and 3 type II, with a total experience of 171 patient-months of followup was associated with "surprisingly few complications when compared with the high incidence of major clinical complications seen in conventional hemodialysis." The actuarial survival rate was 91% at one year and 61% at two years [11]. Recognizing that only a small number of diabetics have been treated by hemofiltration to date, their highly satisfactory survival achieved suggests that hemofiltration be given at least "serious consideration" in future planning for the uremic diabetic.

PERITONEAL DIALYSIS

Compared to hemodialysis, intermittent peritoneal dialysis (IPD) offers the uremic diabetic potential advantages of reduced stress on the cardiovascular system and avoidance of heparin. Unfortunately, in the report of the Toronto Western Hospital experience, only 24% of patients survived two years [12], a finding echoed by a 50% one-year survival at the Mayo Clinic [13]. More encouraging results have been reported by the Toronto team and other groups in the United States, France, and Germany using the newer technique of continuous ambulatory peritoneal dialysis (CAPD) for both type I and type II diabetics [14]. CAPD depends on strong patient cooperation in instilling and draining dialysate under aseptic conditions. Motivated patients can learn to perform CAPD at home within 10 to 15 days.

Employing an in-dwelling Tenckhoff catheter, four two-liter exchanges of dialysate daily, and intraperitoneal insulin, survival at one and two years for type I diabetics was 92% and 75%, respectively [15]. By the third year, however, survival drops to about 50%, approximately the same as for maintenance hemodialysis. Weighing CAPD for the diabetic uremic requires balancing its social advantages, including freedom from a machine and electrical outlets and facility in travel, against the disadvantages of unremitting attention to fluid exchange and constant risk of peritonitis. In 1985, CAPD must join the roster of imperfect uremia therapies, which, like hemodialysis, hemofiltration, and kidney transplantation, prolong life but demand substantial patient and physician participation in the therapeutic regimen for success.

KIDNEY TRANSPLANTATION
Kidney transplantation from a living related donor proffers the greatest opportunity for restoration of health to the uremic diabetic. Patient and graft survival following transplantation of a cadaver donor kidney have continuously improved. Diabetics are now included in the recipient pool for cadaveric kidneys in many but not all American transplant programs. Reluctance to attempt a kidney transplant in a diabetic, a prevalent policy in Great Britain [16], derives from results in the 1970s when poor survival and minimal rehabilitation were usual [17].

Spurred by the pioneering accomplishments of Najarian's University of Minnesota team, a more positive perspective of diabetic transplants has replaced negativism and gloom. As described by Sutherland and associates: "Until 1979, the patient and graft survival rates were less good in diabetic than in nondiabetic recipients. Since 1979, the results in diabetics have been at least equal to those achieved in nondiabetic patients [18]."

PERIOPERATIVE MANAGEMENT
Transplanting a kidney is major surgery. In a diabetic, macrovasculopathy, delayed wound healing, and pendulum swings in the blood glucose level require constant attention, complicating operative management. Blood vessel connection in the diabetic is technically more difficult than in the nondiabetic. Severe atherosclerotic narrowing of the lumen of the hypogastric artery, for example, is discovered during transplant surgery in more than 90% of type I diabetics, necessitating a preanastomotic endarterectomy. Metabolic control preoperatively and postoperatively is accomplished most easily by use of a Biostater, a computer-controlled device integrating intravenous infusions delivered by glucose and insulin infusion pumps attached to a fast glucose analyzer. Few institutions, however, have been able to afford the equipment and personnel costs of establishing automated "feedback" glucose regulation for routine surgical procedures in diabetics.

An acceptable compromise in providing "tight" glucose regulation (plasma glucose level of 60 to 140 mg/dl) for the type I diabetic can be effected by combining frequent finger-stick glucose reagent strip tests with an intravenous insulin infusion (2 to 8 units hourly) as determined by the hourly glucose level. On the day of surgery, intermediate and long-acting insulin is omitted, and an infusion of 100 units of regular insulin in 10% glucose is begun at a rate of 30ml (3 units)/hr. Morning and evening insulin doses (each containing intermediate and regular insulin), can be started as soon as oral feedings are resumed.

A pretransplant conference between anesthesiologist and nephrologist is needed to ensure that diabetic "protective measures" are not ignored in the operating or recovery rooms. During surgery, the patient's head should be raised to prevent elevated intraocular pressure which might precipitate retinal and vitreous hemorrhages. Heel boots prevent ulceration of the feet, a complication of sensory neuropathy, and confinement to bed which can add months to rehabilitation and, more seriously, lead to loss of a leg. An air mattress should be utilized for the same reason, to avoid back and buttocks decubiti. Intravenous fluid therapy in the recovery room, especially during vigorous diuresis, should include the need for insulin whenever glucose is administered.

Posttransplant management of the type II diabetic is little different from that of the nondiabetic. Insulin infusions may facilitate the maintenance of euglycemia during intercurrent infections or the administration of intravenous methylprednisolone for allograft rejection. Once steroid immunosuppression is begun in a patient receiving insulin, distinguishing a type I from a type II diabetic given insulin for ease of regulation may prove impossible outside of a clinical research center. About one-third of newly transplanted diabetics "on insulin," in our experience, cannot be clearly termed type I or II diabetics on the basis of pretransplant studies. When the need for insulin is uncertain, a trial of dietary regulation is appropriate, especially in stable (two weeks posttransplant), obese diabetics, with onset after the age of 35 years.

IMMUNOSUPPRESSION

Whether given azathioprine (5 mg/kg/day tapered to 2.5 mg/kg/day by the second week), plus prednisone (1 mg/kg/day tapered to 0.2 mg/kg/day at one year), or cyclosporine (14 mg/kg/day tapered by one week to 12 mg/kg/day), plus lower doses of prednisone (0.2 mg/kg/day by one month), one-year patient and cadaver graft survival in type I diabetic recipients have reached approximately 92% and 85%, respectively [19]. Other teams have reported less satisfactory results. Speculation as to the variables responsible for the superior Minnesota transplant team's results has focused on their adherence to pretransplant splenectomy, pre- and posttransplant antimicrobial prophylaxis with trimethoprim and sulfamethoxazole, and donor-recipient DR matching. As remarked by Sutherland and colleagues, "No patients with poor matches receive transplants [19]."

Binswanger and associates analyzed the causes of failure in "less successful" transplant programs, concluding that cardiovascular and infectious complications were more prevalent in these series with negative patient selection [20]. Because exclusion of higher risk diabetics might create a recipient pool destined to have a better outcome, Binswanger and associates advocate more complete reporting of information about each recipient, including precise notation of cardiovascular, microvascular, neurologic, and endocrinologic complications at the time of transplant. Furthermore, Vollmer and associates propose that all reports of uremia therapy in diabetic and nondiabetic patients be adjusted by the statistical application of proportional hazard analysis to permit comparisons between centers [21].

Whether cyclosporine will prove to be a quantum improvement in immunosuppression for kidney transplantation or a tradeoff of early benefit for later nephrotoxicity [22] is unclear. In our hands, cyclosporine has virtually eliminated the "rejection crisis," reduced posttransplant hospital stay, and allowed maintenance prednisone doses below 10 mg/day before the end of the first year. Cyclosporine's high annual maintenance cost of $4,000 to $7,000 and reduced allograft function (serum creatinine of 1.5 to 2.0 mg/dl), are worrisome. Like so many other transplant "miracles," cyclosporine over the longer term has added both good news and bad news, with an uncertain final conclusion as to its ultimate place in transplant immunosuppression.

There is a sharp difference between some transplant surgeons as to the wisdom of continuing intrafamilial donor transplantation in general and in the diabetic's family in particular. At one extreme, Starzl, citing his excellent recent results with cyclosporine and cadaveric donor transplants, terms living donor transplants "obsolete [23]." On the other side, Belzer and colleagues, employing a donor-specific transfusion (azathioprine plus prednisone) protocol in which 34% of recipients were diabetic, achieved actuarial patient survivals of 96%, 95%, and 91% at one, two, and three years following transplantation [24]. Commenting on an actuarial graft survival of 94%, 90%, and 85% at one, two, and three years after transplantation, Belzer and colleagues state that "when graft and patient survival, quality of life, rehabilitation, cost, and availability are considered together, living–donor renal transplantation is now the 'gold standard' of treatment for end-stage renal failure." We concur.

Cognizant of the immediate and potential (though unproven) long-term risks to kidney donors [25], we nevertheless conclude that the enhanced quality of life achieved through receipt of a well-matched intrafamilial kidney (as compared with the usual cadaver kidney) warrants the continued use of living donors for the time being. Without exception, to date, renal fellows in our program, who may be regarded as knowledgeable medical consumers able to give informed consent, aver that they would offer themselves as kidney donors should the need arise in their own families.

HYPERTENSION

Management of diabetic kidney-transplant recipients requires attention to specific complications which are far less prevalent in the nondiabetic (table 8–2). Hypertension is as dangerous to the diabetic after a kidney transplant as it was in the pretransplant years of accelerated renal functional decline. In a series of 67 diabetic

Table 8–2. Special concerns in diabetic kidney transplant recipients

1. Control of hypertension
2. Normalization of blood sugar
3. Resumption of voiding capacity
4. Defensive foot care
5. Gastric retention
6. Fecal impaction
7. Protection against retinal hemorrhages
8. Protection against decubiti
9. Profound depression

patients who received a total of 73 kidney transplants at our institution (46 type I and 21 type II), 60 (90%) were hypertensive before transplantation, of whom 52 patients (87%) remained hypertensive posttransplantation [26]. Among the 28 (42%) patients who died, mean blood pressure was significantly higher (110.3mm Hg) than in those who survived (99.8mm Hg), indicating an adverse effect of posttransplant hypertension.

Management of posttransplant hypertension in a diabetic is similar to that of hypertension in the later pretransplant years. Nearly all patients require a combination of a potent diuretic (furosemide) plus a vasodilator (hydralazine, clonidine, methyldopa, prazosin). Resistant hypertension usually responds to captopril [27]. Several of our recipients are being treated with calcium channel blockers (nifedipine) with initially satisfactory results. The exact place for nifedipine in combination with central and peripherally acting vasodilators has yet to be determined. We have not had to resort to the use of minoxidil (hirsutism and fluid retention are serious side effects) in any recipient whose creatinine clearance exceeds 30 ml/min. A typical drug regimen for a patient with a creatinine clearance of 50 ml/in might include: furosemide 40 mg twice daily, and hydralazine 50 mg plus clonidine 0.4 mg thrice daily.

EUGLYCEMIA

Debate over the merit of tight blood glucose regulation polarizes advocates of the genetic and environmental schools of the pathogenesis of diabetic vascular complications [26]. Recent reports of reversal in capillary basement membrane thickening in both type I [29] and type II [30] diabetics consequent to careful glucose regulation provide strong support for the proponents of strict control. Exciting evidence that (at least early) glomerulopathy may be reversible lies in the disappearance of glomerulosclerosis in two cadaveric donor kidneys obtained from a diabetic after transplantation into nondiabetic recipients [31]. Given that euglycemic diabetics have a return to normal macrocyte function, counterregulatory hormone secretion, wound healing, and motor nerve conduction velocity, it appears sensible to advise that extremes of hyperglycemia and hypoglycemia be muted. Until a closed loop (feedback-controlled) implantable insulin pump is

Table 8–3. Effect of self-glucose monitoring on control in uremic diabetics

Age	Therapy	Glucose Range[1] (mg/dl)		Glycohemo-globin[2] (%)	
		Pre-	Post-	Pre-	Post-
35	Transplant	181–350	100–180	—	—
48	Transplant	31–152	100–180	9.0	7.0
37	Transplant	96–314	80–80	9.3	6.8
51	Transplant	280–612	120–120	7.9	7.0
41	Transplant	96–224	110–120	10.5	9.7
54	Hemodialysis	160–375	80–180	12.9	8.1
54	Hemodialysis	78–162	80–120	9.1	6.8
44	Hemodialysis	142–195	150–180	10.8	9.4

1. Using Chemstrip
2. Lowest value during first six months of monitoring

devised, reliance on the patient for repeated daily finger-stick blood glucose measurements is the key to contemporary control regimens. Reliable lightweight glucose meters can be purchased for about $150, and individual reagent test strips cost about $0.50. Effective glucose regulation programs have been constructed using continuous insulin infusions [32], or multiple injections of mixtures of intermediate and regular insulin [33]. Deteriorating renal function adds to the variables in establishing and maintaining euglycemia in the type I diabetic by extending insulin half-life as functioning renal mass decreases with duration of diabetes. For this reason, the insulin prescription should be regarded as subject to modification with changes in diet, renal function, or steroid treatment. There are several equally acceptable protocols for insulin administration, all of which depend on frequent finger-stick blood glucose measurements. Conversion from a single daily insulin regimen to multiple doses guided by finger-stick glucose tests is not difficult. As a start, divide the total daily dose of insulin into two doses—two-thirds prebreakfast and one-third predinner. Subdivide the morning dose into two-thirds intermediate acting insulin (NPH or lente) and one-third regular insulin; the evening dose is equally split between intermediate and regular insulin. Based on glucose levels premeals and in the evening, a third dose of regular insulin before lunch may be required to keep blood glucose concentration in the desired range of 60 to 140 mg/dl.

Adjustments in insulin dose can be made on a rational basis. As examples, hyperglycemia prebreakfast is an indication for more intermediate insulin in the evening, while hypoglycemia predinner can be corrected by lowering the morning dose of intermediate insulin. Expectation of extra calories at an evening party can be managed by prior administration of additional regular insulin. Given these principles, and a method for repeatedly checking actual blood glucose level, the type I diabetic is able to assume charge of his body, a right previously denied by mysterious and seemingly unpredictable alterations in blood glucose concentration. While unexplained excursions of blood glucose level, both high and low, are common, overall improvement in control is usual upon beginning fractional insulin doses. Normalization of the glycosylated hemoglobin concentration (glycohemoglobin) is the best indicator of sustained satisfactory diabetic control. The glycosylated hemoglobin level reflects the mean glucose concentration over the preceding two to three months (life of the red blood cell). Thus, a normal glycosylated hemoglobin integrates transient hypoglycemic episodes with short lapses in control leading to hyperglycemia, to proffer what amounts to a "mean" indicator of diabetic control.

Our use of glycosylated hemoglobin levels in diabetic kidney transplant recipients taught the technique of self-glucose monitoring is shown in table 8–3. Admittedly, the case for strict glucose control is still incompletely documented. Taking into account that euglycemic patients feel better, and welcome the opportunity to take charge of their illness, it seems prudent to err on the side of striving for euglycemia in the hope that retinopathy will be retarded and recurrent glomerulopathy (in the allograft) prevented.

CYSTOPATHY

About one-third of our type I diabetic kidney-transplant recipients have difficulty emptying their bladder either immediately posttransplant or at some later time. During intercurrent illnesses, the diabetic recipient may be unaware of a grossly distended bladder holding 1,000 ml or more of urine. Incomplete bladder emptying

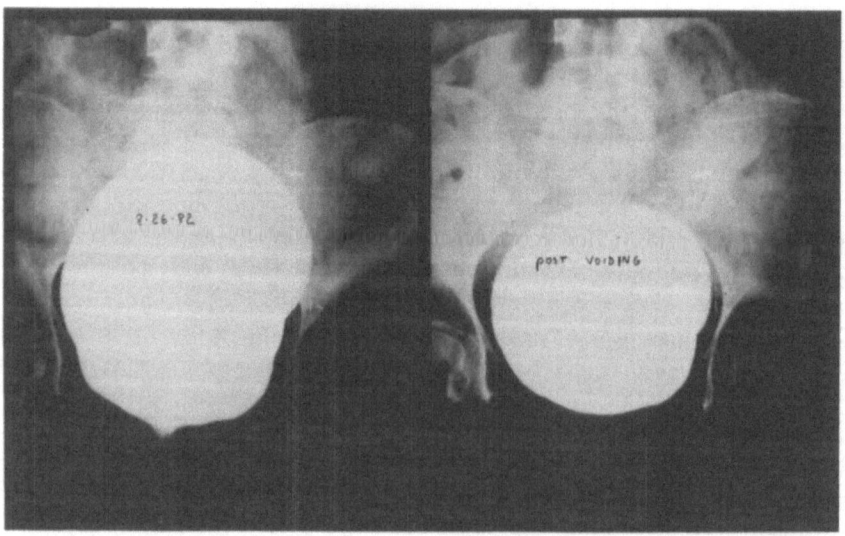

Figure 8–2. Cystopathy in a uremic type I diabetic woman under evaluation for a kidney transplant. A large bladder is evident in the left panel fails to empty postvoiding as shown on the right panel.

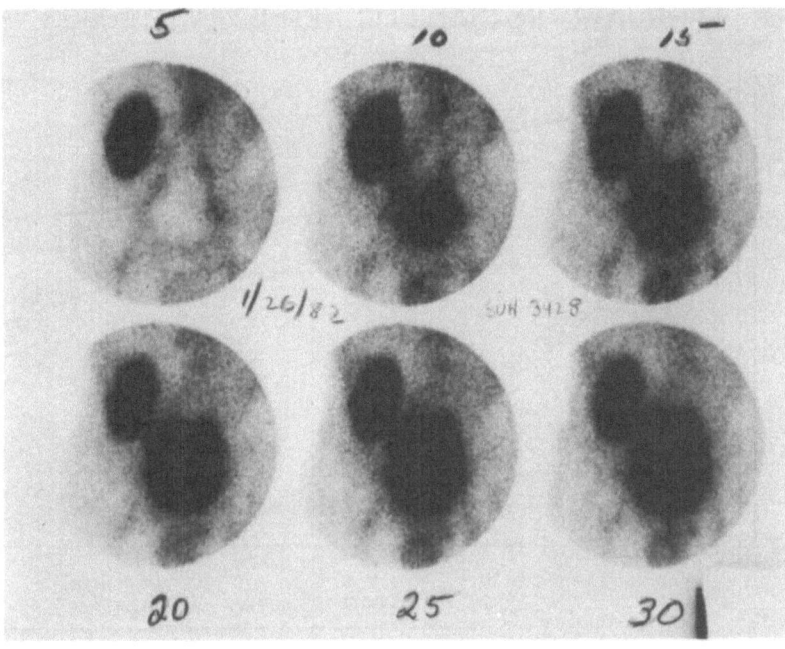

Figure 8–3. This type I diabetic transplant recipient admitted for graft rejection was found to have functional urinary retention due to cystopathy. Bladder capacity was 1,100 ml.

may simulate rejection and must be excluded when an unexplained rise in serum creatinine concentration is taken as heralding a rejection episode. Neurogenic diabetic cystopathy is common in uremic diabetics [34] (figures 8–2 and 8–3). Of 12 consecutive type I prospective kidney transplant recipients evaluated in our center by cystometrograms, 9 (75%) had both an enlarged bladder capacity and a reduced ability to perceive the presence of distention. To maximize bladder function, we urge diabetic recipients to void frequently (at least every two hours when awake, and at least once after retiring for the night), and prescribe urocholine when a residual urine volume in excess of 100 ml is detected.

DEFENSIVE FOOT CARE

Rehabilitation for diabetic kidney-transplant recipients may be slowed or preempted by foot and leg vascular and neurologic disease. Limb amputation has been required in the past for as many as 15% [35] over the short term and one-third of ten-year survivors [36]. We have found that incorporation of routine, sensible, podiatric preventive medicine will preserve feet by allowing "minor" foot ulcers and injuries to be treated before the limb is jeopardized [37]. Every diabetic's feet should be examined at each clinic visit. New shoes, nail-cutting, and worsening sensory neuropathy are all cause for concern. Consultation with a surgeon skilled in the technique of muscle transposition can salvage ulcerated feet otherwise given

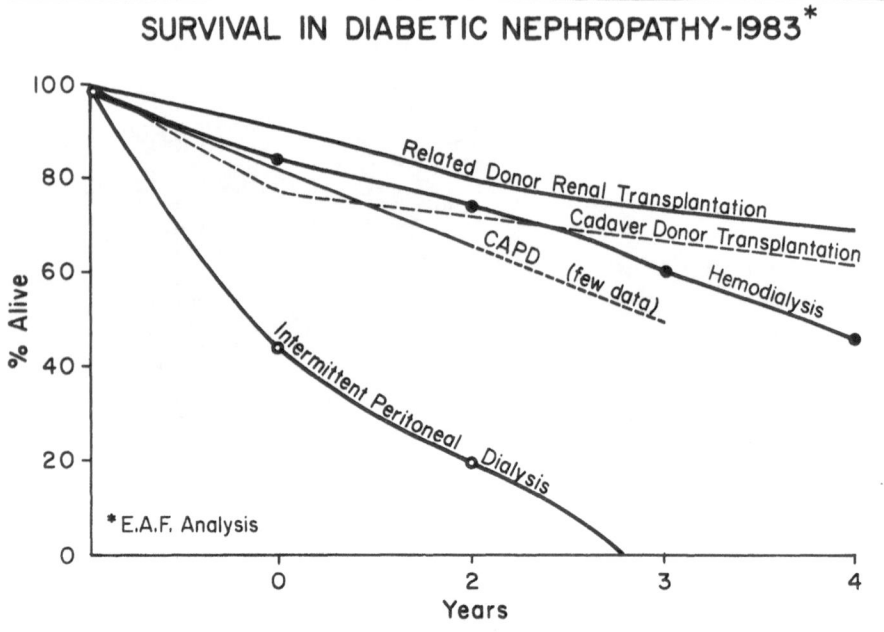

Figure 8–4. Composite presentation of results of uremia therapy in diabetics. Renal transplant recipients evince the best long-term survival. These data suffer from the absence of a controlled prospective study in which each treatment subset is matched for age, sex, and severity of coincident risk factors such as hypertension and cardiovascular disease.

up for lost [38]. The point to be emphasized in diabetic foot care is awareness of the need for the patient to be cognizant of foot integrity every day.

GASTROINTESTINAL MALFUNCTION

The diabetic's gastrointestinal tract does not function normally. Gastroparesis may induce bloating and discomfort while preventing consistent absorption of meals, thereby disturbing exogenous insulin control of blood glucose. Metoclopramide in a dose of 10 mg before meals improves both gastric emptying and the symptoms of gastric stasis in some cases of diabetic gastroparesis [39]. Unless fluid intake is maintained, the rapidly diuresing posttransplant diabetic is at risk of fecal impaction, a preventable complication. Prophylactic prescription of a bowel detergent (Colace) and early intervention with enemas will save the necessity for more vigorous unblocking measures (oil retention enemas and castor oil ingestion). In our experience, bowel integrity is reestablished within one week of satisfactory transplant function.

EYE CARE

By the time that a typical type I diabetic requires uremia therapy, one or more major eye complications have occurred. Because the patient's ophthalmologist may

Table 8–4. Selecting uremia therapy for the diabetic

Advantages	Disadvantages
RENAL TRANSPLANTATION	
• Cures uremia when graft functions	• Steroids complicate control
• Stabilizes retinopathy	• Risk of infectious complication
• Freedom to travel	• Mortality $>$ dialysis
• Reverses neuropathy	• Familial donors risk diabetes
• Best rehabilitation	• Poor survival of secondary grafts
• Long-term survival (>15 years in some cadaveric graft recipients)	• Not applicable to elderly or patients with cardiovascular instability
• Cyclosporine may permit lower dose of steroids	• Glomerulosclerosis can recur
	• 31% limb loss at 10 years
	• Cyclosporine nephrotoxicity
PERITONEAL DIALYSIS	
• Avoids major surgery	• Recurrent pancreatitis
• Minimizes burden on heart	• High mortality
• IP insulin eases glucose control	• Retinopathy may progress
• Adaptable to home care	• Long-term utility unknown
• CAPD 1st-year survival excellent	• Patient boredom and burnout
HEMODIALYSIS	
• Avoids major surgery	• Poor rehabilitation
• Permits care by experienced staff	• Retinopathy may progress
• Available in most countries	• Mortality $=$ to cadaveric graft recipients
	• "Failure to thrive" in about 25% of patients

be at a distance (physical and intellectual) from the transplant floor, it is wise for the renal team to maintain an awareness of what may be harmful to the diabetic eye. Tilting the head below the horizon, straining at stool, repeated severe hypoglycemia, and sustained hypertension are conditions thought to risk retinal hemorrhage. Consultation with an ophthalmologist during posttransplant hospitalization is a sensible step in formulating a strategy to attain maximal rehabilitation.

Collaboration with an eye team proficient in handling uremic diabetics permits performance of vitrectomy and lensectomy at an early date, allo_wign the patient's return to occupational and home responsibilities. In our experience, patients with ambulatory sight at the time of kidney transplantation will retain their vision for at least three or more years should their transplant continue to function, if managed in collaboration with a skilled retina surgeon.

OVERALL CARE

Each diabetic evaluated for uremia therapy requires an individualized plan tailored to the severity of illness and responsive to personal and family wishes. Our current view is that unless a contraindication exists, every potentially rehabilitatable uremic diabetic younger than 55 years should first be offered a kidney transplant. This

Table 8–5. Preferred therapy (1985) for uremic diabetic

Age range (years)	Renal transplant	Peritoneal dialysis	Hemodialysis
18 to 55	1	?4	1
56 to 65	Selected patients	2	2
Over 65 (or presence of intractable heart failure)	3	2	2

1. strongly recommended, especially if family donor available
2. recommended
3. not recommended
4. Insufficient experience is in hand to advise either intermittent peritoneal dialysis or CAPD over a renal transplant as definitive therapy for the long-term management of young type I diabetics who may be rehabilitated by a renal transplant.

thesis is derived from an analysis of treatment results through 1983 (figure 8–4; tables 8–4, 8–5).

Diabetic kidney transplant recipients are fragile patients. Otherwise minor stresses tolerated by nondiabetic uremic patients may precipitate a metabolic or infectious crisis in a diabetic. Schedules for minor surgery, radioactive scans, and posttransplant hemodialyses must take into account the necessity for synchronizing insulin injections and meals. Busy surgeons, X-ray technicians, and ward nurses may resent the required extra time expended on "ordinary" diabetic care. Diabetics trained in self-blood glucose measurement may be forced to confront nurses determined to prescribe insulin doses on the basis of outmoded urine glucose testing. Tears, frustration, and anger all too often confound the health care team's desire to routinize the inexplicable vicissitudes of diabetic management [40].

At our institution, a group of "stable" transplant recipients formed a Diabetic Kidney Transplant Self-Help Group to assist new patients and their families in facing the difficulties inherent in kidney transplantation. Representatives of the group visit new patients, meet with the transplant social worker and dietitian, and serve as a general morale-boosting resource. They are needed, welcomed, and effective.

REFERENCES

1. Friedman EA. Planning therapy for diabetic nephropathy. Diabetic Nephropathy 3:1, 1984.
2. Ma KW, W, Masler DS, Brown DC. Hemodialysis in diabetic patients with chronic renal failure. Ann Int Med 83:215–217, 1975.
3. Carstens SA, Hebert LA, Garancia JC, et al. Rapidly progressive glomerulonephritis superimposed on diabetic glomerulosclerosis—Recognition and treatment. JAMA 247:1453–1457, 1982.
4. Brahams D. The right to be allowed to die. Lancet 1:351–352, 1984.
5. Kaplan AD, Grant J, Galler M, et al. Regional experience with the hemasite no-needle access device. Trans ASAIO 29:369–372, 1983.
6. Goetz FC. Recent progress in the management of end-stage diabetic nephropathy. Clinics in Endocrinology and Metabolism 11:579–590, 1982.
7. Kjellstrand CM, Goetz FC, Najarian JS. Transplantation and dialysis in diabetic patients: an update. In: Diabetic Renal-Retinal Syndrome, Friedman EA, L'Esperance FA Jr. New York: Grune & Stratton, 1980, pp. 345–357.

8. Ramsay RC, Cantrill HL, Knobloch WH, et al. Visual parameters in diabetic patients following renal transplantation. Diabetic Nephropathy 2:26–29, 1983.
9. Ramsay RC, Cantrill HL, Knobloch WH, et al. Visual parameters in diabetic patients on chronic dialysis. Diabetic Nephropathy 2:30–33, 1983.
10. Henderson LW, Silverstein ME, Ford CA. Clinical response to maintenance hemodiafiltration. Kid Int (suppl.) 2:58–63, 1975.
11. Segoloni GP, Pacitti A, Salomone M. Hemofiltration in diabetic uremic patients. Diabetic Nephropathy 3:21–25, 1984.
12. Katirtzoglou A, Izatt S, Oreopoulos DG. Chronic peritoneal dialysis in diabetes with end-stage renal failure. In: Diabetic Renal-Retinal Syndrome, Friedman EA, L'Esperance FA Jr. (eds). New York: Grune & Stratton, 1980, pp. 317–332.
13. Kurtz SB, Wong VH, Anderson CF. Continuous ambulatory peritoneal dialysis—three years' experience at the Mayo Clinic. Mayo Clinic Proc 58:633–639, 1983.
14. Khanna R, Oreopoulos DG. Continuous ambulatory peritoneal dialysis in end stage diabetic nephropathy. In: Diabetic Nephropathy, Friedman EA, Peterson CM (eds). Boston, The Hague: Martinus Nijhoff, 1985, in press.
15. Amair P, Khanna R, Leibel R, Pierratos, A, et al. Continuous ambulatory peritoneal dialysis in diabetics with end-stage renal disease. N Eng J Med 306:625–630, 1982.
16. Cameron JS. The management of diabetic renal failure in the United Kingdom. Diabetic Nephropathy 2:1–2, 1983.
17. Rubin JE, Friedman EA. Dialysis and transplantation of diabetics in the United States (editorial). Nephron 18:309–315, 1977.
18. Sutherland DER, Morrow CE, Fryd DS, et al. Improved patient and primary renal allograft survival in uremic diabetic recipients. Transplantation 34:319–325, 1982.
19. Ferguson RM, Rynasiewicz JJ, Sutherland DER, et al. Cyclosporin A in renal transplantation: a prospective randomized study. Surgery 92:175–182, 1982.
20. Binswanger U, Ermanni S, Keusch G, et al. Diabetic renal failure: where are the limits of treatment success? Diabetic Nephropathy 3:30–32, 1984.
21. Vollmer WM, Wahl PW, Blagg CR. Survival with dialysis and transplantation in patients with end-stage renal disease. New Eng J Med 308:1553–1558, 1983.
22. Meyers BD, Ross J, Newton L, Luetscher J, Perlroth M. Cyclosporine-associate chronic nephropathy. New Eng J Med 311:699–705.
23. Friedman EA, Najarian J, Starzl T, Schreiner GE, Bonomini V, Cameron S, Gurland H, Giordano C, Mignone L, Lesavre P. Ethical aspects in renal transplantation. Kidney Int (Suppl.) 14:S90–S93, 1983.
24. Belzer FO, Glass NR, Miller DT, et al. Should the advisability of live-donor renal transplantation be reappraised? Dialysis & Transplantation 13:26–30, 1984.
25. Hakim RM, Goldszer RC, Brenner BM. Hypertension and proteinuria: long-term sequelae of uninephrectomy in humans. Kidney Internat 25:930–936, 1984.
26. Chou LM, Beyer MM, Butt KMH, et al. Hypertension (HT) jeopardizes diabetic (DM) patients with renal transplants (TX). Abstracts. Amer Soc Artif Int Organs 1985.
28. Cahill GF. Diabetes control and complications. Diabetes Care 6:310–311, 1983.
29. Raskin P, Pietri AO, Unger R, et al. The effect of diabetic control on the width of skeletal-muscle capillary basement membrane in patients with type I diabetes mellitus. N Eng J Med 309:1546–1550, 1983.
30. Camerini-Davalos RA, Velasco C, Glasser M. Drug-induced reversal of early diabetic microangiopathy. New Eng J Med 309:1551–1556, 1983.
31. Abouna GM, Al-Adnani MS, Kremer GD, et al. Reversal of diabetic nephropathy in human cadaveric kidneys after transplantation into non-diabetic recipients. Lancet 2:1274–1276, 1983.
32. Peterson CM, Forhan SE, Jones RL. Self management: an approach to patients with insulin-dependent diabetes mellitus. Diabetes Care 3:82–87, 1980.
33. Levitz CS, Hirsch S, Ross JM, et al. Lack of blood glucose control in hemodialyzed and renal transplantation diabetics. Trans Am Soc Artif Int Organs 26:362–365, 1980.
34. Norlen LJ, Blaivas JG, Gabel H. Cystopathy in patients with severe diabetic nephropathy. Diabetic Nephropathy 2:17–21, 1983.
35. Najarian JS, Sutherland DER, Simmons RL. Renal transplantation in diabetics: the facts. In: Strategy in Renal Failure, Friedman EA (ed). New York: Wiley Medical Publication, 1978, pp. 363–392.

36. Sutherland DER, Bentley FR, Mauer MM, Menth L, Nylander W, Goetz FC, Barbosa J, Ascher NL, Simmons RL, Najarian, JS. A report of 26 diabetic renal allograft recipients alive with functioning grafts at 10 or more years after primary transplantation. Diabetic Nephropathy 3:39–43, 1984.
37. Rausher H, Levitz CS, Butt KMH, et al. Podiatric contribution to limb preservation+ in diabetic renal transplant recipients. In: Diabetic Renal-Retinal Syndrome 2—Prevention and Management, Friedman EA, L'Esperance FA Jr. (eds). New York: Grune & Stratton, 1982, pp. 419–426.
38. Ger R. Consideration in the surgical management of ulcers of the foot in the diabetic patient. Diabetic Nephropathy 3:12–14, 1984.
39. Snape. WJ Jr, Battle WM, Schwartz SS, et al. Metoclopramide to treat gastroparesis due to diabetes mellitus. Ann Int Med 96:444–446, 1982.
40. Piening S. Family stress in diabetic renal failure. Health Soc Work 9:134–141, 1984.

9. PANCREAS TRANSPLANTS IN DIABETIC NEPHROPATHY

DAVID E.R. SUTHERLAND
and
JOHN S. NAJARIAN

Pancreas-transplantation application for the treatment of diabetes mellitus has increased dramatically [1]. More pancreas transplants were performed in the 2 years from January 1, 1982, to December 31, 1983, than during the preceding 16 years [2], following the first transplant performed by Kelly and Lillehei and associates in 1966 [3].

Evidence that the complications of diabetes are secondary to disordered metabolism is very convincing [4]. Many diabetologists make intense efforts to maintain nearly constant euglycemia in diabetic patients [5], but the new techniques of exogenous insulin delivery currently being employed have risks, specifically hypoglycemia [6]. The most physiological approach to maintain euglycemia in the treatment of diabetes is pancreas transplantation. The procedure has had limited application because of immunological and technical problems, but these problems are gradually being overcome, and the number of successful transplants has increased in recent years.

The American College of Surgeons/National Institutes of Health (ACS/NIH) Organ Transplant Registry received information on 57 pancreas transplants in 55 diabetic patients from December 17, 1966, to June 30, 1977, when the Registry closed [7]. Three pancreas transplants, one primary and two secondary, that were performed in 1976 were not reported to the ACS/NIH Registry but were reported to the new International Human Pancreas Transplant Registry [8]. The new Registry has received information on all known cases of pancreas transplantation since July 1, 1977 [1]. The data on vascularized pancreas-transplant cases reported to the Registry from December 17, 1966, through June 30, 1984, are summarized in the following section. The experience at the University of Minnesota, which includes more than one-fifth of the transplants that have been performed [9], are described in a subsequent section.

PANCREAS TRANSPLANT REGISTRY

Number and overall results of pancreas transplantation

Between December 17, 1966, and June 30, 1984, 485 pancreas transplants were performed in 454 diabetic patients at 52 institutions (figure 9–1). Cadaver donors were the source of 445 transplants (414 primary, 29 secondary, and 2 tertiary grafts), and living related donors were the source of 40 primary grafts. Four hundred twenty-five of the transplants (in 400 patients) were performed since July 1, 1977 [table 9–1]. Two patients in the new Registry, one from Lyon and one from Stockholm, had had previous transplants recorded by the ACS/NIH Registry.

Publications from the institutions with the largest and most recent experiences —Minnesota [10, 11], Lyon [12], Stockholm [13], Munich [14], Cambridge [15], Zurich [16], Detroit [17], Wisconsin [18], Birmingham [19], and Cincinnati [20] —include the details on all except their latest cases of pancreas transplantation. The reports published on pancreas transplants from several other institutions are referenced in an earlier comprehensive review article [21].

As of August 1984, 129 patients were listed in the Registry as having functioning grafts. At least 60 had been insulin-independent for more than one year. Thirteen other grafts functioned for more than one year, and then either failed and the patients resumed exogenous insulin, or the recipients died with functioning grafts. The other 343 grafts lost function in less than one year because of either technical complications, rejection, or death of the recipients. All of the grafts that are currently functioning were transplanted since 1978.

The actuarial graft and patient survival rate curves, according to data for all pancreas transplant cases are shown in figure 9–2. The results have improved in recent years as pancreas transplantation became safer. For 60 recipients of 56 grafts transplanted before July 1, 1977, the one-year actuarial graft functional survival rate was 3%, and the patient survival rate was only 39%. In contrast, of the 192 patients who received 205 transplants from July 1, 1977, to December 31, 1982, the one-year graft functional survival rate was 20%, and the one-year patient survival rate was 72%. For cases performed in 1983–84 (219 transplants in 207 recipients), the one-year graft survival rate was 38%, and the patient survival rate was 77%.

Most recipients of successful pancreas transplants are normoglycemic, but the results of the metabolic tests can be quite variable [22,23]. Examples of test result patterns in individual pancreas-transplant recipients are illustrated from the University of Minnesota experience in a following section.

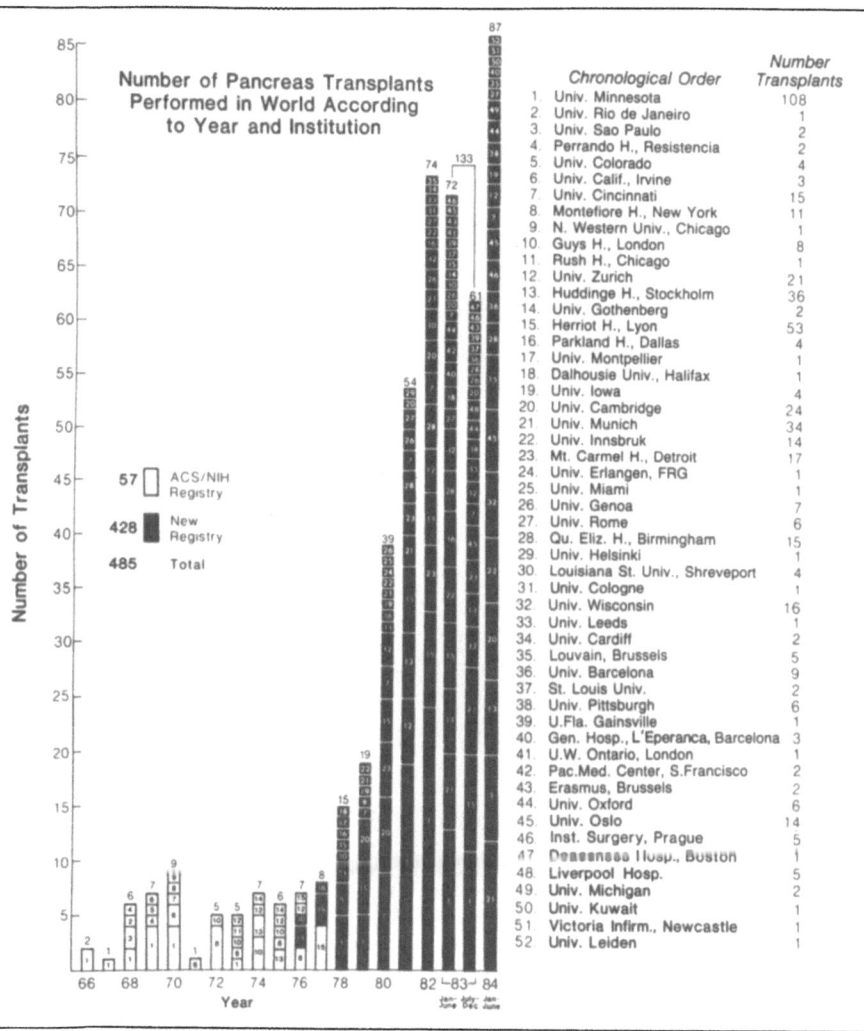

Figure 9–1. Number of pancreas transplants by year and institution reported to the Registries between December 17, 1966, and June 30, 1984. Each institution is assigned a number according to the chronological order by which they did their first transplant (from Sutherland et al, Transpl. Proc., Grune and Stratton, 1985).

Results of pancreas transplantation according to association with or without kidney grafts

Most pancreas-transplant recipients have had diabetic nephropathy and/or other diabetic complications that were far advanced. Kidney transplants have been performed in 322 of the 400 recipients (80%) of 425 pancreas grafts transplanted since July 1, 1977.

Table 9–1. Pancreas transplant experience of individual institutions that performed ≥ 10 cases between July 1, 1977, and June 30, 1984

| Institution | No. tx. (pts) | Reported to be functioning[1] | |
		No.	Months (technique[2])
Univ. of Minnesota	94 (82)	27	57,61,73 (open peritoneal); 15,21,23,31,44 (duct-inj); 8,8,12, 12,13,13,16,16,17,21,25,31,34,36 (enteric)
Herriot Hosp., Lyon	48 (46)	13	3,7,8,10,11,12,16,16,16,20,28,33,41 (duct-inj)
Huddinge Hosp., Stockholm	30 (27)	5	2,6,16,29,33 (enteric)
Univ. of Munich	34 (33)	18	2,2,3,3,3,4,4,5,6,8,12,12,12,13,16, 18,28,38 (duct-inj)
Univ. of Cambridge	24 (23)	9	3,3,5,6,7,7,12,21 (enteric); 60 (duct-inj)
Univ. of Zurich	17	4	3,9,40,49 (duct-inj)
Mt. Carmel Hosp, Detroit	17	2	10,37 (duct-inj)
Univ. of Wisc.	16	8	2,2,3,4,4,8,13,17 (urinary)
Qu. Eliz. Hosp. Birmingham	15	5	3,5,29,35,39 (duct-inj)
Univ. Innsbruck	14 (13)	5	3,4,6,16,17
Univ. Cincinnati	14 (12)	4	5,8,24 (urinary); 32 (duct-inj)
Univ. of Oslo	10	7	2,3,3,4,6,8,9
≤ 10 cases	92 (89)	22	2,3,3,5,5,8,9,10,10,16,21 (enteric); 4,5 (urinary); 2,3,4,6,6,14,18,44 (duct-inj)
Total	425 (400)	129	2–71 months

1. Recipients insulin-independent, assuming continuous function of cases reported to be functioning between June 1984 and August 1984
2. For drainage or occlusion of exocrine secretion

The pancreas-transplant success rates have been approximately the same in non-uremic, nonkidney-transplant recipients and in kidney-transplant recipients (figure 9–3A). The functional survival rates of pancreas grafts transplanted either simultaneously with or after a kidney transplant have also been similar. Actuarial graft survival rates at one year were 31% in recipients of simultaneous kidney transplants, 26% in recipients of previous kidney transplants, and 24% for nonuremic, nonkidney-transplant patients (p > .2). The two recipients of kidney grafts after pancreas transplants lost pancreas graft function before the kidney transplant.

Patient survival rates have been higher in recipients of pancreas grafts alone and in recipients of pancreas grafts after a successful kidney graft than in pancreas transplant recipients of simultaneous kidney grafts (figure 9–3B). Patient survival rates would be expected to be higher in recipients of pancreas transplants alone, since the nonuremic diabetic patients would be more likely to have less advanced

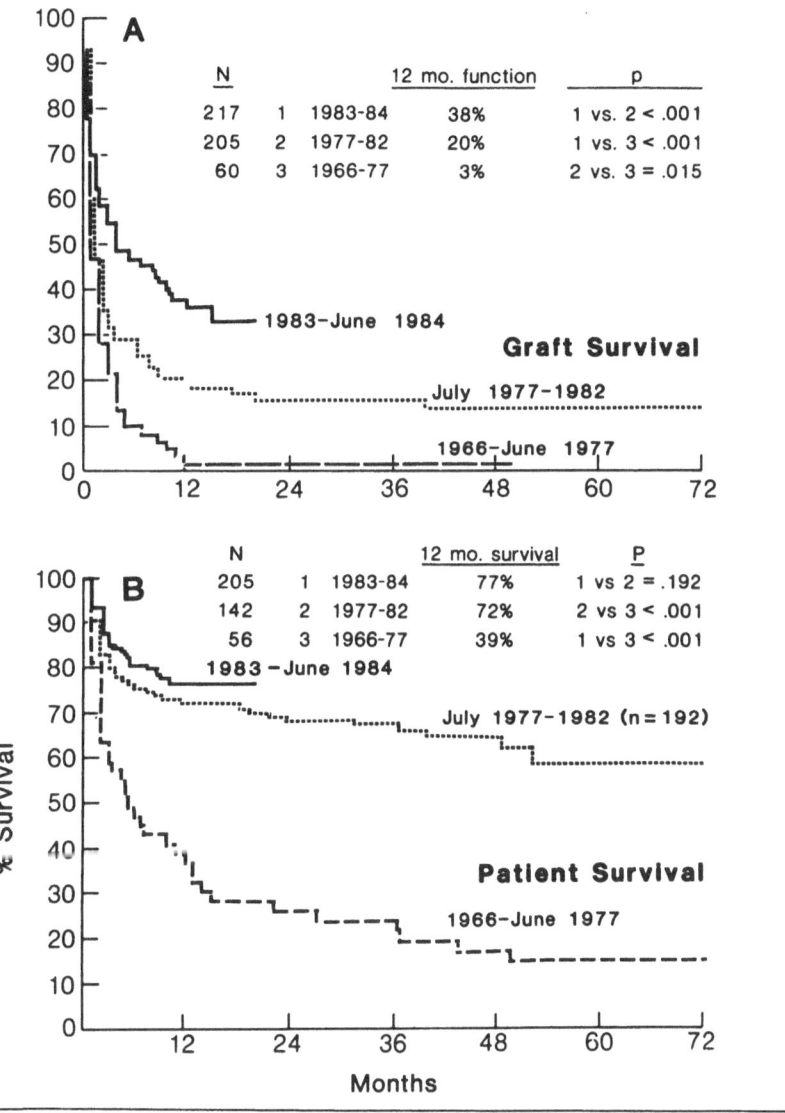

Figure 9–2. (A) Functional graft survival rate for all pancreas–transplant cases, and (B) patient survival for all primary pancreas–transplant cases, reported to the Registry by year of the transplantation up to June 30, 1984 (from Sutherland et al, Transpl. Proc., Grune and Stratton, 1985).

complications than the uremic diabetic recipients. The fact that patient survival rates are also higher in uremic diabetic patients who received a kidney transplant before pancreas transplant than in those receiving both grafts simultaneously, however, suggests that a penalty is paid for synchronous as opposed to dyssynchro-

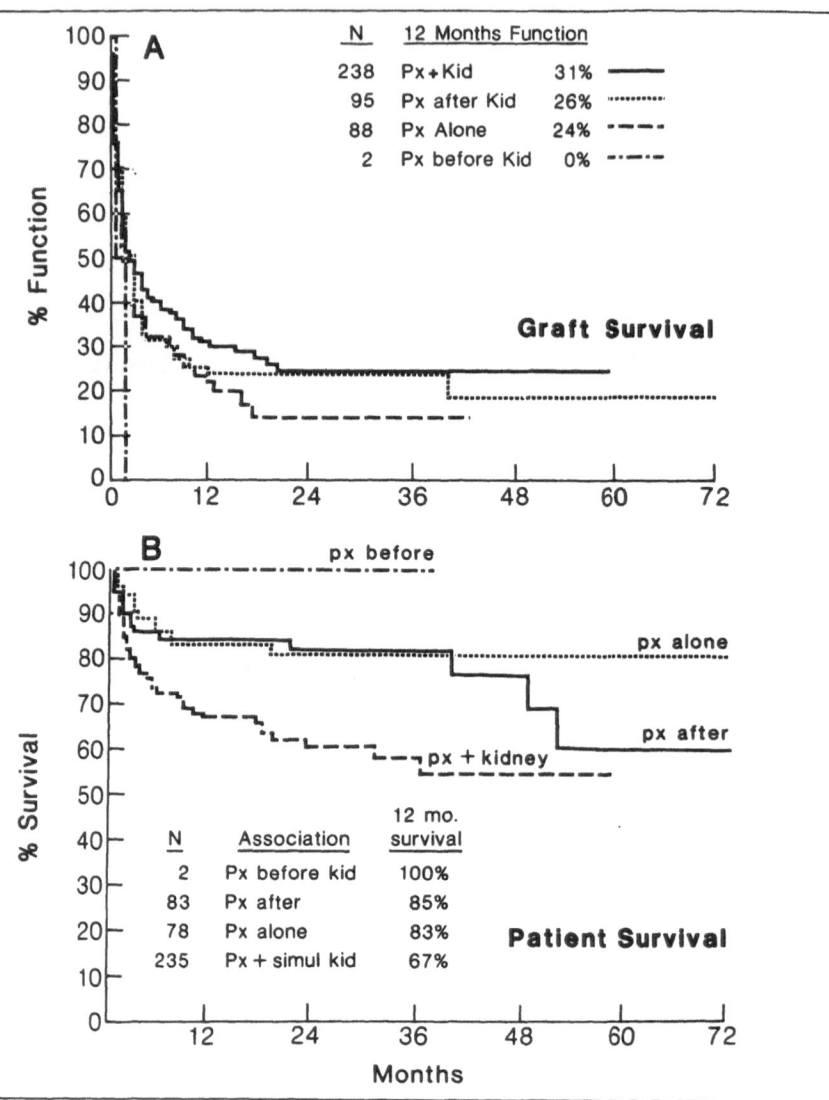

Figure 9–3. (A) Graft survival rates for all pancreas transplants reported to the Registry from July 1, 1977, to June 30, 1984, according to association with kidney transplants; and (B) patient survival rates for recipients of primary pancreas transplants performed during the same time period according to association with kidney transplants (from Sutherland et al, Transpl. Proc., Grune and Stratton, 1985).

nous grafting in uremic diabetic patients. This interpretation is supported by an analysis of graft and patient survival rates according to whether the recipients of pancreas transplants did or did not have end-stage diabetic nephropathy (ESDN). Pancreas graft survival rates were approximately the same in the two categories of recipients (figure 9–4A), but patient survival rates were significantly higher in patients with than without ESDN (figure 9–4B).

There is no evidence that pancreas transplants have improved the kidney transplant results in uremic diabetic patients. Kidney graft functional survival rates, as

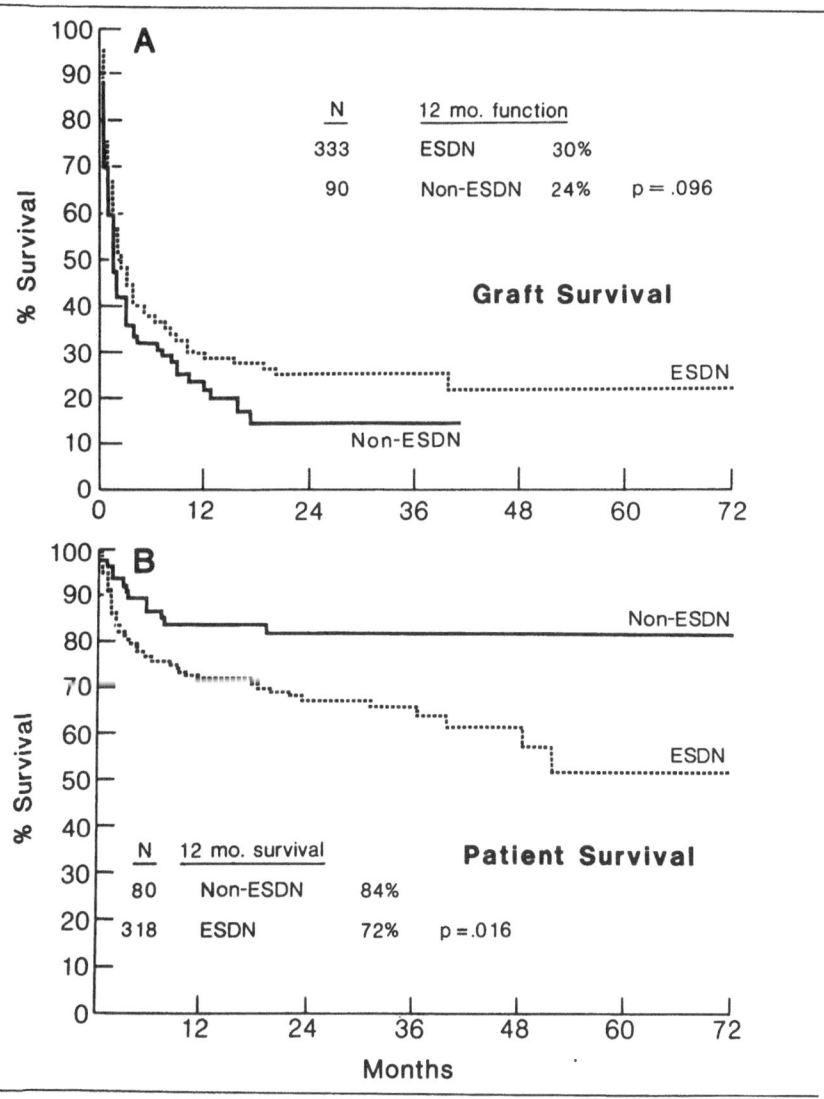

Figure 9–4. (A) Graft survival rates for all pancreas transplants performed between July 1, 1977, and June 30, 1984 in recipients with or without end-stage diabetic nephropathy (ESDN), and (B) patient survival rates for all recipients of primary pancreas transplants performed during the same time period for ESDN and non-ESDN patients (from Sutherland et al, Transpl Proc, Grune & Stratton, 1985).

well as patient survival rates, in pancreas-transplant recipients with ESDN [24] are less than those reported for diabetic uremic recipients of kidney transplants alone [25,26]. Thus it appears that correction of uremia by kidney transplantation is more important and more beneficial than total endocrine replacement therapy in diabetic patients with renal failure.

Results of pancreas transplantation according to surgical technique

A variety of surgical techniques have been used for pancreas transplantation, and are classified according to the method used for duct management (occluded or drained into a hollow viscus). Duct occlusion is accomplished by either ligation or by injection of a synthetic polymer to obliterate the entire ductal system. Duct-drained grafts can be divided into those in which an anastmosis is made to either the gut or to the urinary system (ureter or bladder).

The first pancreas transplant performed was a segmental graft of only the distal portion of the gland [3]. However, in the ACS/NIH Registry encompassing the period from 1966 to 1977 [7], nearly half of those transplanted were whole-organ pancreaticoduodenal grafts [27]. The high technical complication rate of pancreaticoduodenal transplants lead to a near abandonment of this approach by the mid-1970s, and, until recently, the segmental technique was used almost exclusively (figure 9–5). With this approach, the body and tail (approximately 50%) of the pancreas is removed, and the donor celiac axis (or splenic artery) and portal vein

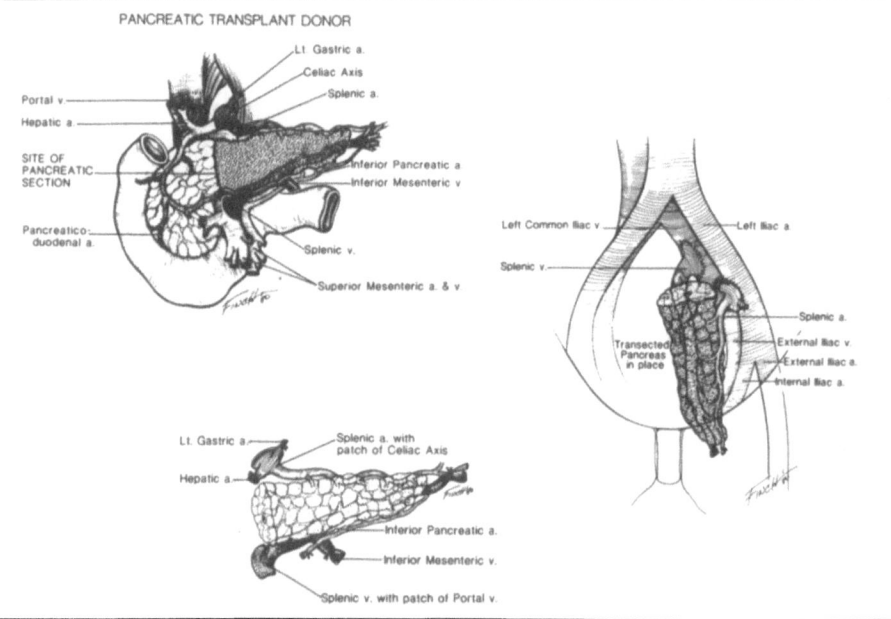

Figure 9–5. Technique of segmental pancreas transplantation. Body and tail are transplanted with anastomoses of splenic vessels of donor pancreas to iliac vessels of recipient (From Sutherland DER, Diabetologia 20:435, 1981, Springer Verlag, Co.).

(or splenic vein) are used for vascular anastomoses, usually to the iliac vessels of the recipient. The recipient's splenic vessels have also been used for anastomoses, resulting in drainage of the graft venous effluence into the portal circulation [28]. The techniques for removal of segmental pancreas grafts from cadaver donors, before [29, 30] or after circulatory arrest [31], have been described.

The segmental approach allows living related donors to be the source of pancreas transplants (figure 9–6) [32]. The splenic artery and vein are ligated in the hilum of the spleen, and the spleen survives on the collateral blood supply [33]. Metabolism remains normal if the donors have normal glucose tolerance prior to hemipancreatectomy [33, 34].

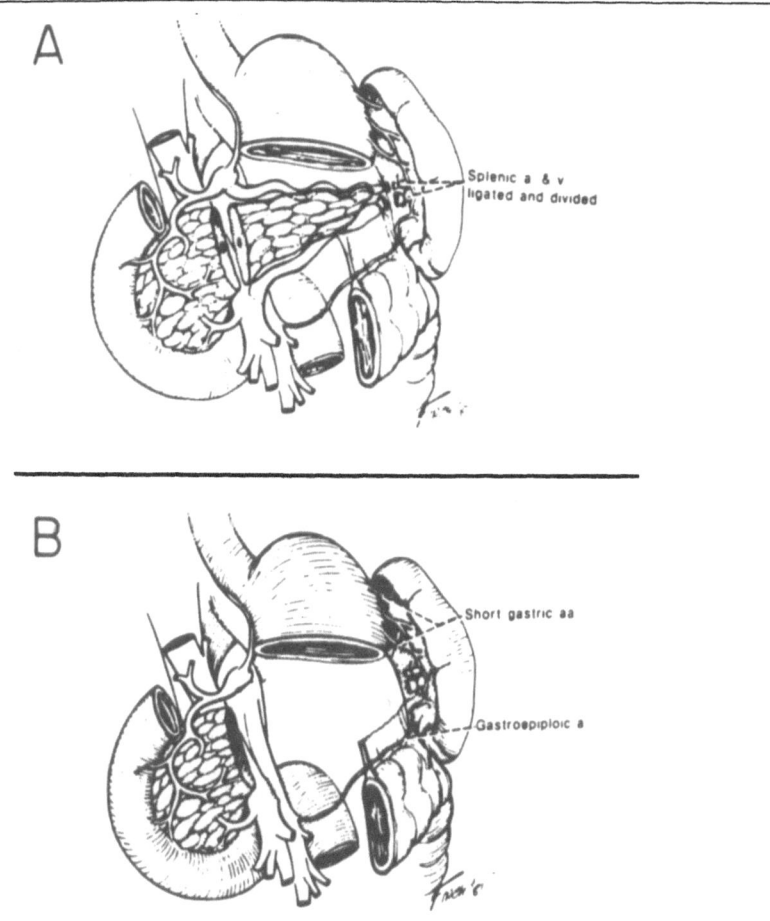

Figure 9–6. (A) Technique of distal pancreatectomy in living related donor for segmental transplantation. (B) Collateral blood supply to the donor spleen is preserved (from Sutherland DER, et al. Pancreas and islet transplantation in diabetic patients with long-term followup in selected cases. In: Diabetic Renal Retinal Syndrome, Prevention and Management, Friedman EA, L'Esperance FA, (ed). New York: Grune & Stratton, 1982, pp. 463–494).

In recent years, there has been a renewed interest in transplantation of the entire pancreas from cadaver donors, with or without the duodenum. The entire duodenum can be transplanted, or the duodenum can be trimmed to just a bubble encompassing the portion that is most intimate with the pancreas [35]. The pancreas also can be meticulously freed from the duodenum so only the Papilla of Vater is left attached, or it can be completely separated so both the common bile duct and pancreatic duct are divided before they enter into the duodenum [36]. The last approach obviates enteric contamination from the donor, and has been used for duct management techniques that do not include drainage into a hollow viscus. The former approach has been exclusively with the viscus drainage techniques. Some pancreas–transplant surgeons have also left the spleen attached to the pancreas graft in order to increase the blood flow through the large splenic vessels [35, 37].

The most important technical issue in pancreas transplantation is the provision made for the management of the exocrine secretions. Several methods have been used. Suppression of exocrine function by polymer injection into the duct [30] has been the most widely used technique; 235 of 425 grafts transplanted since July 1, 1977, were duct-injected (55%). The complication rate for polymer injection remains relatively low; but fibrosis, induced by the injected agent, may involve the islets and lead to graft failure [38]. Duct ligation was used in the first pancreas transplant case [3], but has been used sporadically since July 1, 1977 (11 cases, 3%). The pancreatic duct can also be left open to drain freely into the peritoneal cavity [39], and the secretions are absorbed if the pancreatic enzymes are not activated (19 cases since July 1, 1977, 4%). Pancreatico–enterostomy [40] and pancreaticoductoureterostomy [29] were used in some of the earliest pancreas transplant cases and have regained popularity. A variety of anastomotic techniques have been used, including direct insertion of the pancreatic duct into the bladder [18]. Enteric drainage has been established most often by an intussusception technique for segmental grafts (figure 9–7) and by mucosal to mucosal anastomosis for whole pancreas [41] or pancreaticoduodenal grafts [35]. Pancreatico–enterostomy [13, 42, 43] has been performed in 120 cases and urinary drainage [18, 20, 44] in 37 cases (19 ureter, 18 bladder) since July 1, 1977 (28% and 8%, respectively).

Except for ligation, all methods of duct management have been associated with long-term graft function (figure 9–8A). The one-year actuarial functional survival rates of pancreas transplants since July 1, 1977, were 40% with enteric drainage, 30% with urinary drainage, 26% with duct-injection, and 16% for intraperitoneal open duct; the differences are not statistically significant ($p > 0.1$). The methods of duct management associated with the highest patient survival rates have been ligation and enteric drainage, but again none of the differences is statistically significant (figure 9–8B).

Results of pancreas transplantation according to immunosuppression in the recipients

Azathioprine was used to treat all pancreas-transplant recipients transplanted before June 30, 1977. Since July 1, 1977, azathioprine has been the principal immunosup-

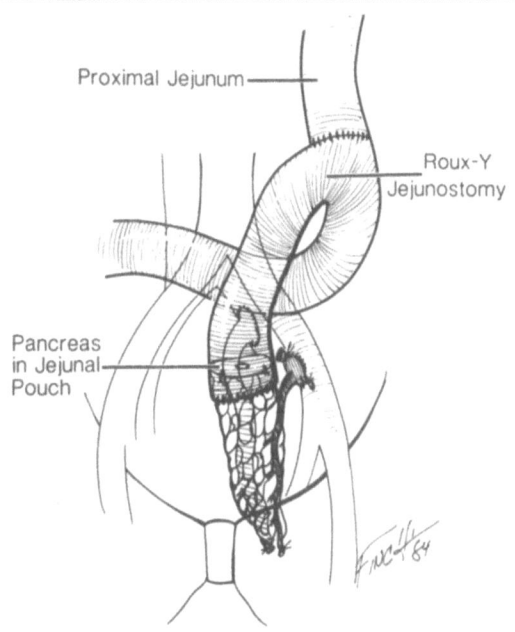

Figure 9–7. Technique for drainage of the segmental pancreas graft exocrine secretion via a Roux-en-Y limb of recipient bowel (from Sutherland DER, Goetz FC, Elick BA, Najarian JS. Pancreas and islet transplantation in diabetic patients with long-term followup in selected cases. In: Diabetic Renal Retinal Syndrome, Prevention and Management, Friedman EA, L'Esperance FA (eds). New York: Grune & Stratton, 1982, pp. 463–494).

pressant in 198 recipients and cyclosporine in 217 recipients of pancreas allografts. An analysis according to immunosuppression showed that the pancreas allograft functional survival rates were significantly higher in all patients treated with cyclosporine than with azathioprine, 37% versus 20% at one year (figure 9–9A). When technically successful transplants only were considered, the one-year pancreas allograft function rates in 189 cyclosporine- and 152 azathioprine-treated recipients were 41% and 26%, respectively (figure 9–9B).

Results of pancreas transplant according to duration of graft preservation
Some of the pancreas grafts were transplanted immediately following removal from the donor. Of cases since July 1, 1977, the interval between removal from the donor and transplantation to the recipient were reported on 225 grafts preserved by hypothermic storage in electrolyte solutions. The functional survival rate was higher for grafts preserved less than six hours than for those stored more than six hours (figure 9–10). A longer storage time was associated with a higher percentage of early (less than three days) graft failures, but late losses were nearly equivalent. At one year the differences in graft survival rates were not substantial, 26% for the <6 hour and 24% for the >6 hour preser-

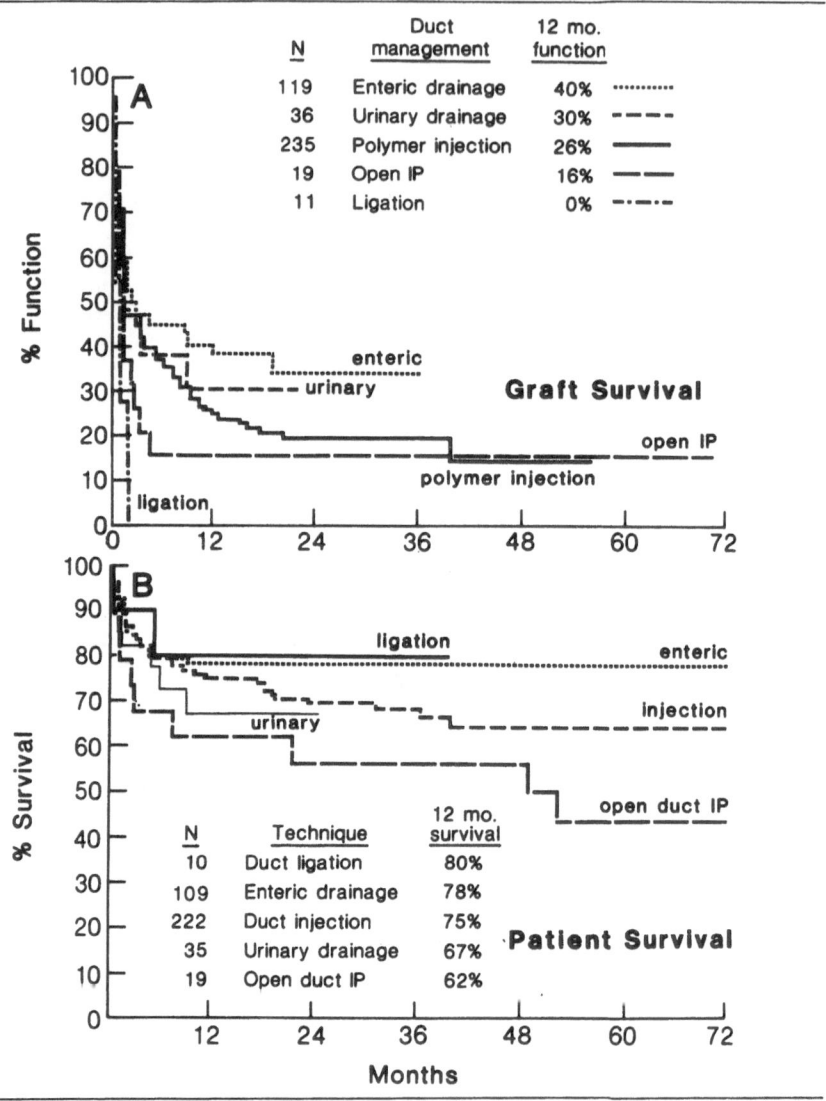

Figure 9–8. (A) Graft survival by duct management technique for all pancreas transplant cases reported to the Registry from July 1, 1977, to June 30, 1984, excluding three cases unclassified due to immediate technical failure; and (B) patient survival rates for recipients of primary pancreas transplants performed during the same time period (from Sutherland et al, Transpl. Proc., Grune & Stratton, 1985).

vation groups. An analysis performed earlier had shown that the immediate function rates were similar for all storage times up to 24 hours [45]. The logistical aspects of pancreas transplantation [46] have been greatly facilitated by the capacity to preserve pancreas grafts.

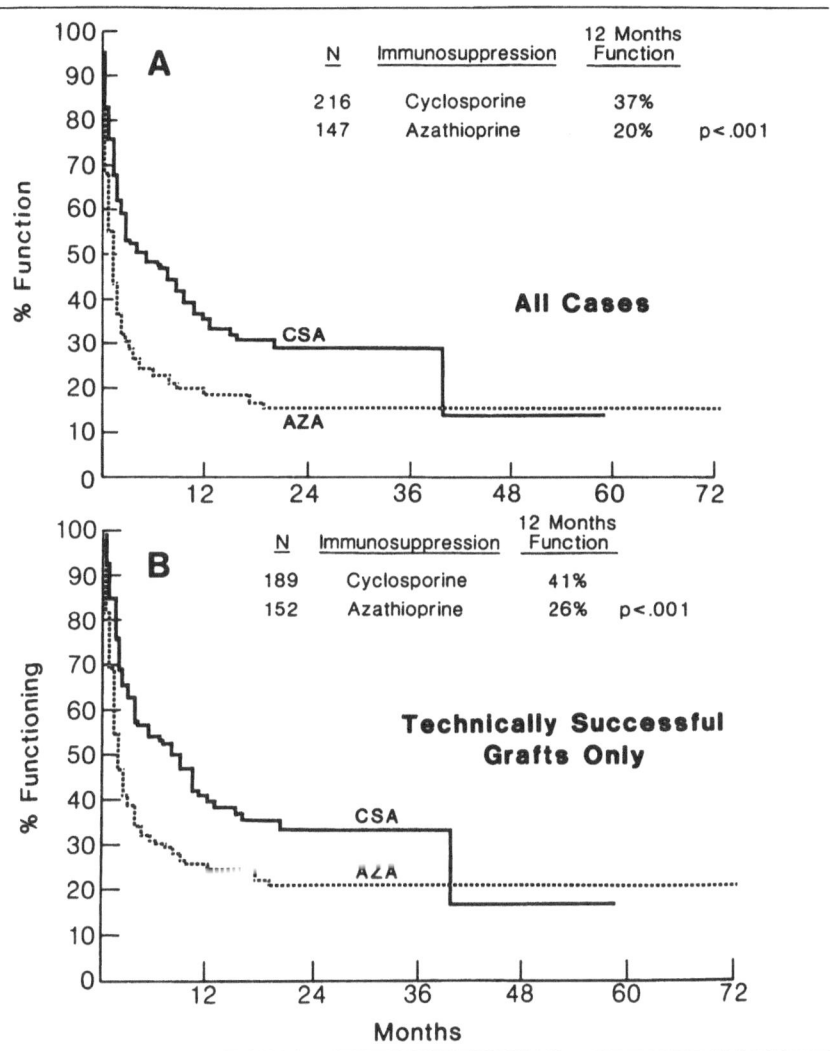

Figure 9–9. (A) Pancreas allograft survival rates according to principal immunosuppressant used in the recipients for all cases reported to the Registry between July 1, 1977, and June 30, 1984, and (B) for technically successful cases only reported to the Registry during the same time period (from Sutherland et al, Transpl. Proc., Grune and Stratton, 1985).

EXPERIENCE WITH PANCREAS TRANSPLANTATION AT THE UNIVERSITY OF MINNESOTA

Immediately vascularized pancreas grafts or free grafts of islet tissue have been transplanted at the University of Minnesota since 1966 [27, 47]. There have been two series of pancreas transplants and two series of islet transplants. No recipients become permanently insulin–independent in either of the islet transplant series (10 cases each) [48, 49].

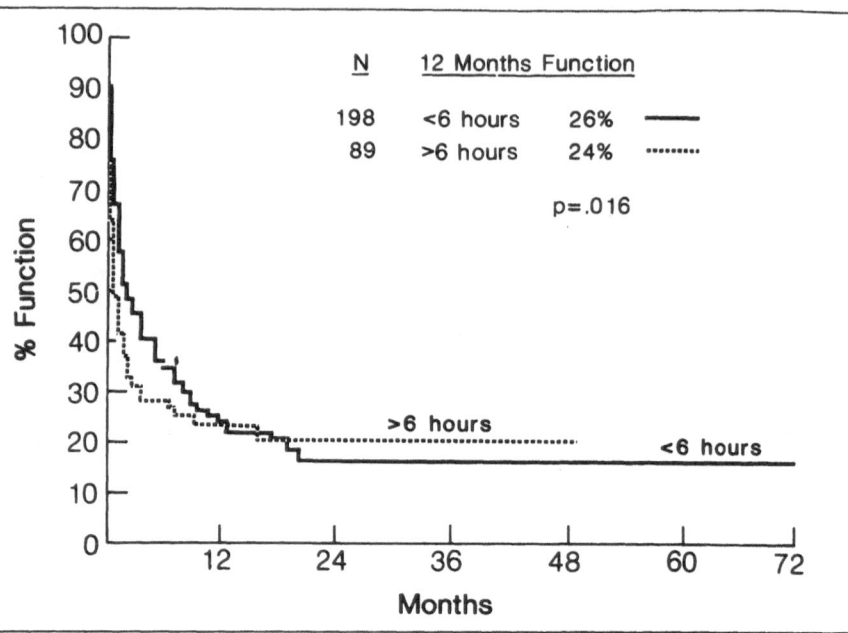

Figure 9–10. Cadaver pancreas graft functional survival rates according to preservation times for cases performed between July 1, 1977, and June 30, 1984 (From Sutherland et al, Transpl. Proc., Grune and Stratton, 1985).

The first series of pancreas transplants was performed between 1966 and 1973 [10], and only one recipient survived for more than a year with a functioning pancreas graft [50]. The most recent series began on July 25, 1978 [39]. As of June 30, 1984, this series included 94 pancreas transplants performed in 82 diabetic patients. The results of this series have been periodically reported [9, 11, 34, 42, 51, 52].

Patient demographics, transplant technique, and immunosuppression

Of the 82 patients who have received pancreas transplants in the most recent University of Minnesota series, 43 had functioning renal grafts (42 allografts, 1 isograft) placed six months to nine years previously for treatment of end-stage diabetic nephropathy. Thirty-nine patients were nonuremic and, at the time of the pancreas transplant, had not received kidney grafts. Of the 94 pancreas grafts, 56 came from cadaver donors (60%) and 38 came from living related donors (40%). Seventy-two grafts were segmental (all of the ones from living related and 32 from cadaver donors), while 22 were the whole pancreas from cadaver donors as previously described [36, 41]. Technical problems were responsible for 24 graft failures (9 thrombosis, 7 infections, 3 inadequate preservation, 3 ascites, 2 bleeding).

The pancreas grafts were placed intraperitoneally. Four different techniques were used for management of the pancreatic duct, but enteric drainage into a Roux-en-Y limb of recipient jejunum is now preferred (table 9–2).

Table 9–2. Outcome after pancreas transplantation in 1978–1984 Minnesota cases according to donor source, technique, and immunosuppression

Technique	No. of txs (rel/cad)	Im.sup.[1] C/A/T	Technical failures	Late loss[2] of function	Grafts no.	Currently functioning[3] duration in Mos
Duct ligated	3 (0/3)	0/3/0	3(100%)	0(0%)	0(0%)	—
Open peritoneal	15 (5/10)	1/14/0	8(53%)	4(27%)	3(20%)	57(A)^c, 61(A)^r, 73(A)^c
Enteric	37 (28/9)	15/9/11	10(27%)	6(16%)	19(51%)	2(T)^r, 2(T)^c, 3(T)^c, 5(A)^r, 5(T)^c, 8(T)^c, 8(T)^r, 12(T)^c, 12(T)^c, 13(A)^r, 13(C)^r, 16(C)^r, 16(A)^r, 17(A)^r, 21(C)^r, 25(C)^r, 31(C)^r, 34(A)^r, 36(C)^r 15(T)^c, 21(A)^r, 23(C)^c
Duct-inj.	39 (5/34)	29/8/1	3(8%)	28(72%)	5(13%)	31(C)^c, 44(A)^r
Total	94(38/56)	45/34/12	24(26%)	38(40%)	27(37%)	2–73

1. All patients except one received prednisone in addition to either Cyclosporine (C), Azathioprine (A), or Triple Therapy (T, combination of cyclosporine and azathioprine).
2. Four patients with technically successful transplants (2 duct-inj., 2 enterically drained) who died with functioning grafts are not included in this column. As of August 1984, 11/56 (20%) cadaver grafts and 16/38 (42%) related were functioning. Of technically successful allografts, 9/17 (53%) treated with Azathioprine, 9/40 (23%) with Cyclosporine, and 9/10 (90%) with triple therapy are functioning.
3. Immunosuppression is indicated in parentheses (C, A, or T), and donor source, cadaver^c or related^r, by superscripts.

We have described previously the immunosuppressive protocols used in our patients [9, 52–54]. For recipients of pancreas allografts, 23 were treated with azathioprine (AZA), prednisone, and antilymphocyte globulin (ALG); 7 were treated with AZA and prednisone only; 9 were treated with cyclosporine (CSA) (and usually prednisone) after an initial course of conventional (AZA, prednisone, ALG) immunosuppression; 36 were treated with CSA and prednisone beginning immediately after transplantation; and 13 patients received a combination of CSA, AZA, and prednisone (triple therapy) (table 9–2). Four patients were switched to AZA after being treated with CSA for the first three to six months posttransplant. One of the patients converted to AZA had no change in graft function and is currently insulin-independent with a functioning graft at > 2 years after transplantation. The other three patients who were switched to AZA had decline of graft function and resumed exogenous insulin two to six months after conversion. In the conventionally immunosuppressed patients, 15 grafts failed for technical reasons, while 7 grafts in the CSA group were lost to technical failure.

Current results of pancreas transplantation at the University of Minnesota

As of August 1984, 27 of 82 patients (33%) had full (22 cases, receive no exogenous insulin) or partial (5 cases, have C-peptide levels above baseline and are no longer ketosis-prone, but require supplemental insulin to maintain normoglycemia) function of their pancreas grafts, and 67 of the patients were alive (82%). Twenty grafts have functioned for > 1 year, and 18 of these are still functioning, the longest for 6.1 years. Sixteen of the 27 currently functioning grafts were obtained from living related donors [34].

In 36 instances the pancreas grafts functioned for 1 to 12 months before hyperglycemia recurred. The recipients than resumed exogenous insulin. Graft biopsies, performed in 16 cases at the time of or a few months after loss of function, showed rejection in 13 instances [54]. In 3 cases (including 2 isografts with insulitis) it appeared that specific beta cell destruction resulted in recurrence of diabetes independent of rejection [42, 55, 56], most likely because of an autoimmune insulitis [54, 55].

When hyperglycemia occurred weeks or months after transplantation, a presumptive diagnosis of rejection was made (24 graft recipients, 10 from related, 14 from cadaver donors). Rejection episodes were treated by either an increase in prednisone dose or by administration of antilymphocyte globulin [9, 52, 53]. Three recipients of cadaver and four recipients of related donor grafts reverted to euglycemia after antirejection treatment and are currently insulin-independent.

Oral glucose tolerance test results and metabolic profiles in most of the insulin-independent patients with functioning grafts are normal or nearly normal [9, 11, 22, 34, 52]. The range of results, however, is quite variable (figure 9–11). A patient whose graft has functioned the longest (now 73 months posttransplant) had normal glucose tolerance test results at two, three, and four years, while the results were slightly abnormal at one and five years (figure 9–11C). The fact that absolutely normal metabolic profiles and glucose tolerance test (both oral and intravenous) results occur in some pancreas-transplant recipients (figure 9–12) shows that the denervated state of the graft or drainage of the venous effluent into the systemic circulation are not by themselves responsible for the abnormalities seen in other recipients.

All of the 38 related donors of segmental pancreas grafts are currently alive. Two donors (5%) required a reoperation; one had a splenectomy and had the pancreatic duct religated at the line of transection. Glucose tolerance test results changed in some donors postoperatively, but the changes were physiologically significant only in one obese donor [33].

Comments

The current pancreas-transplantation protocol at the University of Minnesota has been derived from lessons learned during 128 attempts at endocrine replacement therapy in 109 patients since 1966. The experience includes 20 islet, 12 pancreaticoduodenal, 23 whole, and 73 segmental pancreas transplants. Currently, we offer

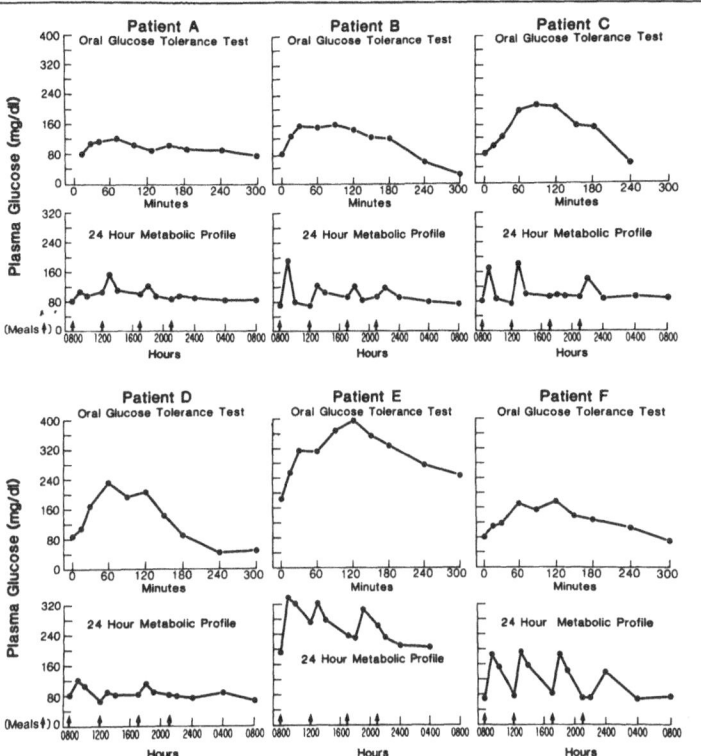

Figure 9–11. Results of metabolic studies (glucose tolerance tests and 24–hour profiles) in the absence of exogenous insulin in six recipients of segmental pancreas transplants functioning at > 12 months, illustrating the variability in response of individual patients. Patient (A), *12 months posttransplant,* has both a normal glucose tolerance test (GTT) results and a normal metabolic profile during a day of normal meals and activity. Patient (B), *36 months posttransplant,* is normal except for a slight hypoglycemic trend at four to five hours during the GTT. Patient (C), at *60 months posttransplant,* has an abnormal GTT with elevated two–hour glucose value, but *is* euglycemic through a day of standard meals and activity. Patient (D), *24 months posttransplant,* has abnormal GTT (with both hyperglycemia and hypoglycemia), but displays a normal 24–hour glucose profile. Patient (E), *36 months posttransplant,* has highly abnormal GTT as well as fasting and postprandial hyperglycemia during a day of normal meals and activity. Patient (F), *12 months posttransplant,* has a normal GTT, but an abnormal profile with elevated postprandial glucose during 24–hour profile (from Sutherland DM, Kendall DM, Goetz, FC, Najarian JS. Pancreas transplantation in man. Diabetes Annual, 1984, in press).

pancreas transplants to patients whose diabetic complications are, or potentially will be, more serious than the possible side effects of chronic immunosuppression. Of the 82 patients transplanted since 1978, 39 were nonuremic, nonkidney–transplant recipients (48%), including 21 of 30 (70%) in 1983 and the first half of 1984. Early and progressive nephropathy, neuropathy, or retinopathy were indications for pancreas transplantation in these patients. Of the 27 patients whose grafts are currently functioning, 15 (56%) had not received previous kidney grafts.

Most of our efforts have been focused on simply achieving an acceptable pancreas

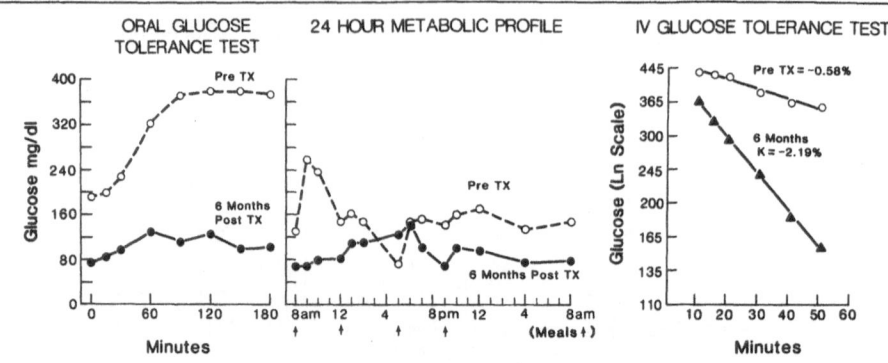

Figure 9–12. Results of metabolic profiles and oral and intravenous glucose tolerance tests before and six months after a segmental pancreas transplant with enteric drainage of the pancreatic duct and systemic drainage of the graft venous effluent. The results after transplantation are entirely normal (from Sutherland et al, Ann. Surg. 200:414, 1984, J. B. Lippincott).

graft functional survival rate with a low morbidity and mortality rate. We now prefer to drain exocrine pancreas secretions into a hollow viscus, and enteric drainage is the most physiologic method.

The diagnosis of rejection can be quite difficult, as noted by other groups [57]. Monitoring of plasma glucose levels at home and early use of a graft biopsy have been the most useful indicators of rejection in our series [9, 54].

The recipients are being closely followed for the effect of the procedure on secondary complications. Unpublished observations on kidney biopsies in two renal allograft recipients, followed for > 4 years following successful pancreas transplantation, suggest that the progression of renal lesions can be prevented and that early lesions may actually regress.

Some aspects of our protocols, including the use of cyclosporine for recipient immunosuppression [53] and pancreaticoenterostomy [42] for management of exocrine function, are similar to those of other groups [13, 43, 58] applying pancreas transplantation to the treatment of diabetes. Our treatment of uremic diabetic patients, however, differs from most groups performing pancreas transplantation. We do not transplant kidney and pancreas grafts simultaneously, since kidney transplants alone will rehabilitate most uremic diabetics [26, 59], and since simultaneous pancreas and kidney grafting does not improve renal graft survival rates [24]. For these reasons, we delay pancreas transplantation until the renal graft is well established, and only perform the procedure in patients whose rehabilitation will be further enhanced by correction of diabetes.

If possible, pancreas transplantation should be performed much earlier in the course of the disease than has been the case for most recipients. Since generalized immunosuppression is required to prevent rejection, this approach is taken only in patients who clearly have, or are developing, serious secondary complications.

In summary, 94 pancreas transplants have been performed in 82 diabetic patients at the University of Minnesota since 1978. Twenty-seven patients currently (August 1984) have functioning pancreas grafts. Twenty patients have had the grafts function one year or more posttransplant. Advances in immunosuppressive therapy, in surgical technique and in patient selection criteria, have been associated with a progressive increase in the success rate of pancreas transplantation at our institution [52].

DISCUSSION

Approximately one-third of the pancreas transplants performed worldwide since 1966 were done in 1983 and the first half of 1984, emphasizing the fact that there has been a renewed interest in pancreas transplantation in recent years. The success rate is steadily improving. Long-term graft function with normal or near-normal glucose metabolism has been sustained in several patients. Ultimately, pancreas transplantation should have the same impact on the treatment of diabetes as kidney transplantation has had on the treatment of end-stage renal disease. Observations in pancreas transplant recipients may also provide information answering many fundamental questions related to the nature of diabetes mellitus [60].

Most pancreas graft recipients have had secondary complications of diabetes that were far advanced prior to transplantation. Ideally, pancreas transplantation should be performed early in the stages of the disease. This approach is being taken, particularly in the recent Minnesota series.

Immune rejection has been the greatest hindrance to successful pancreas transplantation. The use of cyclosporine has been associated with an improvement in the results of pancreas transplantation (figure 9–9). The success rate, however, is still much less than that reported for kidney transplantation [15]. Cyclosporine is still a generalized immunosuppressive agent, and has adverse side effects. Nevertheless, the introduction of cyclosporine has expanded the patient population that can be considered for pancreas transplantation.

Attempts at clinical islet allotransplantation have been unsuccessful [1]. The manipulations that have lead to a relatively high success rate in experimental animals models [61] have not been applied in the clinical situation. Islet transplantation is not simple for the transplant team. It is very difficult to procure a sufficient quantity of viable islet tissue from a single donor pancreas, and techniques to alter the immunogenicity of human islets need to be made practical. If the methods currently being used in animals are effective for human islet isolation and reduction of immunogenicity [62], clinical attempts at islet transplantation should be made although the probability of success is uncertain.

Pancreas transplants are being performed in rigorously selected diabetic patients at this time. Because of the need for generalized immunosuppression to prevent rejection, pancreas transplantation has been restricted to patients whose secondary complications of diabetes are, or predictably will be, more serious than the potential side effects of antirejection therapy. Patients who require or who have had a kidney transplant, and who are obligated to immunosuppressive therapy, meet this criteria. However, some nonuremic, nonkidney-transplant patients are also in this category, such as those with preproliferative retinopathy and who are thus at great risk for loss of vision.

If it becomes possible to abrogate specific immune response in humans and if the risks of transplantation are minimal, the limiting factor will be the availability of donor pancreases. This problem can be solved. More than 5,000 kidney transplants are done in the United States each year [63]. The incidence of new cases of type I diabetes in the United States has been estimated to be 10,000/year, and less than half of the patients with the disease develop serious complications [64].

The current kidney transplant rate, thus, is the same as the yearly incidence of complication prone type I diabetes. Unfortunately, only a small proportion of potential donors are currently used as a source of organs [65]. However, there is no inherent reason to believe that donor procurement will be any more difficult for pancreas transplantation than for kidney transplantation. Measurement of insulin-like growth factors [67] or of joint stiffness [66] might identify diabetic patients who are at high risk to develop secondary complications. It should be possible to also identify diabetic patients who have impaired counterregulatory mechanisms and who are at high risk for hypoglycemic reactions while on insulin pump or other intensified insulin therapy regimens [6]. Patients with these characteristics [6, 66, 67] are the ones who will derive the most benefit from a successful pancreas transplant. A sufficient supply of pancreases from cadaver and related donors should be available for this select group.

In conclusion, pancreas transplantation has become increasingly effective for the treatment of human diabetes. Islet transplants have been successful only in the laboratory. Unless islet yield can be improved and methods to reduce immunogenicity can be made practical, pancreas transplantation is the only method of total endocrine replacement therapy in diabetes that can succeed. Pancreas transplantation potentially could be applied on as large a scale as renal transplantation. Eventually, pancreas transplantation may be routinely performed at a stage sufficiently early to prevent the development of diabetic nephropathy, and supersede kidney transplantation in the management of complication prone diabetic patients.

ADDENDUM

Two pancreas transplants, one performed at Institution No. 37 (preserved < 6 hours, transplanted after a previous kidney, with enteric drainage in an azathioprine-treated recipient) in the last half of 1983, and one at Institution No. 40 (preserved > 6 hours, transplanted simultaneously with a kidney, and drained into the urinary system of a cyclosporine treated recipient), were reported to the Registry after August 1, 1984, the date of this analysis, and were not included in the calculations for figures 9–2 through 9–5 and 9–8 through 9–10. Both failed within six weeks of transplantation for technical reasons, so their exclusion does not alter the results reported.

ACKNOWLEDGMENTS

Janet Sanders prepared the manuscript. Martin Finch and associates, Department of Biomedical Graphics, University of Minnesota prepared the illustrations. David

Kendall compiled data and performed statistical analyses. Dr. Frederick C. Goetz was an integral member of the pancreas transplant team at the University of Minnesota, and was responsible for the metabolic studies in the recipients.

REFERENCES

1. Sutherland DER, Kendall D. Clinical pancreas and islet transplant registry report. Transpl Proc 17:307–311, 1985.
2. Sutherland DER. Pancreas and islet transplantation registry data. World J Surg 8:270–275, 1984.
3. Kelly WD, Lillehei RC, Merkel FK, Idezuki Y, Goetz FC. Allotransplantation of the pancreas and duodenum along with the kidney in diabetic nephropathy. Surgery 61:827–837, 1967.
4. Brownlee MC, Cahill GF. Diabetic control and vascular complications. In: Atherosclerotic Reviews, Vol. 4, Paoletti R, Gatto AM (eds). New York: Raven Press, 1979, pp. 29–70.
5. Ungar RH. Meticulous control of diabetes: benefits, risks and precautions. Diabetes 31:479–483, 1982.
6. White N, Skor DA, Cryer PE, Levandoski PA, Bier DM, Santiago JV. Identification or Type I diabetic patients at increased risk for hypoglycemia during intensive therapy. N Engl J Med 308:485–491, 1983.
7. Gerrish EW. Final Newsletter, American College of Surgeons/National Institutes of Health Organ Transplant Registry, June 30, 1977.
8. Sutherland DER. International human pancreas and islet transplant registry. Transpl Proc 12 (No. 4, Suppl. 2):229–236, 1980.
9. Sutherland DER, Goetz FC, Najarian JS. 100 pancreas transplants at a single institution. Ann Surg 200:414–438, 1984.
10. Lillehei RC, Ruiz JO, Acquino C, Goetz FC. Transplantation of the pancreas. Acta Endocrinol 83 (Suppl. 205):303–320, 1976.
11. Sutherland DER, Goetz FC, Najarian JS. Recent experience with 89 pancreas transplants between 1978 and 1983. Diabetologia 27:149–153, 1984.
12. Dubernard JM, Traeger J, Bosi E, et al. Transplantation for the treatment of insulin-dependent diabetes: clinical experience with polymer-obstructed pancreatic grafts using Neoprene. World J Surg 8:262–266, 1984.
13. Groth CG, Tyden G, Lundgren G, et al. Segmental pancreas transplantation with enteric exocrine diversion. World J Surg 8:257–261, 1984.
14. Land W, Illner WD, Abendroth D, Landgraf R. Experience with segmental pancreas transplants in cyclosporine treated diabetic patients using Ethibloc for duct obliteration. Transpl Proc 16:729–732, 1984.
15. Calne RY, White DJG. The use of cyclosporine in clinical organ grafting. Ann Surg 196:-330–337, 1982.
16. Baumgartner D, Largiader F. Simultaneous renal and intraperitoneal segmental pancreatic transplantation: the Zurich experience. World J Surg 8:267–269, 1984.
17. Toledo-Pereyra LH. Pancreas transplantation. Surg Gynecol Obset 157:49–56, 1983.
18. Sollinger HW, Cook K, Kamps D, Glass NR, Belzer FO. Clinical and experimental experience with pancreaticocystostomy for exocrine pancreatic drainage in pancreas transplantation. Tranpsl Proc 16:749–751, 1984.
19. McMaster P, Michael J, Adu D, et al. Experience in human segmental pancreas transplantation. World J Surg 8:253–256, 1984.
20. Munda R, First MR, Webb CB, Alexander JW. Clinical experience with segmental pancreatic allografts. Transpl Proc 16:692–694, 1984.
21. Sutherland DER, Goetz FC, Najarian JS. Pancreas transplantation. Clin Endocrin & Metabol 11:549–578, 1982.
22. Sutherland DER, Najarian JS, Greenberg BZ, Senske BJ, Anderson GE, Francis RS, Goetz FC. Hormonal and metabolic effects of an endocrine graft: vascularized segmental transplantation on the pancreas in insulin-dependent patients. Ann Int Med 95:537–541, 1981.
23. Pozza G, Traeger J, Dubernard JM, Serdri A, Pontiroli AE, Boss E, Malik MC, Ruitton A, Blanc N. Endocrine responses of type I (insulin-dependent) diabetic patients following successful pancreas transplantation. Diabetologia 24:244–248, 1983.
24. Sutherland DER, Kendall D. Pancreas transplant registry data. Transpl Today 2:56–67, 1985.
25. Standards Committee of the American Society of Transplant Surgeons. Current results and expectations of renal transplantation. J Am Med Assoc 246:1330–1331, 1981.

26. Sutherland DER, Morrow CE, Fryd DS, Ferguson RM, Simmons RL, Najarian JS. Improved patient and primary renal allograft survival in uremic diabetic recipients. Transplantation 34:-319–325, 1982.
27. Lillehei RC, Simmons RL, Najarian JS, et al. Pancreatico-duodenal allotransplantation: experimental and clinical experience. Ann Surg 172:405–436, 1970.
28. Calne RY. Paratopic segmental pancreas grafting: a technique with portal venous drainage. Lancet 1:595–597, 1984.
29. Gliedman ML, Gold M, Whittaker J, Rifkin H, Soberman R, Freed S, Tellis V, Veith FJ. Clinical segmental pancreatic transplantation with ureter—pancreatic duct anastomosis for exocrine drainage. Surgery 74:171–180, 1973.
30. Dubernard JM, Traeger J, Neyra P, Touraine JL, Tranchant D, Blanc-Brunat, N. A new method of preparation of segmental pancreatic grafts for transplantation: trials in dogs and in man. Surgery 84:633–639, 1978.
31. Bjorken C, Lundgren G, Ringden O, Groth CG. A technique for rapid harvesting of cadaveric renal and pancreatic grafts after circulating arrest. Brit J Surg 63:517–519, 1976.
32. Sutherland DER, Goetz FC, Najarian JS. Living related donor segmental pancreatectomy for transplantation. Transpl Proc 12 (No. 4, Suppl. 2):33–39, 1980.
33. Chinn P, Sutherland DER, Goetz FC, Elick BA, Najarian JS. Metabolic effects of hemipancreatectomy in living related graft donors. Transplant Proc 16:11–17, 1984.
34. Sutherland DER, Goetz FC, Najarian JS. Pancreas transplants from related donors. Transplantation 38:625–633, 1984.
35. Starzl TE, Iwatsuki S, Shaw BW, et al. Pancreaticoduodenal transplantation in humans. Surg Gynecol Obstet 159:265–272, 1984.
36. Sutherland DER, Chinn PL, Elick BA, et al. Maximization of islet mass in pancreas grafts by near total or total whole organ excision without duodenum from cadaver donors. Transplant Proc 16:115–119, 1984.
37. Sollinger H, Hoffmann R, Belzer F. One year experience with pancreatico–cystostomy in human pancreas transplantation. Transpl Proc 17: 1985, in press.
38. Blanc-Brunat N, Dubernard JM, Touraine JL, et al. Pathology of the pancreas after intraductal neoprene injection in dogs and diabetic patients treated by pancreatic transplantation. Diabetologia 25:97, 1983.
39. Sutherland DER, Goetz FC, Najarian JS. Intraperitoneal transplantation of immediately vascularized segmental pancreatic grafts without duct litigation: a clinical trial. Transplantation 28:-485–491, 1979.
40. Groth CG, Lundgren G, Arner P, Cellste H, Hardstedt C, Lewander R, Ostman J. Rejection of isolated pancreatic allografts in patients with diabetes. Surg Gynecol & Obstet 143:933–940, 1976.
41. Sutherland DER, Ascher NL, Najarian JS. Pancreas transplantation. In: Manual of Organ Transplantation, Najarian JS, Simmons RL, (eds). New York: Springer-Verlag, 1984, pp. 237–254.
42. Sutherland DER, Goetz FC, Elick BA, Najarian JS. Experience with 49 segmental pancreas transplants in 45 diabetic patients. Transplantation 34:330–338, 1982.
43. Calne RY, White DJG, Rolles K, et al. Renal and segmental pancreatic grafting with drainage of exocrine secretions and initial continuous intravenous cyclosporin A in a patients with insulin-dependent diabetes and renal failure. Brit Med J 285:677–680, 1982.
44. Gil-Vernet JM, Fernandez-Cruz L, Corolps A, et al. Clinical experience with pancreaticopyelostomy for exocrine pancreatic drainage and portal venous drainage in pancreas transplantation. Transpl Proc 17:342–345, 1985.
45. Sutherland DER. Current status of clinical pancreas and islet transplantation with comments on need for and complications of cyrogenic and other preservation techniques. Cryobiology 20:-245–255, 1983.
46. Florack G, Sutherland DER, Chinn PL, et al. Clinical experience with transplantation of hypothermically preserved pancreas grafts. Transplant Proc 16:153–155, 1984.
47. Najarian JS, Sutherland DER, Matas AJ, Steffes MW, Goetz FC. Human islet transplantation: a preliminary experience. Transpl Proc 9:233–236, 1977.
48. Sutherland DER, Matas AJ, Najarian JS. Pancreatic islet cell transplantation. Surg Clinics of No Amer 58:365–382, 1978.
49. Sutherland DER, Matas AJ, Goetz FC, Najarian JS. Transplantation of dispersed pancreatic islet tissue in humans: autografts and allografts. Diabetes 29 (Suppl 1):31–44, 1980.

50. Sutherland DER, Goetz FC, Carpenter AM, et al. Pancreatico–duodenal grafts: clinical and pathological observations in uremic versus nonuremic recipients. In: Transplantation and Clinical Immunology, Vol. X, Touraine JL, et al. (eds). Amsterdam: Excerpta Medica, 1979, pp. 90–195.

51. Sutherland DER, Goetz FC, Rynasiewicz JJ, Baumgartner D, White DC, Elick BA, Najarian JS. Segmental pancreas transplantation from living related and cadaver donors: a clinical experience. Surgery 90:159–169, 1981.

52. Sutherland DER, Goetz FC, Kendall DM, Najarian JS. Effect of donor source, technique, immunosuppression and presence or absence of end stage diabetic nephropathy on outcome in pancreas transplant recipients. Transpl Proc 17:325–330, 1985.

53. Sutherland DER, Chinn PL, Goetz FC, et al. Experience with cyclosporine vs. azathioprine for pancreas transplantation. Transplant Proc 15:2606–2612, 1983.

54. Rynasiewicz JJ, Sutherland DER, Ferguson RM, et al. Cyclosporin A for immunosuppression: observations in rat heart, pancreas and islet allograft models and in human renal and pancreas transplantation. Diabetes 31 (Suppl. 4):92–108, 1982.

54. Sibley RK, Mukai K. Pathological features in 29 segmental pancreas transplants in 27 diabetic patients. Lab Invest 48:78A, 1983.

55. Sutherland DER, Sibley RK, Chinn PL, et al. Identical twin pancreas transplants: reversal and recurrence of pathogenesis in type I diabetes. Clin Res 32 (2):561A, 1984.

56. Sibley RK, Sutherland DER, Goetz FC. Recurrence of type I diabetes mellitus in pancreatic allografts and isografts. Lab Invest 50:54A, 1984.

57. Secchi A, Pontiroli AE, Traeger J, et al. A method of early detection of graft failure in pancreas transplantation. Transplantation 35:344–348, 1983.

58. Traeger J, Bosi E, Dubernard JM, et al. Thirty months experience with cyclosporine in human pancreatic transplantation. Diabetologia 27:154–156, 1984.

59. Sutherland DER, Bentley FR, Mauer SM, Menth L, Nylander W, Goetz FC, Barbosa J, Ascher NL, Simmons RL, Najarian JS. A report of 26 diabetic renal allograft recipients alive with functioning grafts at 10 or more years after primary transplantation. Diabetic Neprhopathy 3:39–43, 1984.

60. Barker CF, Naji A, Perloff LJ, Dafoe DC, Bartlett S. Invited commentary: an overview of pancreas transplantation—biologic aspects. Surgery 92:113–137, 1982.

61. Faustman D, Hauptfeld V, Lacy P, Davie J. Prolongation of murine islet allograft survival by pretreatment of islets with antibody directed to Ia determinants. Proc Natl Acad Sci USA 78(8):5156–5159, 1981.

62. Clark WH. (ed.) Proceedings of a workshop on preventing the rejection of transplanted pancreas or islets. Diabetes 31 (Suppl. 4):1–116, 1982.

63. Health Care Financing Administration (IICFA) Office of Special Programs. End-Stage Renal Disease Program Medical Information System, Facility Survey Tables, Department of Health and Human Services, USA, HCFA. January 1–December 31, 1981.

64. West KM. Epidemiology of diabetes and its vascular lesions. New York: Elsevier, 1978.

65. Bart KJ, Macon EJ, Whittier FC, Baldwin RJ, Blount JH. Cadaveric kidneys for transplantation. A paradox of shortage in the face of plenty. Transplantation 31:379–387, 1981.

66. Rosenbloom AL, Silverstein JH, Lezotte DC, Richardson K, McCallum RN. Limited joint mobility in childhood diabetes mellitus indicates increased risk for microvascular disease. N Eng J Med 305:191–194, 1981.

67. Merimee TJ, Zapf J, Froesch ER. Insulin-like growth factors. Studies in diabetes with and without retinopathy. N Engl J Med 309:527–530, 1983.

10. PRESERVATION OF THE COMPROMISED FOOT IN DIABETIC NEPHROPATHY

THOMAS A. EINHORN

Lower limb amputation is an ever-present fear for the diabetic patient. Levine has stated that 10% of all hospitalizations for diabetics are caused by infection, and that 25% of these involve the foot [1]. Should amputation of a lower extremity be performed, 42% of diabetics will lose their contralateral limb within two years, and 56% within three to five years [2].

The fundamental problems compromising the diabetic foot are vascular insufficiency and peripheral neuropathy. The vascular disease is a result of reduced blood flow in the tibial and popliteal arteries (as opposed to the femoral and iliac arteries in nondiabetics). Complaints of intermittent claudication and pain at night signal the onset of this condition. The neuropathy results in perforating ulcers due to unperceived pressure, and decreased perspiration leading to skin cracks and fissures (potential for infection). Loss of vibratory sense, position sense, and foot drop indicate an existing neuropathic process. Thus, as peripheral neuropathy permits small irritations and calluses to progress to perforating ulcers, neurovascular insufficiency reduces blood supply and prevents wounds from healing [1]. In the diabetic renal transplant recipient, the problem of wound healing may be further compounded by the use of immunosuppressive agents such as glucocorticoids [3–5] azathioprine [5], and cyclosporine A [6], depressing the early inflammatory and cellular phases of wound repair and increasing the propensity for infection.

Although the incidence of lower limb amputation after renal transplantation has been reported as high as 17% [7], recent advances in the management of the diabetic

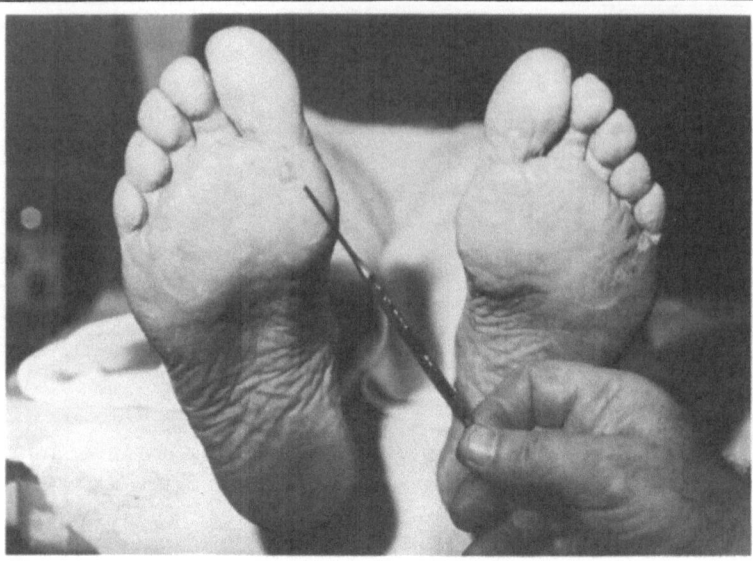

Figure 10–1. The lesion initially presented as a small (1 cm diameter) full-thickness defect over the first metatarsal head.

foot provide a new surgical technology. The results achieved in a large series of diabetic feet have been outstanding [8, 9]. Success is dependent upon a team effort and an aggressive approach toward the problem.

The day-to-day management of the diabetic foot requires the participation of the patient, podiatrist, primary physician, and when necessary, a home-care attendant. The goals of management include optimum metabolic control, prevention of mechanical skin irritation by a poorly fitted shoe, foot hygiene including both mild washing and meticulous drying, and the constant trimming of nails and calluses. It is widely held that the initiating event in a diabetic foot ulcer is direct pressure either by the shoe or an unattended callus. Prevention is certainly the key to management. It must be remembered, however, that the ability of the patient to participate effectively in prophylactic measures can be severely impaired if vision is suboptimal. For this reason, visits to the physician should be frequent; and at the earliest sign of skin irritation, a home-care attendant should be strongly considered when economically feasible.

Once a lesion has developed, be it in the form of mild irritation with peripheral cellulitis or advanced gangrene, a rational plan of treatment should be instituted immediately. With few exceptions, this should begin with admission to the hospital. The fundamental steps of treatment will then involve: (1) optimum control of blood glucose; (2) nutritional assessment and intervention if needed; and (3) surgical evaluation and treatment based upon a step-by-step protocol.

Control of blood glucose is often difficult in the presence of an infected wound. Careful monitoring utilizing an intravenous insulin pump may be required as a

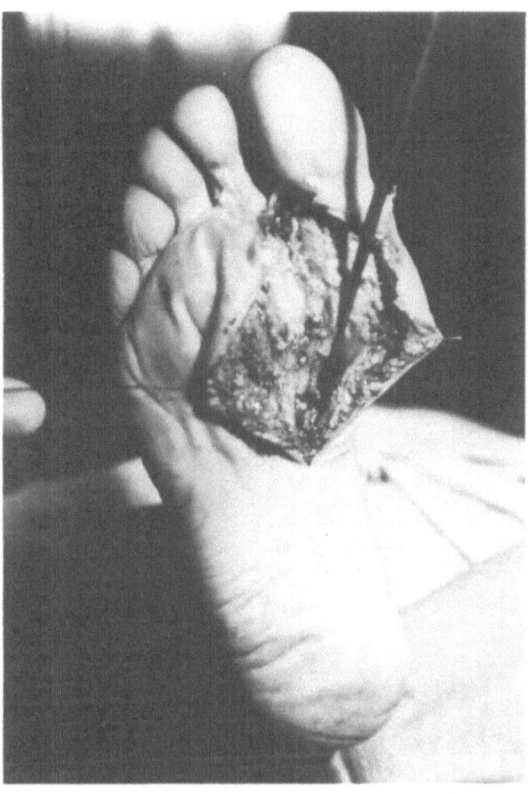

Figure 10–2. Serial debridements of the small ulcer resulted in a large, nonhealing wound involving most of the plantar surface of the forefoot.

temporary measure. Nutritional assessment has repeatedly been shown to be important in optimizing wound healing in the diabetic [10, 11, 12]. The impaired humoral and cell-mediated immunity that accompanies protein-calorie malnutrition increases susceptibility to infection [13]. A simple method for assessing nutritional status utilizes routine parameters obtained on admission blood studies. A serum albumin level of less than 3.5 grams per deciliter, or a total lymphocyte count of less than 1,500 cells per cubic millimeter, or both, are accepted as evidence of preexisting malnutrition [14, 15]. The total lymphocyte count is determined by calculating the product of the white blood cell count and the percentage of lymphocytes on the differential count (i.e., total lymphocyte count = white blood cell count $\times$ percentage of lymphocytes [cells per mm^3]). Once a state of malnutrition has been shown, a carefully designed program of nutritional repletion should be instituted. This will involve a joint effort on the parts of the primary physician and a member of the nutritional support staff.

The surgical protocol begins with a classification system to which all feet can be assigned. The system utilized at the State University of New York, Downstate

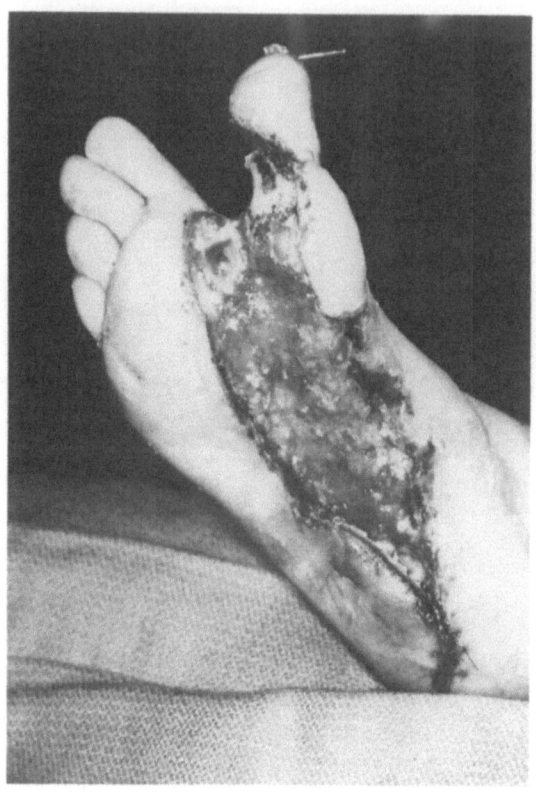

Figure 10–3. Surgical reconstruction of the forefoot was begun by detaching the origins of the abductor hallucis and flexor hallucis brevis muscles and transposing them distally. An attempt was made to preserve the great toe by performing a partial proximal phalangectomy, shortening the distance needed for the muscle transposition and covering the distal-most parts of the wound.

Medical Center, is shown in table 10–1. A plan of treatment can then be designed commensurate with the grade of the lesion:

Grade I. Treatment of Grade I lesions involves redistribution of weight-bearing forces and extrinsic pressures. The method of redistributing pressure often in-

Table 10–1.

Grade I—Superficial irritation
Grade II—Superficial ulcer with cellulitis
Grade III—Deep ulcer with cellulitis but no osteomyelitis
Grade IV—Deep ulcer with osteomyelitis
Grade V—Gangrene

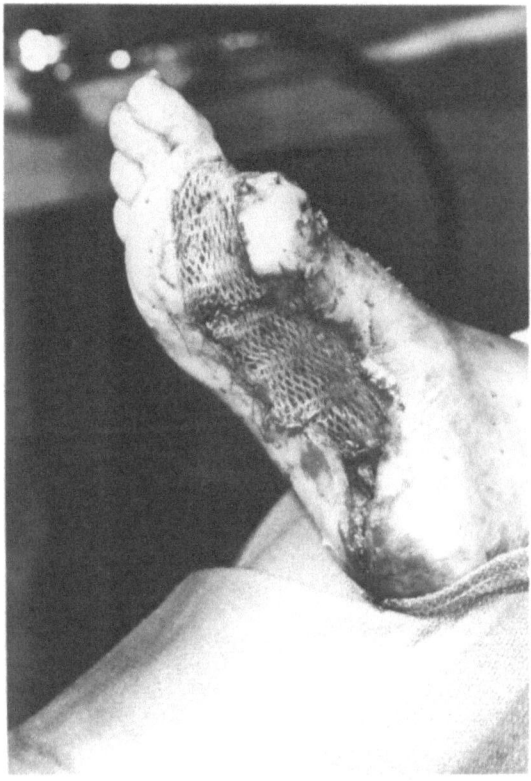

Figure 10–4. The muscle transposition was successful but only as far distal as the first metatarsal head. The great toe could not be salvaged and was disarticulated through the metatarsal-phalangeal joint. A meshed (1.5 to 1) split-thickness skin graft was applied to the remainder of the wound.

volves the use of custom orthotic shoe inserts. If the area of irritation is on the lateral or dorsal aspects of the foot, a slipper or cut-out shoe eliminating all direct pressure on the lesion can be useful.

Grade II. Treatment of Grade II lesions includes that described for Grade I with additional attention directed to the care of the superficial wound. This involves the introduction of antibiotic therapy, followed by sharp debridement and wet-to-dry dressing changes. Antibiotic therapy should be directed toward treating a polymicrobial infection. After obtaining aerobic and anaerobic cultures as well as drawing serum creatinine and blood urea nitrogen levels, the following agents can be used:

1. Oral therapy: amoxicillin in combination with cavulonic acid (a B-lactamase inhibitor).
2. Intravenous therapy: cefoxitin (up to 12 gms per day), or an aminoglycoside in combination with either clindamycin or metronidazole. Blood urea nitro-

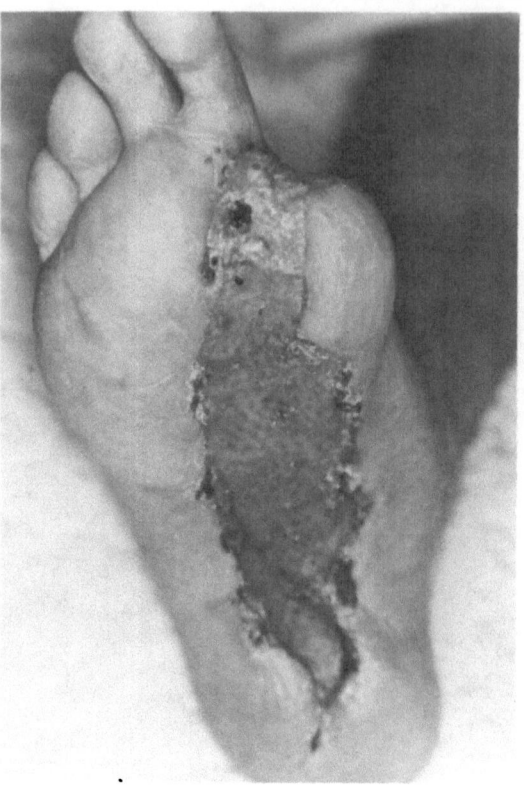

Figure 10–5. The skin graft was successful as demonstrated by this photograph taken three weeks after surgery. Weight bearing with the aid of a custom-molded shoe orthotic was begun at six weeks.

gen and serum creatinine levels should be carefully monitored to avoid iatrogenic deterioration of the already compromised kidneys or renal allograft.

At this point, a vascular evaluation including a Doppler examination is indicated. Based on the Doppler examination, an Ischemic Index is calculated by dividing the dorsalis pedis or posterior tibial pulse pressure (mm Hg) by the brachial pulse pressure. If the Ischemic Index is less than 0.45, vascular bypass surgery to improve distal blood flow should be considered [1]. This may possibly increase the chances of success for wound healing. Once a satisfactory vascular status is established or obtained, wet-to-dry dressing changes, three times per day is begun. If this is not sufficient to promote adequate granulation, enzymatic debridement with trypsin containing agents can be employed. After each dressing change, an ace bandage is applied in such a way as to prevent edema but not compromise blood supply. Attention to prevention of edema cannot be overemphasized.

In many cases treatment of small Grade II lesions, as outlined above, will result in slow but spontaneous wound healing. When well-granulating wounds are too large for spontaneous closure, a meshed, split-thickness skin graft should be applied. We have found that a graft thickness of $15/1,000$ of an inch, and a mesh ratio of 1 to 1.5 are the optimum specifications for skin grafts in diabetic wounds. This provides a graft that is thin enough to "take" in a poorly vascularized bed, and permits drainage of edema fluid. After the graft is inset into the bed of granulation, it is covered with a sterile cotton and mineral oil stent. No sutures are required. Instead, attention should be directed toward obtaining skin-to-wound contact in all areas. The patient is then confined to bed rest with the foot slightly elevated (one pillow is sufficient). After one week, the operative dressing is removed. Follow-up care then involves light sterile dressings and application of an ace bandage until full epithelialization is achieved. Weight bearing directly on the graft is not permitted until six weeks following full epithelialization. Prior to weight-bearing, a complete gait and force-plate analysis of ambulatory dynamics should be performed. This information is then utilized to construct an orthotic shoe insert redistributing weight-bearing forces and unloading pressure from the graft site.

Grade III. Treatment of Grade III lesions differs from Grade II in the method of surgical care only. In these wounds, a large defect is present, and an adequate source of fibroblasts for granulation tissue is absent. For this reason, a local muscle transposition is utilized to reconstruct the foot. This involves origin detachment of one or more of the small muscles of the foot with implantation of the detached ends into the lesion [8, 9]. This method not only covers the defect with viable muscle tissue but also promotes granulation from the depths of the wound as a result of the high capillary density in the transposed muscle [8]. The wound is then treated with a split thickness skin graft and is managed postoperatively as described for Grade II treatment. Occasionally, a Grade II lesion can present as a Grade III defect after extensive surgical debridement. Figures 10–1 through 10–5 illustrate a typical case where a small ulcer over the first metatarsal head resulted in an infected nonhealing wound. Although amputation was recommended, extensive debridement, muscle transposition, and split-thickness skin grafting resulted in a functional, weight-bearing foot.

Grade IV. When osteomyelitis is present, treatment must begin with removal of all infected and necrotic bone and soft tissue. Since a return to ambulation (as opposed to a cosmetic result) is the goal of foot care, amputation of the toes and metatarsals should be performed when necessary. Foot reconstruction is then achieved by leaving the wound open and reinspecting it in 48 to 72 hours. At that time, a decision should be made as to whether a delayed primary closure could be performed or if further wound care followed by skin grafting is needed. If the wound remains recalcitrant to treatment, further debridement or restrictions may be required.

Grade V. While gangrene has previously been thought to be an indication for foot amputation, this is not always the case. When the extent of the lesion involves less than the entire foot, radical resection of all necrotic tissue, followed by a similar approach as that outlined in Grade III and IV lesions, often proves successful.

While the above scheme of care provides hope for preservation of the diabetic-nephropathic foot, it should be remembered that function is the most important result of treatment. Amputation at an appropriate level is often preferable to heroic surgical procedures involving prolonged hospitalizations and excessive physical and emotional stresses. Each patient requires an individual plan of care which is tailored to his or her physical, emotional, and socioeconomic needs.

REFERENCES

1. Levin MC, O'Neal LW. The diabetic foot, Levin ME, O'Neal, LW (eds). St. Louis: C.V. Mosby Co., 1977.
2. Levin ME. The diabetic foot. J Am Podiatry Assoc 66:825–839, 1976.
3. Goforth P, Gudas CJ. Effects of steroids on wound healing: a review of the literature. J Foot Surg 19:22–28, 1980.
4. Shamberger RC, Devereux DF, Brennan MF. The effect of chemotherapeutic agents on wound healing. Int Adv Surg Oncol 4:15–58, 1981.
5. Goldberg M, Lima O, Morgan E, Azabe HA, Luk S, Ferdman A, Peters WJ, Cooper JD. A comparison between cyclosporin A and methylprednisolone plus azathioprine on bronchial healing following canine lung autotransplantation. J Thorac Cardiovasc Surg 85:821–286, 1983.
6. Efron G. Cyclosporine A impairs wound healing in rats. J Surg Res 34:572–575, 1983.
7. Peters C, Sutherland DER, Simmons RL, Fryd DS, Najarian JS. Patient and graft survival in amputated vs. non-amputated diabetic primary renal allograft recipients. Transplantation 32:-498–503, 1981.
8. Ger R. Muscle transposition in the management of perforating ulcers of the forefoot. Clin Orthop. 175:186–189, 1983.
9. Ger R. Considerations in the surgical management of ulcers of the foot in the diabetic patient. Diab Nephr 3:12–14, 1984.
10. Cannon PR, Wissler RW, Woolridge RL, Benditt EP The relationship of protein deficiency to surgical infection. Ann Surg 120:514–525, 1944.
11. Mullen JL, Gertner MH, Buzby GP, Goodhart GL, Rosato EF. Implications of malnutrition in the surgical patient. Arch Surg 114:121–125, 1979.
12. Dickhaut SC, DeLee JC, Page CP. Nutritional status: importance in predicting wound healing after amputation. J Bone Joint Surg 66(A): 71–75, 1984.
13. Bistrain BR, Blackburn GL, Sherman M, Scrimshaw NS. Therapeutic index of nutritional depletion in hospitalized patients. Surg Gynec and Obstet 141:512–516, 1975.
14. Seltzer MH, Fletcher HS, Slocum BA, and Engler PE. Instant nutritional assessment in the intensive care unit. J Parent and Ent Nutr 5:70–72, 1981.
15. Shetty DS, Jung RT, Watrasiewicz KE, James WPT. Rapid-turnover transport proteins: an index of subclinical protein energy malnutrition. Lancet 2:230–232, 1979.

11. MANAGING THE DIABETIC RENAL-RETINAL SYNDROME DURING PREGNANCY

CHARLES M. PETERSON
and
LOIS JOVANOVIC

Classification of Pregnancies Complicated by Diabetes

Pregnancy may occur in women who have preexisting diabetes mellitus, or diabetes may occur de novo during gestation. In the former instance, the diabetic woman is labelled as having pregestational diabetes, and in the latter instance the diabetes is classified as gestational. Pregestational diabetes is further subdivided according to whether the woman has lost residual islet cell function with a quantitative loss of B cell tissue and low circulating insulin levels (type I) or whether there is residual islet cell function with circulating insulin but qualitatively abnormal insulin secretion with insulin resistance (type II).

Gestational diabetes occurs during pregnancy and generally disappears following delivery of the infant. The peak onset of gestational diabetes falls between 27 and 30 weeks. For this reason, the risk of congenital malformations in the infant of the gestational diabetic woman appears to be no different than that of the nondiabetic population [1].

The White classification of diabetes in pregnancy (delineated by Priscilla White), includes prognostic factors for mother and fetus [3]. White tabulates diabetes's impact on pregnancy alphabetically, according to increasing presumed clinical severity and risk to the fetal maternal unit (table 11–1). Of note is that both renal disease and retinal disease were felt to carry a poor prognosis, and a separate category was created when the two risk factors existed together: the RF classification recently termed a renal-retinal syndrome by Friedman and L'Esperance.

Table 11–1. White classification

Class	Description
A	Glucose tolerance test abnormal; no symptoms, euglycemia maintained with treatment by diet but without insulin
B	Adult onset (age 20 or older) and short duration (less than 10 years)
C	Relatively young onset (age 1–19) or relatively long duration (10–19 years)
D	Very young onset (age less than 10) or very long duration (20 years or more) or evidence of background retinopathy
E	Pelvic vascular disease (determined by x-ray)
F	Renal disease (creatinine clearance less than 80 ml/min)
R	Proliferative retinopathy
RF	Both renal disease and proliferative retinopathy
G	Multiple failures in pregnancy
H	Arteriosclerotic heart disease
T	Pregnancy after renal transplantation

Tables 11–2 and 11–3 summarize the prognostically bad signs during pregnancy and the Pyke classification [4]. Both of these classifications recognize that renal disease or infection imports a poor prognosis for the pregnancy.

The literature substantiates the thesis that coexistence of renal disease and pregnancy is usually associated with a high rate of fetal wastage. A normal gestational course is rare when preconception serum creatinine is greater than 3.0 mg/dl and/or the blood urea nitrogen (BUN) is greater than 30 mg/dl. In a 10-year study, McKay reported no fetal survivor when the BUN exceeded 60 mg/dl[5]. Kitzmiller and associates also addressed the issue of perinatal outcome in pregnancies complicated by diabetic nephropathy [6]. In 36 patients with nephropathy, spon-

Table 11–2. Prognostically bad signs during pregnancy

1. Clinical pyelonephritis (Culture positive urinary infection with temperature over 39° centigrade)
2. Precoma or acidosis (venous bicarbonate less than 17 mEq/liter)
3. Pregnancy-induced hypertension
4. Neglectors

Table 11–3. Pyke classification

Type of diabetes	Description
Gestational diabetes	Diabetes that starts during pregnancy and goes away after the pregnancy
Pregestational diabetes	Diabetes that began before conception and continues after the pregnancy
Pregestational diabetes complicated by vascular disease	Retinopathy, nephropathy, pelvic vessels, or peripheral vascular disease

taneous abortion occurred in 4, and elective abortions in 5, while the rest delivered live infants after 27 weeks' gestation. Of the 26 live births, all survived their perinatal period. Little information is available regarding the course of the renal disease in the mothers.

RATIONALE FOR EUGLYCEMIA DURING PREGNANCY

Our own experience, and that of others, with programs for diabetic pregnant women based on the premise that establishing euglycemia as reflected by blood glucose measurements performed by the patient, indicates that a modified classification may be warranted (table 11–4). Preliminary studies suggest that problems associated with each stage of gestation (table 11–5) can be avoided if glucose is normalized before, during, and after gestation [7–12].

NATURAL HISTORY OF MATERNAL RENAL FUNCTION DURING NORMAL AND DIABETIC PREGNANCY

Few studies have been performed on the influence of pregnancy on diabetic renal disease if normoglycemia is achieved throughout gestation. We have had the opportunity to follow 105 diabetic women with studies of renal function prior to gestation, at 5 weeks' gestation, between 38–40 weeks' gestation, and at 6 weeks postpartum [13, 14]. Proteinuria was absent in the 49 White class B patients and the 34 White class C patients. Proteinuria of greater than 150 grams per 24 hours occurred during gestation in 2 of 14 White class D patients with backround retinopathy or White class R patients who had pregestational proteinuria of 100

Table 11–4. Modified classification of Jovanovic and Peterson

1. Good metabolic control documented: fasting blood glucose 55–70 mg/dl, mean 84 mg/dl, postprandial less than 140 mg/dl
2. Less than optimal control
   2.1. Not documented
   2.2. Documented outside recommended guidelines
3. Hypertension
   3.1. Good metabolic control
   3.2. Less than optimal metabolic control

Table 11–5. Problems associated with maternal hyperglycemia by trimester

First trimester	Second trimester	Third trimester
Malformations	Hypertrophic cardiomyopathy	Hypoglycemia
Growth retardation	Polyhydramnios	Hypocalcemia
Fetal wastage	Erythremia	Hyperbilirubinemia
	Placental insufficiency	Respiratory distress
	Preeclampsia	Macrosomia
	Fetal Loss	Hypomagnesemia
		Intrauterine demise

and 140 mg/24 hours. All eight women in White classes F or RF showed proteinuria greater than 250 mg/24 hours prior to gestation. In all eight, proteinuria increased during gestation, but in only two cases did proteinuria exceed 1.5 grams per 24 hours. Peak proteinuria in these two cases was 11 and 9 grams per 24 hours in the third trimester. Postpartum proteinuria returned to prepartum values in all cases. Therefore, pregnancy did not appear to have an adverse effect on maternal proteinuria except in persons with preexisting proteinuria. Even in the presence of preexisting proteinuria, pregnancy-induced rises in proteinuria appear transient and reversible postpartum if euglycemia was maintained throughout gestation.

Creatinine clearance during gestation showed markedly different patterns of response between the different White classes. In White class B patients, the pregestational creatinine clearance was 91 $\pm$ 14 S.D. ml/min which rose significantly to 140 $\pm$ 15 ml/min at 5 weeks, and then decreased to 110 $\pm$ 20 ml/min at 38–40 weeks and 98 $\pm$ 8 ml/min postpartum similar to the response reported in normal pregnant women [15–19].

White class C women had a mean pregestational creatinine clearance of 87 $\pm$ 10 ml/min that rose to 127 $\pm$ 14 ml/min at 5 weeks, 124 $\pm$ 16 ml/min at 38–40 weeks, and decreased to 102 $\pm$ 12 ml/min postpartum. Although not statistically significant, these women with longer duration diabetes appeared to have a slightly blunted rise in creatinine clearance in the first trimester. Nevertheless postpartum creatinine clearance actually increased somewhat when compared to pregestational values.

Women in White class D, with background retinopathy, and class R had elevated pregestational creatinine clearance values of 111 $\pm$ 15 ml/min, which rose to 127 $\pm$ 10 ml/min at 5 weeks, and showed an even further increase to 145 $\pm$ 16 ml/min at 38–40 weeks. Creatinine clearance in these groups actually decreased to more normal values of 101 $\pm$ 10 ml/min postpartum when compared with pregestational values.

Even more impressive were the changes in creatinine clearance in White classes F and RF. These women had a mean creatinine clearance of 65 $\pm$ 7 ml/min prior to gestation, a value significantly lower that that seen in the other groups. This group also showed a rise in creatinine clearance throughout pregnancy to 95 $\pm$ 17 ml/min at 5 weeks, and 104 $\pm$ 18 ml/min at 38–40 weeks. Six weeks postpartum, creatinine clearance was 84 $\pm$ 17 ml/min, a value significantly ($p < 0.01$) increased when compared to pregestational values.

Thus, the renal response to gestation varies with White class during pregnancy complicated by diabetes mellitus. Increasing duration of diabetes appears to lead to an initial increase in creatinine clearance as seen in the White classes D and R which, with further passage of time, results in decreased creatinine clearance as observed in White classes RF and F. In no White class did pregnancy superimposed on diabetes lead to deterioration in renal function postpartum in terms of proteinuria or creatinine clearance. In fact, in each White class, postpartum creatinine clearance appeared to normalize when compared with pregestational testing.

NATURAL HISTORY OF MATERNAL OCULAR STATUS DURING NORMAL AND DIABETIC PREGNANCY

To date, few prospective studies of ocular status have been performed in diabetics during gestation since the advent of techniques for achieving and maintaining normoglycemia throughout gestation. Furthermore, it is current practice, at most centers, to treat underlying ocular pathology prior to advising conception. Therefore, few data are available analogous to the above data on renal function. Our own experience suggests that the risk of pregnancy initiating clinically important ocular pathology is negligible, and that the risk of worsening established diabetic eye disease can be minimized if careful surveillance is instituted [14].

APPROACHES TO NORMALIZING BLOOD GLUCOSE THROUGHOUT GESTATION

A number of approaches to normalizing blood glucose throughout gestation have been published [4, 6–12, 20, 21]. Inherent to the success of these programs is the monitoring of self-blood glucose determinations by the patient before and after meals and at times of potential low or high blood glucose values. In our experience, a creatinine clearance as low as 40 ml/min does not affect the 24-hour insulin requirement. First trimester insulin requirements remain at 0.7 units/Kg/24 hours rising to 0.8 units/Kg/24 hours at 26 weeks, 0.9 units/Kg/24 hours at 32 weeks, and 1.0 units/Kg/24 hours after the 36th week of gestation. Blood glucose monitoring before and one hour after each meal allows the patient to maintain and document blood glucoses in the normal range. Glucosylated hemoglobins may be used to verify normality at monthly intervals.

The goal of nutritional therapy during gestation is to maintain optimum maternal and fetal nutrition. It is also felt that optimum nutrition avoids maternal ketonuria. Weight gain during gestation should be 12.5 Kg to term. These goals can be attained even in the presence of renal disease with a diet prescribed at 30 kilocalories/Kg present pregnant weight. Dietary composition during gestation is targeted at 40% carbohydrate, 40% fat, and 20% protein. Breakfast can only comprise about 12% of daily caloric intake due to the increased glucose intolerance seen in the morning, which appears to be potentiated by pregnancy.

CONCLUSION

As programs of improved maternal glucose control have resulted in improved outcome of pregnancies associated with diabetes, an increasing number of diabetic women are contemplating pregnancy. Women with a diabetic renal-retinal syndrome now consider establishing families. Recent reports document the view that normalization of maternal blood glucose levels throughout gestation is associated with neonatal morbidity and mortality not differing from the nondiabetic population. The effect on the mother of pregnancy with maintained euglycemia has been less well studied.

We believe that diabetic renal disease does not progress during normoglycemic gestation and may even improve as reflected by normalization of creatinine clearance postpartum when compared to pregestational values. Anatomical correlates of these physiological observations remain to be documented. The influence of normoglycemic pregnancy on diabetic ocular disease, however, remains to be studied, but frequent ophthamologic surveillance combined with modern treatment appears to avoid deterioration in the ocular status of diabetic women during pregnancy. Long-term studies in diabetics relating the postpartum course of renal or retinal disease have not been performed. Therefore, while the prognosis for pregnancy in diabetes appears excellent for mother and infant, the long-term responsibility of parenthood must be emphasized to the couple especially in the presence of maternal renal or retinal pathology.

REFERENCES

1. National Diabetes Data Group. Classification and diagnosis of diabetes mellitus and other categories of glucose intolerance. Diabetes 28: 1039–1057, 1979.
2. Neufeld ND. Gestational diabetes and congenital anomalies. In: Diabetes and Pregnancy: Teratology, Toxicology, and Treatment. Jovanovic L, Fuhrmann K, Peterson CM (eds). New York: Praeger, 1985, in press.
3. White P. Diabetes mellitus in pregnancy. Clinical Perinatology 1: 331–339, 1974.
4. Jovanovic L, Peterson CM. Diabetes and pregnancy. In: Principles of Obstetrics, Kaplan RM (ed). Baltimore: Williams and Wilkins, 1982, pp. 168–180.
5. McKay EV. Pregnancy and renal disease: a ten-year survey. Australia and New Zealand J. of Obstet and Gynecol 3: 21–27, 1963.
6. Kitzmiller JL, Brown ER, Philippe M. Diabetic nephropathy and perinatal outcome. Am J Obstet and Gynecol 141: 741–744, 1981.
7. Jovanovic L, Druzin M, Peterson CM. Effect of euglycemia on the outcome of pregnancy in insulin-dependent diabetic women as compared with normal control subjects. Am J of Med 71: 921–927, 1981.
8. Coustan DR, Berkowitz RL, Hobbins JC. Tight metabolic control of overt diabetes in pregnancy. Am J of Med 68: 845–852, 1980.
9. Roversi GD, Gargiulo M, Nicolini U, Pedretti E, Marini A, Barbarani V, Peneff P. A new approach to the treatment of diabetic pregnant women. Am J of Obstet and Gynecol 135: 567–576, 1979.
10. Adashi EY, Pinto H, Tyson JE. Impact of maternal euglycemia on fetal outcome in diabetic pregnancy. Am J of Obstet and Gynecol 133: 268–274, 1979.
11. Miller JM. A reappraisal of "tight control" in diabetic pregnancies. Am J of Obstet and Gynecol 147: 158–162, 1983.
12. Fuhrmann K, Reiher H, Semmler K, Fischer F, Fischer M, Glockner E. Prevention of congenital malformations in infants of insulin-dependent diabetic mothers. Diabetes Care 6: 219–223, 1983.
13. Jovanovic , and Peterson CM. Is pregnancy contraindicated in women with diabetes mellitus? Diabetic Nephropathy 3: 36–38, 1984.
14. Jovanovic L, Chang S, and Peterson CM. The interaction of pregnancy and diabetic renal/retinal disease. Diabetes 32: 28A, 1983.
15. Davison JM, Dunlop W, Ezimokhai M. Twenty four hour creatinine clearance during the third trimester of normal pregnancy. Brit J of Obstet and Gynecol 87: 106–109, 1980.
16. Davison JM, Noble MDB. Serial changes in 24-hour creatinine clearance during normal menstrual cycles and the first trimester of pregnancy. Brit J of Obstet and Gynecol 88: 10–17, 1981.
17. Davison JM. Changes in renal function and other aspects of homeostasis in early pregnancy. J of Obstet and Gynecol of the Brit Commonwealth 81: 1003–1006, 1974.
18. Ezimokhai M, Davison JM, Philips PR, Dunlop W. Non-postural serial changes in renal function during the third trimester of normal human pregnancy. Brit J of Obstet and Gynecol 88: 465–471, 1981.

19. Sims EAH, Krantz K. Serial studies of renal function during pregnancy and the puerperium in normal women. Obstet and Gynecol 44: 1764–1774, 1958.
20. Peterson CM, and Jovanovic L. The diabetes self care method. New York: Simon and Schuster, 1984.
21. Jovanovic L, Fuhrmann K, Peterson CM. (eds). Diabetes and pregnancy: teratology, toxicology and treatment. New York: Praeger, 1985.

12. NURSE TO NURSE: NURSING ROLE IN DIABETIC NEPHROPATHY MANAGEMENT

LINDA S. COHEN

Many health professionals are unaware of the devastating impact diabetic ne-phropathy has on its victims (patients and their families). These mainly young and middle-aged adults have experienced multiple losses and impairments affecting various bodily functions, which often lead to anxiety, despair, and defeat at a time in their lives when careers are beginning to develop, or they are raising a family, or buying a house. Now, instead of moving ahead with their lives, roadblocks are encountered, and fear abounds. There is the fear of the unknown, incapacitation fears, fear of pain, fear of abandonment by loved ones, fear of more complications, and fear of lost control of an illness that is "running wild." There are life-saving decisions to be made now, many specialists with whom to engage, new information to absorb, and tests to endure.

How can the health-care team meet the enormous needs of these individuals in a caring, efficient, and professional manner? One thing is certain: no one component of the health-care team can provide all the necessary interventions and support required by this complex group of patients in order for them to travel through the various stages of diabetic nephropathy and work toward maximal rehabilita-tion. Energy must be expended to allow for ongoing communication with patients and their families. Collaboration among the health-care team members is essential if they are to provide the multiple types of support for these people, as well as for members of the team themselves. This chapter presents our approach when dealing with diabetic nephropathic patients and their families.

Patients with diabetic nephropathy are managed by a team. Each patient is viewed as also having present or potential extrarenal complications of diabetes, requiring that our team have expertise in both diabetes and renal diseases.

The renal team usually sees diabetic patients between 15–20 years after the onset of diabetes. These patients bring with them the positive and negative adjustment patterns relating to their disease. Examples of poor adjustment patterns include:

1. Inactivity and overdependence on family members or the health-care team;
2. Over independence and denial of realistic dangers with increased risk-taking activities;
3. Withdrawal and resentment;
4. Denial of possible complications to a point of not following their health maintenance;
5. Manipulation by taking advantage of their disease to gain attention.

It has been our experience that these poor adjustment patterns are severe barriers that must be overcome in order to attain optimal rehabilitation.

As diabetic nephropathy is a chronic disease that has periods of crisis and resolutions on a continuum, it is more advantageous for the health-care team to work with active, informed, and involved patients and their families on an ongoing basis. Often patients can be their own most valuable resource (detecting and reporting physical and mental changes, knowing the range of key laboratory values, speaking up should care be inadequate or confusing, e.g., drugs, tests, medical, surgical or nursing attention, etc.). Support and encouragement of such involvement is mandatory for a true partnership to evolve allowing for the best possible outcome.

Listening to patients when first evaluated is instructive: "I never knew diabetes had anything to do with my kidneys, no one ever told me"; "I knew diabetes had something to do with the kidneys, but I never realized just what the kidneys do or how serious it was." Unfortunately, these comments are typical of the poor understanding uremic diabetics have of their illness. The genesis of the diabetic's misinformation lies in their inadequate prior relationship with health professionals. Frequently, the uremic diabetic's first presentation of kidney disease as a life threat comes during his/her first interview with our team—years after the actual onset of nephropathy.

No two diabetics are identical. Each, upon developing nephropathy, comes with his or her own unique qualities (physical, psychological, social, cultural, financial, and coping abilities). In analyzing an individual patient, it is helpful to divide the course of kidney involvement in diabetes into three stages requiring different interventions. For ease in use, the nurse educator's role is given in tabular form (table 12–1).

Table 12–1. Nurse-educator's role in diabetic nephropathy

Stage of nephropathy	Appropriate intervention
ASYMPTOMATIC KIDNEY IMPAIRMENT	
Proteinuric	1. Educate
Azotemic	2. Closely monitor kidney function
Hypertensive	3. Prevent further damage
	4. Supportive team approach
SYMPTOMATIC KIDNEY IMPAIRMENT	
Hypertensive	1. Educate-uremia therapy
Nephrotic	2. Prevent further damage
Uremic	3. Closely monitor kidney function
	4. Plan uremia therapy
PATIENTS RECEIVING UREMIA THERAPY	
Hemodialysis	1. Education
Peritoneal dialysis	2. Prevent further damage
Kidney transplant	3. Closely follow chemistries
	4. Change therapy if desired or needed

ASYMPTOMATIC KIDNEY IMPAIRMENT

Education of diabetic

To understand and ultimately "accept" his afflictions, the diabetic who is still asymptomatic may benefit from learning about the normal kidney and its functions. Concepts to cover (through discussion and visual aides) presented at the patients' level are:

1. Everyone normally has two kidneys, each weighing approximately a third of a pound. The size of a fist, kidneys are located in the back with the bottom of the kidney falling just below the lowest rib.
2. Blood is pumped by the heart and is carried to the kidneys. The blood delivered to the kidneys has delivered nutrients or food to other parts of the body, and has picked up waste products in return. These waste products in large quantities are toxic and must be removed.
3. The renal arteries bring blood to the kidneys, where it is filtered and then returned (cleansed) to the circulation by the renal veins.
4. The kidney contains nephrons (1 million in each). Nephrons are the basic filtering units of the kidney. Kidneys can filter 200 or more quarts of blood each day. The filtered material, urine, is drained from the kidney to the bladder. When the bladder contains a certain volume, a signal is sent to the brain and one feels the urge to urinate.
5. Major functions of the kidney:
   (a) Regulates fluid balance in the body. By reabsorbing or excreting water, the kidneys adjust to the level of fluid intake. When little water is ingested (in

the desert, for instance), most of the water filtered in the kidney is conserved and a dark, concentrated, scanty urine is a normal response.

(b) Eliminates waste products, drugs and toxins;

(c) Releases hormones that help control blood pressure;

(d) Releases a substance which stimulates the bone marrow to manufacture red blood cells;

(e) Helps maintain bone integrity by making an active form of Vitamin D which promotes absorption of calcium in the bowel during digestion.

6. Facts about diabetic nephropathy:

(a) Of type I diabetics 40% develop renal failure in a mean of 20 years from onset. (Data are not available on the type II diabetic, but a substantial proportion will develop renal failure.)

(b) Diabetics are 17 times more likely to develop renal failure than nondiabetics.

(c) At the onset of renal failure 97% of diabetics have retinopathy, and many will have lost vision.

CLOSELY MONITOR KIDNEY FUNCTION

Explain to patients all laboratory results and tests so that they can assume control and follow their own improvement, stability, or progression of disease.

Urinalysis.

Proteinuria is generally the first clue that the diabetic patient has kidney problems. The amount of protein excreted in the urine can be determined by obtaining a 24-hour urine collection which is then tested for protein. There is normally a small amount of protein present in the urine (up to 50 milligrams daily) and amounts in excess of this indicate disease.

Blood urea nitrogen (BUN).

This is a waste product that results from the body's breaking down protein food sources. A functioning kidney should remove this waste product, and its level is indicated by a blood test. A normal BUN is 8–20mg/100 ml (8–20 mg%). However, several factors might elevate this value, falsely suggesting kidney impairment. For example: an elevated BUN occurs in dehydration, internal bleeding, or in patients receiving steroid medications. A normal BUN level can also occur in a person with impaired renal function. For example: anorexia, avoiding protein intake, or not eating at all can result in a normal BUN in a person with kidney disease.

Creatinine.

This is one of the waste products of muscle breakdown or metabolism. Since muscles produce energy, even when they are at rest, creatinine is continually produced, which normally is then filtered and eliminated by the kidneys. The creatinine level in blood is not usually altered by diet or activity, though heavy meat eaters may have a transient rise for several hours after a meal. The normal serum creatinine value for a man is about 0.7 to 1.4 mg/100 ml and for a woman is 0.6 to 1.2 mg/100 ml. The creatinine does not rise above normal until 70% of renal function is lost.

Glomerular filtration rate (GFR).

This measures the rate at which certain substances are cleared from the blood by filters (glomeruli) in the kidneys. Creatinine clearance (C_{cr}) is approximately equal to the GFR and provides a good assessment of kidney function. To determine the creatinine clearance, a urine specimen is collected over 24 hours, or over some other timed interval, and one blood sample is taken during the same period. C_{cr} is the volume of blood cleared of creatinine in one minute (normal 90 to 160 ml/min depending on the age, sex, and size of the patient). The creatinine clearance can assess the current state of the kidneys, and the repeated serum creatinine levels can tell the direction of changes.

Hematocrit (Hct).

This is the percentage of the blood made up of red blood cells. A normal hematocrit is approximately 40% to 45%, and is higher in men than in women. People with chronic renal failure have a lower than normal Hct because of their kidney disease. If it becomes too low, a blood transfusion may be required. *Renal insufficiency* occurs when the GFR is about 25% of normal. *Uremia* occurs when the GFR is less than 5–10% of normal. It is between these stages that most patients develope symptoms of kidney disease. (See table 12–2).

PREVENT FURTHER DAMAGE

A diabetic who has proteinuria, increased BUN, or increased creatinine needs protection from any further insults to his remaining kidney function. For example:

Table 12–2. Correlation of creatinine clearance with signs and symptoms of uremia

Creatinine clearance	Signs and symptoms
Above 60 ml/min.	None
30–59 ml/min.	Subtle changes; impaired critical decision making ability; altered judgment; mild anemia; increased parathyroid hormone.
15–29 ml/min.	Reduced exercise tolerance; anorexia; restless legs; restricted affect; anemia; bone pain; pruritis.
5–15 ml/min.	"Sick all the time"; cold; nauseated; depressed; restless; reversed sleep pattern; waves of nausea; "metallic" taste.
2–5 ml/min.	Moribund; constantly bedridden; pericarditis; colitis; emesis; bleeding.
Below 2 ml/min.	Death

Dyes.

Contrast media dyes used for intravenous pyelograms (IVP), gallbladder x-rays, and/or computerized tomography (CAT scan), are known to decrease blood flow to the kidneys and may be directly toxic. The longer the contrast agents remain in the blood, the greater the chances for additional damage to the kidneys. This may accelerate the need for chronic uremia therapy. If studies employing contrast agents must be performed, the following may prove helpful: schedule the test or procedure in the morning so the patient does not have to be NPO (nothing by mouth) for a long period of time, which lessens the chance of dehydration; maintain hydration (intravenously) as well as providing a diuretic to help the kidneys excrete the dye; check lab values as well as urine output daily.

Urinary tract infection.

This can occur in a diabetic because of a neurogenic bladder which results in urinary stasis. Signs of neurogenic bladder are: large amounts of urine output during a single urination; residual urine in the bladder (decreased urine output, feeling full after urination, loss of urine after a cough). We advise diabetics to void at frequent, regular (hourly) intervals and to practice hygienic cleansing after a bowel movement. Urinary infection is treated promptly once detected by urine culture; the effectiveness of therapy is determined by re-culture after treatment. Urinary catheters should be avoided. The diabetic's risk of infection by catheter is increased because of a weaker immune response. We therefore catheterize only when absolutely necessary using careful sterile technique. Current evidence suggests that intermittent catheterization is less likely to cause infection than is an in-dwelling catheter.

Nephrotoxic drugs.

Drugs such as aminoglycosides should be avoided. If used, frequent monitoring of blood levels of the drug, plus monitoring of serum creatinine, blood urea nitrogen, and urine output are indicated to detect early kidney injury.

High blood pressure.

This is harmful to the kidneys and is a major cause of kidney failure in itself. Diabetics are at increased risk for development of high blood pressure because of blood vessel disease, and because of fluid overload as kidney function deteriorates. By controlling the blood pressure, diabetics may conserve as much as 9 ml/min of GFR per year, thereby forestalling the onset of uremia. Blood pressure can be controlled by medications, low salt diets, exercise, and relaxation techniques. Self-monitoring of blood pressure enables the patient to take a more active role in this effort by facilitating adjustments of medication and diet.

Blood glucose.

The positive effects of normalizing the blood glucose for diabetics dependent on insulin (type I) are discussed elsewhere. The majority of newly referred diabetics to our service have been diabetic for more than 15 years. However, living with a chronic illness such as diabetes does not guarantee that the patient or his physician is knowledgeable or capable of managing his disease optimally. It is a disservice to the new patient to assume that he/she understands proper diabetes management, even though it has previously been taught. Diabetics need to be educated and reeducated.

Essential points to cover in patient education about glucose regulation

Discussion of diabetic pathophysiology can range from simple to complex, based on the desire and capabilities of the patient. Many diabetics, despite years of insulin therapy, lack basic diabetes information and are unable to answer simple questions such as: "What is diabetes? What is insulin? Where does it come from?"

The diabetic or his family must continuously and accurately measure blood glucose levels. Reliability of these measurements will be improved by reviewing the technique of monitoring, including: proper use, calibration and care of the selected meter, and the handling of test strips. A protocol for monitoring the patient's schedule, recording results, interpretation of results, and translation of glucose values into changed insulin doses should be constructed to suit each patient.

Special attention should be devoted to instruction on insulin type, onset of action, and peak effect for that individual. We also review how to mix and administer (pump or injection) insulin. A team dietitian teaches the basics of diet and a schema for matching food, insulin, and activity, while addressing the patient's nutritional requirements, taste, culture, and financial capabilities (see table 12–3).

Table 12–3. Topics covered in instruction in glucose regulation

1. Food groups

TYPE	PEAK ABSORPTION
Simple carbohydrates	15–30 minutes
Complex carbohydrates	30–60 minutes
Fats	90 minutes (may delay absorption of protein and carbohydrate)
Protein	2 hours

2. Variables raising blood glucose
   Decreased activity
   Emotional stress
   Infection
   Reduced insulin
   Some medications (steroids)
   Increased food intake
3. Variables reducing blood glucose
   Increased activity
   Increased insulin
   Declining renal function
   Decreased food intake

SUPPORTIVE TEAM APPROACH

An asymptomatic patient needs help with ongoing prevention of further complications, as well as aggressive intervention when necessary. As kidney function deteriorates, the patient feels sicker and becomes more frightened, while the health-care team becomes larger and more complex. Individuals and their families must be (and feel that they are) an integral part of the team in order for the supportive services to be utilized maximally. The team is illustrated in figure 12–1.

Illustrative case i

Age: 58
Married, one child, supportive family
Retired school teacher with zest for life
Motivated and knowledgeable with regard to management of diabetes
Complications: Diabetic nephropathy (proteinuria), hypertension, diabetic retinopathy, peripheral neuropathy.

Mrs. L, a type I diabetic for 49 years, has been followed by the renal team for five years and is an active participant in her health care. Regulation of blood glucose is achieved by monitoring her sugars with a reflectance meter, and by adjusting her NPH and regular insulin requirements based on blood sugar values. Hypertension is managed by combining a vasodilator (clonidine) and a diuretic

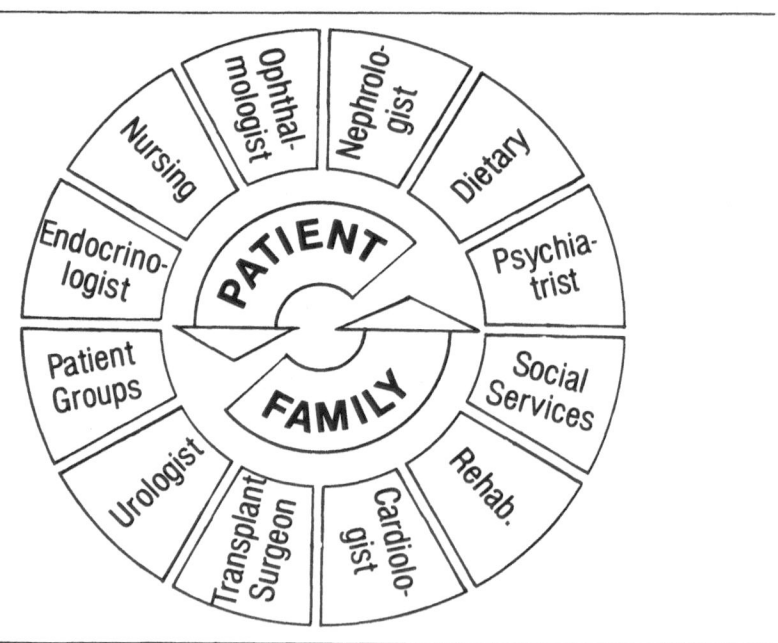

Figure 12–1. Few disorders rival diabetic nephropathy in the requirement for integrating multiple professional talents in order to attain rehabilitation. Key to the team structure is a satisfactory resolution to the interaction between patient and his family.

(furosemide), aided by self-monitoring of blood pressure at home. She is under the close care of an ophthalmologist who has expertise in diabetic retinopathy. (She has undergone laser therapy and a vitrectomy.)

Intervention is ongoing—education on diabetic management and prevention of complications, and updating her knowledge is a primary concern. The patient's blood chemistries are closely followed (creatinine ranges from 1.7–2.5 mg/dl), and she is supported by doctors and nurses for ongoing problems and needs. One of her desires, which had not been met for many years, was addressed recently— piercing her ears. Although this was not part of diabetic nephropathy management, it was extremely important for this woman who had wanted her ears pierced since she was a child. If we are sincere about meeting the needs of our patients, we must go beyond the usual medical/surgical views.

SYMPTOMATIC KIDNEY IMPAIRMENT

Uremia effects all the systems of the body. Clinical manifestations of renal insuffi- ciency upon various body systems depend on underlying renal and systemic pathol- ogy, degree of renal dysfunction, and the age of the patient. It is known that diabetics are sicker at a lower creatinine level than nondiabetics, primarily due to their decreased capacity to produce creatinine secondary to reduced muscle mass, and other organ failure. These associated changes create stress and anxiety in patients and their families. These stresses are amplified in the uremic diabetic because of the following:

Nephropathic diabetics rarely feel well. They are depressed, nauseated, fre- quently vomiting, and have decreased work tolerance. Increasing effort is needed to perform daily activities (work, household chores); climbing stairs and/or walk- ing can be difficult or even impossible; peripheral motor neuropathy usually worsens; there may be alternating diarrhea and constipation compounded by gas- troparesis. All of the above factors, along with decreased insulin catabolism by failing kidneys, result in worsening blood glucose control, despite effort on the patient's part. "I can't remember the last time I felt well. When will I feel like I used to?"

Forced alteration in life style. As uremia progresses, the patient is unable to perform usual tasks, posing a threat to professional and social life. There is dimin- ished alertness, escalating lethargy, and diminishing libido. The patient may appear bewildered and of low intelligence. New information is difficult to absorb. At- tempting to assess intellectual and emotional capacity of a patient met for the first time poses a great challenge because of all the new and sometimes frightening information he or she is asked to absorb. Financial problems arise from reduced income, both of the patient and other family members who lose time from work to care for, or accompany, the patient to increasingly frequent medical visits. Plans for the future, even leisure-time activities, become difficult, partly because of limited funds but also because of the inability to predict when, if ever, the patient will be feeling well again.

Family Crisis. The first two circumstances set the groundwork for family crisis.

In addition, patient and family are bombarded by new information to learn, and stressed by future uncertainty and immediate fear. Maintaining customary intrafamilial roles can be difficult. The patient's self-esteem may be challenged, especially if the ill member was the dominant person in the household, and roles must now change in order to meet the changing needs and capabilities of the family.

Fear of Death. As these patients have lived with their diabetes for 15 years or longer, they are now not only confronted with progression in their illness but also faced with making life-saving decisions. It is a frightening time, as death is more of a reality than ever before.

INTERVENTION: SYMPTOMATIC KIDNEY IMPAIRMENT

Education

Uremia therapy education provides patients and families with the means to gain some control, and to make intelligent choices based on sound knowledge. The tools for uremia therapy education include:

1. Meeting of the health-care team by both the patient and family. (It is important that all members of the family be told, and hear, the same information.) Explanations should include risks, benefits, inherent complications, followup procedures, medications, and cost.
2. Touring treatment facilities offering home hemodialysis, satellite hemodialysis, peritoneal dialysis, and kidney transplantation.
3. Formal lectures by the health-care team for patients, families, and friends.
4. Meeting other patients who have had successful and unsuccessful experiences.
5. Reviewing options in therapy (see table 12–3).

Choosing uremia therapy depends upon several factors:

1. Patient preference—"I've been on hemodialysis for eight years. I'm afraid of having a kidney transplant, so I'll stick with this even though I am unable to do what I used to do."
2. Physician bias—"My doctor said that a kidney transplant was my best option for the best rehabilitation possible. I want to go back to work, so I chose to have a transplant."
3. Resources available—"Where I come from they only offered hemodialysis." Or, "Where I come from they only had CAPD."
4. Ignorance of available options by patient and/or health-care team—"I wanted to go on home hemodialysis, but my doctor said it was impossible because I was a diabetic, so I went to a hospital that offered home hemodialysis and kidney transplants for diabetics." Or, "My doctor said because I was a diabetic, CAPD was the only therapy that would be suitable."
5. Contraindications to specific therapies—These include hemodialysis (symptomatic cardiovascular disease, difficult or absent vascular access), peritoneal dialy-

sis (multiple abdominal surgical procedures with adhesions, previous diffuse peritonitis, paralytic ileus), and kidney transplant (unwilling to take life-long medications with known side effects).

Prevent further target organ damage

It is crucial at this time to work closely with the ophthamalogist, while maintaining normal blood glucose and blood pressure values. In addition, patients who have received laser therapy should follow the precautions described in table 12–4.

Monitor kidney function

Initiation of uremia therapy depends on both objective (blood chemistry) and subjective (symptom) criteria.

Plan for uremia therapy

If planning for hemodialysis.

Tasks include placement of vascular access, exploring home dialysis and arranging for training, exploring satellite facilities within the patient's community and arranging for placement.

If planning for peritoneal dialysis.

Tasks include placement of peritoneal catheter and scheduling for training.

If planning for kidney transplant.

In the case of a living related donor, it is important to create access for either form of dialysis, and to screen donors medically, surgically, and psychologically. Evaluate tissue compatibility, arrange for donor-specific blood transfusions.

In the case of a cadaveric donor, arrangements must be made to create access for either form of dialysis, type tissue, place on cadaveric waiting list, send monthly bloods to tissue typing lab, nondonor-specific blood transfusions (amount varies with the institution). Because of the multiple specialists involved in caring for

Table 12–4. Current options for uremia therapy

Kidney transplant
   Living related, living unrelated, cadaveric

Hemodialysis
   Home dialysis, satellite facility, hospital ambulatory unit

Peritoneal dialysis
   IPD (intermittent peritoneal dialysis), CAPD (continuous ambulatory peritoneal dialysis), CCPD (continuous cyclic peritoneal dialysis)

No uremia therapy
   Death will occur if the institution does not have the resources or the patient chooses not to have life-prolonging treatment.

---

diabetics becoming uremic, there is a high risk of inadvertently delivering fragmented care; confrontation between patient and staff sometimes results from conflicting advice or proposed regimens. In order to prevent this, collaboration and communication must be ongoing throughout all levels of nephropathy. Interdisciplinary meetings involving the various specialists are crucial, as are small meetings with the involved specialist and the patient and his family. Problems we have encountered while working with such a large team include:

1. Assuming another health-care team member has provided the patient and family with needed information, while that member made the same assumption. As a consequence, the patient is uninformed, confused, and angry, generating a needless waste of time and energy.
2. Patients desiring another opinion within the health-care team, but made to feel disloyal, guilty, or frightened. As a result, the patient is unsatisfied, frustrated, and afraid, while possibly receiving inadequate care. We support the patient's right to any care desired consistent with reasonable practice. A primary physician (the patient's doctor) should know and plan all aspects of therapy, acting as an ombudsman for the patient to the team.

Illustrative case ii: symptomatic nephropathy

Age: 28
Married, three children
Profession—Electrician
Uninformed regarding diabetes management and complications, frightened, unmotivated to persue prevention and health promotion.
Complications: Progressive diabetic nephropathy, diabetic retinopathy, diabetic gastoparesis, neuropathy, hypertension, peptic ulcer disease.

Mr. N, a type I diabetic of 20 years' duration, was referred from another institution for long-term planning nine months ago. At that time, his creatinine was 2.0 mg/dl, his blood pressure 160/100 mm Hg, and he had frequent episodes of nausea and vomiting. Intervention thus far: education involving kidney disease and options; optimal diabetes management (placed on split doses of NPH and regular insulin twice daily, self-monitoring of blood glucose with reagent strips, matching diet with his lifestyle to achieve normoglycemia and to maintain optimal nutritional intake). Normalization of blood pressure with a vasodilator (clonidine) and a diuretic (furosemide). Referred to opthamalogist specializing in diabetic retinopathy (proliferative retinopathy, required photocoagulation). Placed on metaclopramide, for diabetic gastroparesis, and advised to eat small frequent meals. As Mr. N's creatinine has climbed from 2.0–3.6 mg/dl, a vascular access was placed (fistula) in preparation for hemodialysis. Because Mr. N. lacks an intrafamilial donor, he was scheduled for tissue typing and blood transfusions in preparation for an anticipated cadaveric donor kidney transplant within a year.

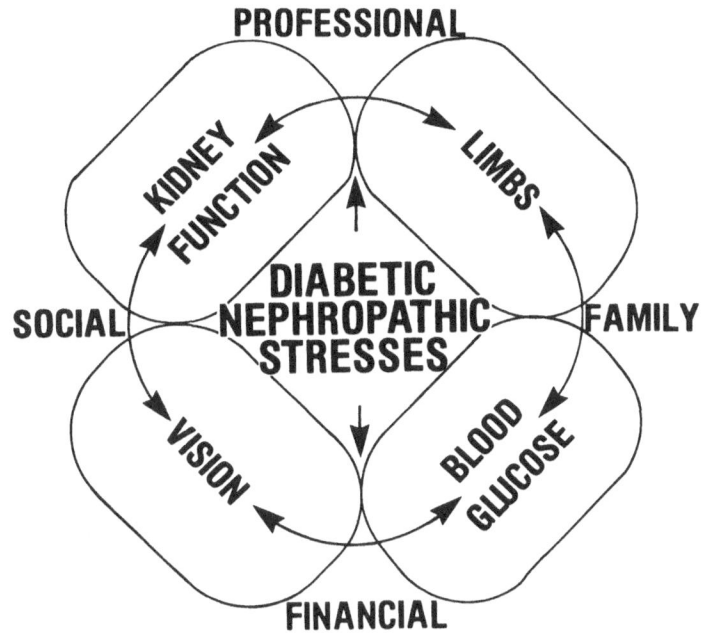

Figure 12–2. The diabetic with failed kidneys must rapidly shift focus from impending medical problem to another. While attending various clinics to preserve sight, limbs, and renal function, the often harried patient must maintain satisfactory relations with spouse and family.

It has been difficult for the patient and his family to absorb new information, while meeting "confusing" specialists (nephrologist, nurses, vascular and transplant surgeon, podiatrist, ophthalmologist, tissue-typing personnel, dietitian, social worker). Serious choices had to be made during five hospitalizations (primarily for dehydration related to nausea and vomiting). Frequent absences from work, while meeting the high cost of medications, transportation, and medical visits, as well as the high cost of raising a growing family, are constant stresses. However, it is more advantageous for the patient, family, and staff to address these difficulties on an ongoing basis, rather than in a crisis situation.

RECEIVING UREMIA THERAPY
Prevent further damage
Each uremia treatment is associated with unique risks, necessitating that patients be educated to prevent, detect, and possibly treat these problems.

To illustrate the point:

1. CAPD can induce peritonitis, catheter infections, and/or occlusion, and migration of the catheter from pelvic region. Inadequate dialysis may be complicated by fluid retention/depletion, hypertension/hypotension, muscle wasting, or respiratory distress.

Table 12–5. Precautions following retinal laser therapy in diabetics

1. Sleep with the head of the bed raised 15° to 20°.
2. Control coughing with cough syrup or other medications. Do not stiffle a sneeze, since this raises the pressure in your eyes to high levels.
3. Avoid bending, straining, and heavy lifting.
4. Do not rub eyes, since this may disrupt blood vessels inside the eyes.
5. Refrain from use of nose drops, sprays, or inhalators which contain ephedrine or adrenalin, as these may raise blood pressure and predispose eye to hemorrhage.
6. Use Colace, a stool softener, if constipated (straining increases pressure).
7. Avoid altitudes over 8,000 feet (decrease in oxygen in the air); predisposes to eye hemorrhage.

2. Hemodialysis poses the risk of vascular access problems, technical complications including air embolism and hemorrhage, bacterial or viral contamination (transmission of hepatitis), and progressive uremia.

3. Kidney transplantation raises the threat of rejection, increased cancer incidence, recurrence in the transplant of renal disease, and a steroid-induced change in physical appearance (acne, obesity). For the diabetic, steroids add the problem of deteriorating glucose regulation.

In addition, uremic diabetics may have multiple and prolonged hospitalizations for a variety of reasons. The nephropathic diabetic often has special problems during hospitalization. Diabetics undergoing uremia therapy have a long history of illness and usually a lower tolerance to the many stresses of being an in-patient. Further adding to stress for the diabetic is the control that is taken away during hospital admissions. For example, the patient no longer determines his insulin dose and the time it is administered, or the choice of food and the time it is served. Any problems in these areas can leave an already drained patient ripe for confrontation with staff, and sometimes the patients are labeled "difficult." We have found it helpful in some situations for patients to continue their own glucose monitoring (after nurses assess the patient's capabilities), thereby advising the staff to suggested insulin requirements. On the other end of the spectrum, difficulties may arise when an uninformed or undisciplined diabetic is hospitalized. Undereducated yet "demanding" diabetics may place diabetic management on the "back burner." They present a need to be educated regarding blood glucose monitoring, diet, prevention with regard to preserving limbs, eye care, and prevention and prompt treatment of infection, producing a difficult chore during an acute illness.

Uremic diabetics also have major obstacles to overcome in order for them to achieve maximal rehabilitation. Figure 12–2 portrays the four major threats confronting these individuals on a daily basis, which are dealt with by fear, hope, and sometimes denial. Notice that surrounding these identified threats are other aspects of daily life that face us all. Because of the devastating impact of diabetic nephropathy, these stresses are magnified (table 12–5).

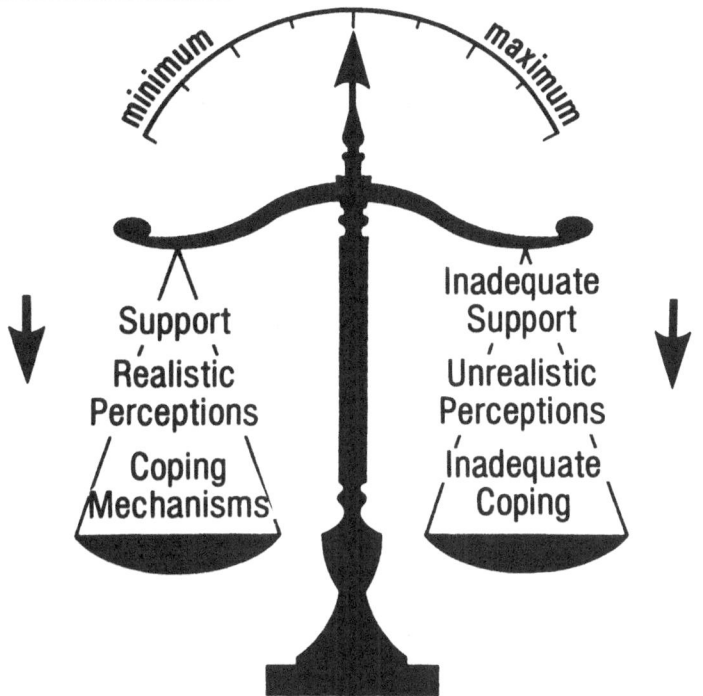

Figure 12–3. Forces acting on the psychologic balance of the diabetic with progressive kidney disease are shown.

Closely follow chemistries

With each uremia therapy, lab values (objective), plus subjective feedback, are essential to determine: (1) efficacy of treatment—determines kidney transplant function or adequate clearance of toxins and fluid during dialysis; (2) correct medication—type and dose of insulin, immunosuppressives, antihypertensives, fluid intake; (3) change in prescription—dialysate, dialyzer, immunosuppression, or uremia therapy.

Change in uremia therapy

There are patient-determined choices in uremia therapy. Informed patient consumers ask, "What is the best treatment for me medically, psychologically, financially, and socially?" One therapy might be utilized initially (CAPD, for example) until it is no longer feasible (peritonitis), and then another pursued because it has advantages the patient needs or desires. As each option in therapy improves with time, and patients become more involved and aware of their choices, matching the individual with the appropriate therapy proves easier for patients and their families.

Table 12–6.

1. Divorce: Husband could not deal with the stress of having a chronically ill spouse whose cushingoid appearance embarassed him.
2. Alcoholism: Because of emotional difficulties, this patient goes on regular drinking binges. (Patient had a cadaveric kidney transplant nine years ago, as well as bilateral below-the-knee amputations.)
3. Overprotection by family: Enables a blind nephrotic patient to take a passive approach toward her rehabilitation. (She prefers to sit home all day and avoid getting training.)
4. Illness in other family members: Diabetic transplant recipient's spouse dies of cancer; failed kidney-transplant recipient's husband dies suddenly of a heart attack.
5. Isolation: Private room was granted to a woman as a benefit, whose husband was a physician at the institution where she was receiving care. This kept her isolated from other patients, and she was denied the supportive experience patients with similar problems give one another.
6. Financial: Difficulty in coming to the hospital for regular visits because of transportation expenses; inability to buy drugs, syringes, braces, special shoes, etc.
7. Depression: "I don't want to live like this—blind, unable to walk, unable to drive, etc."

Illustrative case iii: on uremia therapy

Age: 36 years

Engaged to be married, supportive relationship

Profession—Engineer

Knowledgeable regarding diabetes management and prevention, uninformed regarding uremia therapy options.

Independent

Complications: diabetic nephropathy (receiving CAPD), diabetic retinopathy, diabetic gastroparesis, neurogenic bladder.

Ms. R, a type I diabetic for 27 years, is a small-framed woman who had been on CAPD for two weeks when referred because of failure to improve. As she became progressively weaker, she had to leave her job which had been extremely important to her because of professional, financial, and social rewards and positive self-esteem. Ms. R was informed that CAPD was the only treatment for diabetics in kidney failure. She made telephone inquiries in areas outside her state, and eventually came to us for help. At first, Ms. R was angry (low tolerance to the difficulties of being hospitalized); frightened (away from home with new people to meet); and confused (conflict in information regarding appropriate therapy for diabetics: "I was told hemodialysis and transplantation are not good for diabetics"). This setting was indeed a difficult one in which to have a therapeutic relationship begin.

The intervention, it was decided, centered on providing up-to-date information and options in uremia therapy; gaining vascular access for hemodialysis; meeting with other patients who had had varied experiences with various modes of therapy. Ms. R was advised to pursue a kidney transplant for maximal rehabilitation.

(Hemodialysis provided Ms. R with adequate chemistries, but her appetite deteriorated, and she was tired and depressed nearly all of the time.) Tissue-typing was performed on Ms. R and her possible family donors. She was referred to an ophthalmologist for her proliferative diabetic retinopathy and began laser therapy.

On the day of her scheduled living-related transplant, her donor, an uncle, was found to be unacceptable because of the discovery of renal artery stenosis. At this same time, Ms. R's mother had such a stressful reaction to this news that she had to be admitted to the cardiac intensive care unit because of a possible myocardial infarction. Fortunately, another family member proved suitable and willing to donate her kidney the next week. The patient's posttransplant course was complicated by a rejection episode which responded to an increased dose of cyclosporine, and a neurogenic bladder, which responded to urecholine, and frequent voiding. Two months after her transplant, she went back to her home state where she resumed full-time employment. Ms. R had difficult physical and emotional problems which required support from a variety of nursing staff (hemodialysis, transplant, educator, and transplant coordinators), as well as the social worker and dietitian, to help her in her process of obtaining maximum well-being. She has recently married a childhood sweetheart.

SUMMARY

In summary, we advocate intensive education of the diabetic. Our goal is to have each patient informed and involved in his/her own care. Assuming control, each patient facilitates a healthy adjustment to unavoidable stresses. Figure 12–3 portrays the necessary components for patients to cope adequately with these ongoing threats. It is recognized that adequate uremia therapy does not guarantee a diabetic's overall health and well-being. Examples of some of the problems that these individuals experience are described in table 12–6. Azotemic diabetics need continuing medical, nursing, social service, dietary, and emotional support (prior to, during, and after uremia therapy is initiated). Uremic diabetics and their families (and staff) face enormous stress, and all require appropriate outlets and support to function effectively. Finally, satisfaction generated by rehabilitation of uremic diabetics can be rewarding and fulfilling.

SELECTED BIBLIOGRAPHY

1. Chambers J. Nursing care of the diabetic patient with renal disease. Nephrology Nurse 4:16–18, 1983.
2. Chambers J. Save your diabetic patient from early kidney damage. Nursing 83 13:5–63, 1983.
3. Conway P. The diabetic transplant patient—special considerations. American Assoc of Nephrology Nurses and Technicians J 8:23–26, 1981.
4. Friedman E. Diabetic nephropathy: strategies in prevention and management. Kidney Internat 21:780–791, 1982.
5. Friedman E, L'Esperance F (eds.) The diabetic renal-retinal syndrome. New York: Grune & Stratton, 1980.
6. Friedman EA, L'Esperance F (eds). Diabetic renal retinal syndrome prevention and management. New York: Grune & Stratton, 1982.
7. Gorman D, Anderson J. Initial shock: impact of a life-threatening disease and ways to deal with it. Social Work in Health Care 7:3 (Spring): 37–45, 1982.

8. Guthrie D. Psychosocial side of diabetes and its complications. The Diabetes Educator 3:24–28, 1982.
9. Lancaster L. Renal failure: pathophysiology, assessment and intervention. Nephrology Nurse 5:30–38, 1983.
10. Levine S. Nutritional care of patients with renal failure and diabetes. J of the Amer Dietetic Assoc 81:261–267, 1982.
11. Llewelyn S, Fielding G. Adapting to illness. Nursing Mirror April: 28–29, 1983.
12. Lewis S. Pathology of chronic renal failure. Nursing Clinics of N Amer 16:501–513, 1981.
13. McCarthy J. Diabetic nephropathy. Amer J of Nursing 82:2030–2034, 1981.
14. Mogensen CE Hypertension in diabetes and the stages of diabetic nephropathy. Diabetic Nephropathy, 1:2–7, 1982.
15. Siegal B, Levine M. Structural family theory applied to diabetic renal transplantation. Diabetic Nephropathy 1:17–19, 1982.
16. Weiner R. Observations of a diabetic, hypertensive physician following renal transplantation. Diabetic Nephropathy 1:20–21, 1982.

13. PATIENT TO PATIENT

MILDRED FRIEDMAN

Research in diabetes, research in transplantation, research in uremia, research in any medical area is truly important when its results reach the patient. The quality of life resulting from this research is what it's all about. Treatment for the diabetic and for the diabetic whose kidneys and eyes have failed has changed drastically since I became diabetic 20 years ago. With the advent of techniques that permit tight control of blood glucose levels and medications for controlling blood pressure, there is hope that the outlook for diabetics who maintain near-normal values for these two factors will have a brighter future than might have been possible previously. It is expected that some of the complications due to this illness can be avoided and some made better. It is certainly true that a feeling of well-being is accomplished by the regulation of these elements.

Before the discovery of insulin, diabetes was not treated effectively except with diet. Now we have various kinds of insulin, oral medications, and diet to handle the different types of loss of natural blood sugar control and other manifestations of metabolic imbalance. Until a few years ago the common complication of uremia in the diabetic was nearly always fatal. Now there are several forms of dialysis as well as kidney transplantation to handle renal failure. Retinal disease, going hand-in-hand with kidney disease, often led to blindness in the type I (insulin-dependent) diabetic. Today there is laser therapy and vitrectomy to counteract the previously unavoidable loss of sight. Cataract surgery can restore vision lost due to clouded lenses. Those who suffer from the renal-retinal syndrome (simultaneously occurring kidney and eye disease) have the potential of many years of sighted life. It is heartening to be living today and look back on what might have been. If those who are uremic diabetics now had been afflicted 10 years ago, they would probably be dead. Living through these conditions and their treatment is not easy, but to those who have had good results it is worth the discomfort and pain, the depression and despondency. This chapter will be written from the viewpoint of one patient who has had the experience of undergoing all of the listed eye treatments, being hemodialyzed, and receiving a kidney transplant. I am that patient.

No one chain of complications is typical for the diabetic. Difficulties seemingly can occur in any order and at any time. The list can include kidney failure, loss of vision, amputation, high blood pressure, strokes, bowel problems, CNS problems, and foot problems. Living with this chronic disease as an informed patient involves learning and using a technique for evaluating the blood sugar level. There are at least four kinds of test strips and several meters available for determining the blood sugar value within minutes of obtaining a drop of blood. The choice of which setup to use probably depends on what method is favored by the physician in charge of the patient but should be influenced by other considerations as well. For instance, some meter readouts are more legible to the person with low-vision, while test strips read without a meter must be compared with color swatches on the strip bottle—a difficult chore for either the visually impaired or color blind. In applying self-glucose monitoring, cost used to be a factor ($.50 a strip, four times a day—meters may be priced at as much as $200) but now, if ordered by a diabetes specialist, the materials may be covered by Medicare and Medicaid.

Introduced to the idea of sticking one's own finger to make it bleed, each of us wonders whether or not we can repeatedly hurt ourselves. Having done this a minimum of three times a day for nearly five years I can assure the reader that the use of an automatic lancing device (I use the Autolet; see Peterson's chapter), which controls how far into the finger the needle will go, makes self-testing possible indeed. It really does not hurt except occasionally. A worry about infection was with me for the first few years, but I have never had any of these sites become infected. My fingers do not keep me from knitting, crocheting, sewing, or typing. Another aspect of modern blood glucose control that probably does not occur to the professionals is the fear of embarrassment when doing finger sticks in public (i.e., at a restaurant). Over the years I have done it many times and will state that few people notice except those at your own table. Insulin injections can be taken under nonprivate circumstances without making a fuss.

Having gotten used to sticking one's fingers and determining the level of sugar in the blood, one must learn what to do with the information obtained. Keeping a log of blood sugar values and amounts of insulin administered two to four times each day lets one take an educated guess as to what dose of the medicine should be used. Multiple insulin injections seem to be the best way to control the sugar (see Peterson's chapter). Insulin pumps are available, but they are not within my experience and so I will not discuss them. Again, there is the worry that one can't administer three shots a day. With the new, very fine needles, there is usually no pain. Their disposability and the resulting lack of need to sterilize results in a gain of time. The testing of blood sugar and administration of insulin is best done half an hour before each meal. Looking at their own records and deciding insulin dosages puts patients in charge of regulating their disease. It lets them see at a glance when the insulin requirement has changed. Record-keeping becomes a way of life —an important way of life.

Nearly all uremic diabetics are hypertensive. High blood pressure can be a disaster for anybody, especially the diabetic, by causing strokes, heart attacks, and worsening of the renal-retinal syndrome. Records of blood pressure control should be kept. There are pressure-measuring devices, costing as little as $50, that can be easily handled by the individual.

Bringing all these written facts (which can be in one notebook) with you at your appointment time makes the doctor's job easier and more scientific—a boon to you both.

The low-vision patient has been mentioned earlier in this chapter. The prospect of becoming one brings moments of terror. "How far will it go?" you ask. The ophthalmologist tries to find out about your specific case by taking a series of pictures of your retinas after injecting a dye to see where they are leaking blood. This test hurt me due to the brilliance of the camera flash on my dilated and light-sensitive eyes. My retinas (the place in the back of the eye where images are formed) had not yet bled enough to obscure sight but required laser therapy. A laser is a concentrated beam of light which can be used to cauterize what it is aimed at. The eye doctor directs the laser into the eye through the pupil. A large contact lens is first put on the eye to neutralize the power of the eyeball to position itself. An ordinary focusing light beam is aimed through the contact lens and the laser is fired. You see a flash of light. As many as 2,000 laser burns may be given to each eye. It was done for me in a series of five sessions for the left eye and five more for the right. After about the third sitting the process began to hurt. That is, each "shot" hurt. There was no lasting pain. Each treatment made me tired, depressed, and very sensitive to light.

The struggle to stop oncoming blindness was a time of high hope, hope that I would not lose my sight and that the progression of diabetic eye disease was being halted. Then my eyes began to bleed. It takes very little blood to obscure vision, I am told. "What do see when your eye bleeds?" you might want to know. There were two things that signaled hemorrhage. One course of eye hemorrhage was characterized by a few small dark spots suddenly appearing, spiraling, and over several hours disappearing, leaving the vision cloudy like looking through multiple layers of transparent curtains. Another time there was a sheet of blood, red and slowly flowing upward, that left no doubt as to what it was. I am sure that other patients could give other descriptions of eye bleeds. The chance of having that blood reabsorbed, thus returning vision, was a gamble, and so I spent many months living nearly blind.

Normal people have trouble understanding how you feel: crossing streets when you can't tell whether that thing you see moving, is a bus; finding a cab when you can't identify one; crossing streets in the middle of crowds because you can't tell what color the light is; buying items without knowing what their prices are; giving up reading because you can't make out big print with a magnifying glass; and just plain filling up your time when you don't know what to do. There is another aspect. Your new handicap does not show on the outside. People looking at you do not know that you are nearly blind and so do not make any compensation for you. You get no mercy from the stranger. Depression sets in. It is my thought that this despair could be helped if the ophthamologist's offices had a listing of what is available for the low-vision patient, what books, what stores, what organizations. Blind people are promptly put in touch with what is at their disposal, an action often not taken for the partially sighted. The period of losing sight was a difficult time to live through, and when they told me that the blood would not clear, I would need an operation—a vitrectomy—to let me see again, I panicked.

Explanations of what this vitrectomy involved were given to me. The fluid in the middle of the eyeball is called the vitreous humor. Blood sitting in this vitreous, not being absorbed, stops the light from passing through the eye and getting to the retina; therefore, you can't see. The operation is done by cutting a small hole in the eyeball, going in and removing this fluid and fibers which have formed, and replacing it with saline solution. Local or general anesthesia can be used. I chose local and worried about what I was going to see. Nothing, is the answer. I felt the first shot of anesthetic like you feel at the dentist's, except in a different spot, and then, no feeling while I heard the doctors talking and working. The hospital stay was brief, four days. There was no pain. An eye patch was worn outdoors and for sleeping. The sight was greatly improved. As is not rare, the eye bled again. Same story—except that this time they decided also to remove the cataract on that eye. There are several ways to provide aids to the patient who has lost the ability to focus due to lensectomy (removal of the clouded lens—cataract). Spectacles are acceptable to many, and an implanted plastic lens (sewn in at the time of surgery) or an extended wear contact lens (the kind that does not need to be removed daily) take care of the rest. Implants are not usually used on diabetics because of a risk of irritation and bleeding, so I was scheduled for the other kind. However, there is usually a wait of several months until the eye is ready for testing for the lens prescription. Here you are, not bloody but nevertheless out of focus, i.e., still with rotten sight. After the necessary time I was given the lens and could see again. A similar series of events happened to the other eye. Was it worth it? Yes! Yes! Yes! With the aid of reading glasses I can read all but the smallest print and am driving again. There has been no progression of disease for two years. A medical miracle was performed!

While all this was happening my kidneys were deteriorating. A lot of protein appeared in my urine and my creatinine value was elevated. Creatinine is one of the nitrogen-containing waste products that the normal kidney filters out, and the amount present in the blood is used as an indicator of how that organ is functioning. Fatigue and lethargy were increasingly part of my day. Every morning I would spend a few minutes retching, bringing up nothing, and not being left with a feeling of nausea. When it was over, it was over—no lasting effect. There was often a bad taste in my mouth but it was not associated with this last symptom. Coldness frequently made me uncomfortable. Shaking chills would occur. Climbing steps was torture. I had no desire to do anything and often thought how nice it would be to just not wake up the next morning. There was not enough sleep to satisfy me.

One winter night I realized that what I thought was the flu was not getting any better although two weeks had passed—I just felt awful. Admission to the hospital was necessary the following day. Diagnosis—uremia. Treatment—hemodialysis. Question—whether I would accept it or choose to die. That decision must be made quickly, within days. Death is not so far away. Not deciding is making a decision. You remember the goodness of life, you hope for a return to it, or you do not. Hope stays with most of us no matter how bad things seem. It is: ". . . the thing with feathers that perches in the soul," according to Emily Dickinson. The staff repeated over and over that rehabilitation was possible, that I would feel better, and so I decided to try hemodialysis.

Fortunately I was too sick to be aware of the discomfort of having needles inserted in my groin (for dialysis it is necessary to remove and return your blood to your body, and here it was done with the femoral veins which are at the inside tops of your thighs) and being told not to move for four hours. In subsequent dialyses (which took place three times a week and lasted about four hours each) I became knowledgeable about the discomforts but slept through most of each treatment. I found that I was exhausted for the rest of the dialysis day as well.

One of my most serious problems was what to eat. The dialysis patient is on a very restrictive diet and regimen. Sodium and potassium intake, one is told, must be rigorously controlled as must the intake of fluid. I could grasp that idea, but combining these new limitations with the usual diabetic diet in my state of mental dullness was too much for me to handle. A combined diabetic-dialysis diet was not available at our institution. I felt so constrained that I imagined that there were six things left for me to eat, all broiled, and none interesting. (This led to my construction, when my mind was working again, of a diabetic-renal diet based on the food exchange system and printed in big print which you can see in appendix A.)

Another problem was the hours necessary for dialysis. Not only the time on the machine but the time transporting me to and from the artificial kidney center. Although I wasn't using these moments constructively, I still felt them slipping away needlessly.

During the period of this therapy the doctors decided to construct a fistula in my arm. One of the original problems preventing the people who first wanted to use the artificial kidney for the treatment of chronic (long-lasting) kidney disease was the necessity of entering the patient's bloodstream repeatedly. This poking of holes in the arteries and veins resulted in clotting, leaking, and infection, leading to the impossibility of using these sites again. A fistula is a way around that problem. An artery and a vein in my forearm were connected, shunting the blood flow from the artery into the vein. The veins in the arm with the fistula became larger than normal with the help of exercise (squeezing a ball or a pair of socks repeatedly). The result was a thin scar about 3 inches long with an increased pulse in the veins under the skin. An interesting side effect occurs when my arm is in a certain position under my pillow. I can hear the beat—a soothing way to fall asleep!

I was told that transplantation was the preferred method of treatment for diabetics, that we seemed to do better with a new kidney. A series of decisions had to be made: living related donor or cadaver (dead person); if living related—who? Is your life important enough to possibly jeopardize another human being's? How much at risk will they be with only one kidney? How old should the donor be? Maximum age? Minimum age? What should their mental state be? Retarded? Senile? You listen to what the professionals have to say, decide, ask the potential benefactor (giving them a whole set of feelings, anxieties, and guilts), and wait to see if their tissue type matches yours (done by comparing parts of the blood).

You match well enough. The operation is scheduled, and you go through with it. Several hours in the recovery room and there you are—a transplant recipient. In the hospital it is required that you measure your fluid intake and output. Intake is easy. You can see the glass or cup. Output is harder if your vision is gone. The markings on the measuring cup just aren't there for you.

You will live the rest of your life waiting to learn what your creatinine value is because a raised creatinine value signals returning uremia and failure of the transplant. You'll know what your other blood values are but that's the dramatic one. You may go through rejection with its attendant medications, some of which (antithymocyte globulin or antilymphocyte globulin) involve being tied to an IV (intravenous tube) for five or so hours a day for two weeks. Ever tried to wheel an IV stand over the door saddle into a bathroom? Leaves a lot to be desired. There is the usual trouble with IV's: getting them put in, having them infiltrate (leak into the tissue), and the pain that occurs every once in a while at the site after they have been removed. Troubles? Yes, but one great thing—you can eat again, anything that the "normal" diabetic can eat.

With all this accomplished you go home to deal with the problems. I didn't have much pain; I healed well, but there are complications due to the medications. My experiences being on imuran (azathioprine) and prednisone are probably different from those who are being immunosuppressed with cyclosporine. The similarities have to do with living as an immunosuppressed individual. One dreads catching a cold or getting an infection. Infections often are difficult to heal in a diabetic but can be much worse when the body's natural defenses are cancelled out.

The sword of rejection will dangle over your head for the rest of your life. Any new physical sensation is thought of in those terms. Is this really a hangnail or an early sign? Problems exist for the diabetic transplant recipient, but the renewal of life can be exhilarating. Almost immediately after the operation I experienced a return of mental alertness and now, almost five years later, look back and see a return of my former personality. I have reentered the world and am involved and doing.

Of course I have not dealt with all the diabetic or transplant complications possible. While I have had serious foot infections, I have not had an amputation or gastric disorders, to name a few of the potential problems. Neuropathy (that pins-and-needles sensation in the limbs which goes along with numbness) is present but happily it has improved, not disappeared, since the transplant.

The whole experience of dealing intimately and often with health-care people raises complex questions. I do not have the answers to such problems as what you do when your spouse and/or family can't take the strain anymore. You must recognize that there is a tremendous strain on them. Suppose you can afford to pay for your medical expenses but doing so will deprive your family (cyclosporine is very costly)?

In an attempt to allow involved patients to discuss these and many other questions and to help by relating our personal experiences for them, the diabetic transplant patients at Downstate Medical Center have formed the Diabetic Renal Transplant Self-help Group. (Figure 13–1 shows the second meeting.) We are trying to aid others and their families in coming to terms with problems of daily living both in the hospital and at home. We attempt to answer the questions that are felt to be too trivial to ask physicians such as: What is a lens? What does a fistula look like? The group has helped me greatly—by enabling me to share my fears, thoughts, and moods with people who have gone through similar adventures.

A major problem to deal with in the diabetic renal-retinal syndrome is depression. This frustrating condition is a fact of life for both the patient and their loved ones (family or friends). The patients are helped by attaining partial control of their disease and destiny. Self-medication and self-diabetic control helps. Having people to speak with who understand is important. Other families who have gone through similar experiences benefit newly afflicted families by sharing.

What the future holds for any diabetic uremic is unknown. We each must take advantage of the day before us and be glad that research in the areas that affect us has made that day possible.

Here are some common questions for which my answers may help. If you don't find your concern addressed here, write to us and maybe it will be included in a future edition of this book. It will certainly educate the author.

1. I've been diabetic for many years but don't understand the exchange system for eating. How do I get help?

If you don't know a nutritionist or dietitian ask your doctor for the name of one and get in touch. Have it explained as many times as necessary. Get a diabetic cookbook. There are some available in big print, such as *The Elegant Touch Cookbook: Gourmet Cooking for the Diabetic* by Marjorie Zats and Karen Ruben (Jonathan David Company, 540 Taft Street, N.E., Minneapolis, MN 55413; $9.45). They usually have a written description. Try it. It's not as confusing as it sounds.

2. My doctor and podiatrist insist that I wear closed, oxford-style shoes and closed slippers. Aren't they awful?

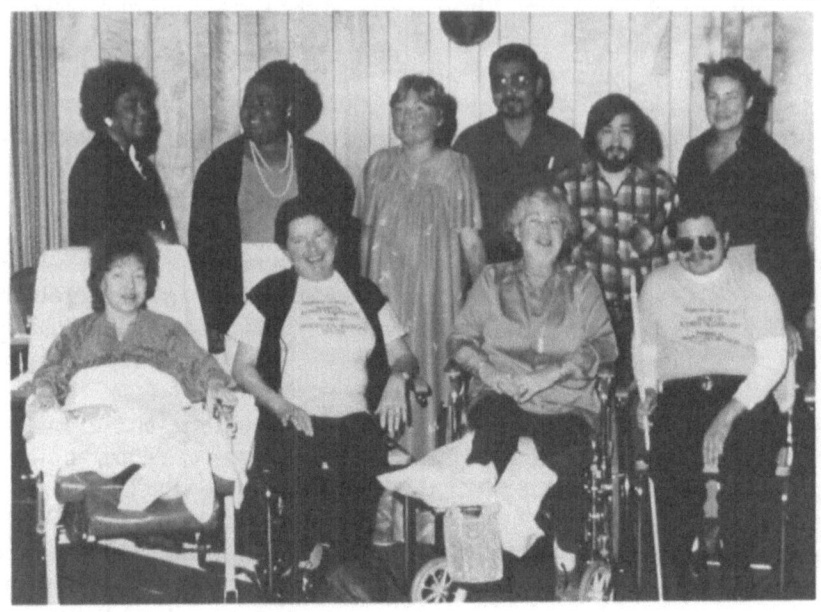

Figure 13–1. Founding members of Downstate Medical Center Diabetic Kidney Transplant Self-help Group. Of 10 patients pictured, 2 are blind in both eyes, 2 are legally blind in one eye, and all have undergone ophthalmic intervention (laser photocoagulation and vitrectomy). The author is second from the left in the front row.

Yes, they're as ugly as can be, but there are several ways around the problem, and it is necessary to follow their instructions to keep your feet. Injuries to the diabetic foot are a cause for serious worry for several reasons. The damage is often not felt by the person with neuropathy until it is infected. Infections in the diabetic foot often do not heal promptly because of decreased circulation and because the high-blood sugar caused by the infection makes the wound a near-perfect place for bacteria or fungus to grow. This can lead to amputation. Therefore, an ounce of prevention is worth the proverbial pound of cure. Wear the ugly shoes. Many women do find them more acceptable when worn with slacks. Another attack on their looks is to combine them with dark stockings. I don't mind how they appear with skirts when I use black hosiery (with black shoes—blue would go with blue). Seamless, round-toe, flexible sole, low-heel boots in which your feet don't slip around are good, too. I go to shoe stores at uncrowded times, explain to the manager that I have neuropathy, and ask for their best salesperson. It works—and I find I get a good fit plus the understanding that I will bring my purchase back if my podiatrist does not approve.

3. I have some questions that I want to ask my doctor but he won't take the time to answer me. What do I do?

Explain pleasantly and politely to him that he is there to serve you, that you are paying him. If he doesn't change, change doctors. ("He" can also be "she.")

4. I want a kidney transplant but my doctor says "No" and won't discuss it with me.

Insist on knowing why, and if you get an unsatisfactory answer, change doctors or communicate with another one. I know that if you live in a small town or in an area where there is only one renal center available to you, you may feel trapped. The mail or the telephone gives you an "out."

5. My kidney doctor and my endocrinologist (diabetes specialist) don't seem to agree on what my diet should be. Are there special food restrictions for people with failing kidneys?

Yes, there are but *what* they are depends on what stage of kidney failure you are at and what treatment you are receiving. Tell them you are confused and ask them to decide together what you should do. If you do not understand how to follow their directions, get in touch with a nutritionist or dietitian. Your diabetic diet is always important in your care.

6. What do I do if I need my doctor at a strange time (middle of the night, weekend)?

You should ask ahead of time how you will contact him, what phone numbers are available, and who will cover his practice when he is not available.

7. I always forget some of the things I want to ask the doctor, the nutritionist, the podiatrist, anybody. Help!

Write them down beforehand and don't forget your glasses at appointment time.

8. How do I decide which treatment is right for me?

Dr. Friedman thinks that the decision as to which treatment you will accept for your kidney failure is one made with thought and care at the appropriate time. I feel that this is really decided beforehand. We are influenced by media stories, accounts we hear from others, our doctors' attitudes (which may be unspoken), and many other inputs. Then the result is a decision made ahead of time. How did you come to your verdict? Let us know.

9. I have a question I want to ask but don't want to make an appointment and make a visit. What do I do?

Use the phone—with respect. A short, to-the-point call should be an annoyance to no one. If you are the last of a long string of calls asking the same thing or if you ramble on you may be a bother. Don't be.

14. IS DIABETIC NEPHROPATHY PREVENTABLE?

ELI A. FRIEDMAN

Stating the Problem

In 1975 Goodman and Schung reported the incidence of diabetes mellitus in North America to be approximately 1.5% to 2.5% [1]. Depending on diagnostic criteria employed, an additional 3% of Americans (total 5% to 6%) are diabetic. The financial toll imposed by diabetes on the health-care system is enormous. About one-third of hospitalized patients on a medical service are diabetic. More than one-quarter of new dialysis and kidney-transplant patients are diabetic. The cost of diabetic care can be measured in terms of the macrovascular and microvascular complications resulting from long-term diabetes, especially nephropathy and retinopathy.

Based on accumulating knowledge of its pathogenesis, however, there is reason for optimism in the quest for prevention of diabetic microvasculopathy. Evidence, derived from study of the streptozotocin-induced diabetic rat, subsequently confirmed and extended in human recipients of kidneys obtained from nondiabetic donors [2], strongly indicates that diabetic glomerulopathy is a consequence of ambient hyperglycemia, rather than genetic predisposition. Furthermore, Abouna and associates have recently shown that diabetic glomerulopathy may regress when the nephropathic kidney is transplanted into a nondiabetic but uremic recipient [3].

If this "environmental hypothesis" is proven correct, it follows that medical regimens aimed at establishing sustained euglycemia might prevent glomerulopathy as well as other microvascular complications of diabetic hyperglycemia. Longitudinal study of the effect of type I diabetes on the kidney has identified a sequence of glomerular hyperfiltration—associated with microalbuminuria in those likely to develop clinical nephropathy [4, 5]—followed by proteinuria and, ultimately, renal insufficiency. Concurrent histopathological findings indicate that intensifying occlusion of glomerular capillaries (glomerulosclerosis) as a function of the duration of type I diabetes. Equivalent information detailing the course of nephropathy in type II diabetes is lacking, mainly due to imprecision in timing the onset of hyperglycemia, which may be present without signs or symptoms for a decade or longer [6]. Glomerulosclerosis is the characteristic microangiopathic lesion and is the most clinically significant form of renal damage encountered in both type I and type II diabetes [7].

PATHOGENESIS OF GLOMERULOPATHY

The mechanism by which hyperglycemia causes microangiopathy in diabetic glomeruli is poorly understood. As hypothesized by Ainsworth and associates, morphologic alterations in diabetic glomerulopathy might be mediated by immunologic, biochemical, and/or functional factors [8]. It is probable that the pathogenesis of glomerular basement membrane and mesangial changes may be different [9]. Hyaline arteriolar lesions, characteristic of diabetic glomerulosclerosis, may result primarily from hyperlipidemia—a result of abnormal carbohydrate metabolism—and hypertension.

Experimental diabetes in rats, induced by alloxan or streptozotocin, will cause thickening of the glomerular mesangium, and crescent-shaped or nodular hyaline deposits within glomeruli, after four to six months of hyperglycemia. Immunofluorescent studies in the induced–diabetic rat disclose concomitant IgG, IgM, and C3 deposition in the mesangium [10]. Although the glomerular pathology of diabetic nephropathy in animals does not perfectly mimic changes in humans, there are striking similarities [10].

Type I diabetics have large kidneys with greater than normal glomerular diameter and capillary surface area. Renal plasma flow and glomerular filtration rate are supernormal for the first decade of insulin dependence [11]. Alterations from normal, observed in the diabetic kidney during the first decade of insulin use, in addition to increased overall length and weight include: glomerular enlargement, glomerular basement membrane thickening, hyaline arteriolosclerosis, intercapillary glomerulosclerosis, and proximal convoluted tubular basement membrane thickening [12]. None of these morphologic changes has been directly tied to hyperglycemia or perturbations in glomerular and tubular function [13].

On the other hand, in streptozotocin-induced-diabetic rats, kidney weight increases within the first few days after onset of hyperglycemia [14]. Initially, glomeruli enlarge at a more rapid rat than does the entire kidney. Subsequently, after about 10 days, glomerular growth rate slows [15]. There is a positive correlation between kidney size, and glomerular filtration rate (GFR) and renal plasma flow (RPF) [16]. Hyperglycemia, per se, appears to be important to the genesis of raised GFR and RPF [17, 18]. Type I diabetics exhibit an elevated RPF and a consequent increase in transglomerular ultrafiltration coefficient. It has been hypothesized, therefore, that increased kidney size in type I diabetics reflects alterations in determinants of GFR, such as RPF, which in turn are increased by hyperglycemia [16]. As viewed by Ditzel and his colleagues, glomerular hemodynamics are controlled by a tubuloglomerular feedback which, in the diabetic, is augmented by increased water and sodium reabsorption, leading to decreased tubular pressure, increased effective filtration pressure, and accentuated autoregulatory glomerular flow, culminating in an elevation in GFR [19]. Brenner and his colleagues, based on studies of single nephrons in induced–diabetic rats, propose that an increased GFR in diabetic rats or humans is associated with higher glomerular pressures, causing proteinuria and direct direct injury (focal sclerosis) to the glomerulus [20].

Albuminuria, a cardinal sign of clinical diabetic nephropathy, may also be seen in newly diagnosed type I diabetics. Viberti and his associates demonstrated the efficacy of insulin treatment and good glycemic control in promptly reducing subclinically elevated albumin excretion in nonazotemic type' I diabetics [21]. Enhanced glycemic control effected by intraperitoneal insulin administration has been reported by Stephen and associates to reduce "established" proteinuria in type I diabetics with mild renal insufficiency [22]. In this context, regulation of hyperglycemia is one method of slowing the progression (preventing) of diabetic glomerulopathy.

IMPORTANCE OF HYPERTENSION
The majority of diabetics with clinical nephropathy, as in the series of Keen and his associates, manifest significant hypertension [23]. It is generally believed that high blood pressure is the result, rather than the cause, of the nephropathy. Once present, hypertension unquestionably accelerates the inexorable decrease in renal function typical of diabetic nephropathy. Mogensen demonstrated that the rate of decline in glomerular filtration rate in diabetic nephropathy is positively correlated with diastolic hypertension [24]. Hypertension is often an early sign of worsening renal function in the type I diabetic [25]. The hypertensive diabetic has low plasma renin activity and low aldosterone levels [26]. Subsequently, hypertension accelerates loss of GFR in the later stages of diabetic nephropathy [24]. GFR decline in diabetics with nephropathy, and moderately increased blood pressure, can be slowed by antihypertensive treatment [27]. As much as 9 ml/min of creatinine clearance can be preserved per year of effective antihypertensive therapy. It follows that treatment for the nephropathic diabetic should include control of hypertension, thereby forestalling (preventing for a time) renal failure.

PREVENTION OF DIABETIC GLOMERULOPATHY
Diabetic glomerulopathy begins in the mesangium. Mesangial function and morphology are sensitive to alterations in the metabolic environment [28, 29]. Insulin treatment [30, 31] or pancreatic transplantation [32] prevents or reverses early glomerular lesions in streptozotocin–induced–diabetic rats, emphasizing the rela-

tionship between metabolic control and nephropathy. The fact that diabetic glomerulopathy recurs in kidney transplants obtained from nondiabetic donors can only be construed as an argument favoring the "environmental hypothesis" for the genesis of diabetic nephropathy. Reversal of recurrent glomerulopathy by a successfully functioning pancreas transplant affords compelling testimony supporting the thesis that diabetic glomerulopathy is not an inevitable consequence of long-term diabetes.

Fairness and balance require the admission that no carefully controlled studies of the effects of strict glucose control on the onset or progression of diabetic glomerulopathy have been reported. Barbosa challenges the inference that human diabetic glomerulopathy is causally related to hyperglycemia as "premature and counterproductive" [33]. Indeed, few well-structured, prospective controlled studies of the effect of "strict" glucose regulation on the course of "early" diabetic microvasculopathy have been completed. Until the past three years, ethical and practical concerns have restricted human trials of islet or whole or partial pancreas transplants to prior recipients of renal allografts already requiring immunosuppressive drugs to sustain their renal grafts [34, 35, 36].

Animal experimentation leads convincingly to the conclusion that diabetic microvasculopathy is preventable, if hyperglycemia is controlled. Like, for example, reported reversal or prevention of spontaneous diabetes in the BB Wistar rat with antilymphocytic serum [37]. Laupacis and associates have shown prevention of otherwise lethal hyperglycemia with cyclosporine treatment in the same animal model [38]. By dietary restriction of caloric intake in spontaneous diabetic db/db mice, Lee and his associates enhanced insulin sensitivity (possibly a result of increased receptor number) and restored euglycemia, thereby preventing development of diabetic nephropathy [39]. Further to the point are the findings of Rasch in diabetic rats, in which glomerular morphology of diabetic animals in good control remained normal, whereas rats in poor diabetic control developed glomerular changes characteristic of diabetic glomerulopathy [40].

Extrapolation from the induced hyperglycemic rat to human diabetic nephropathy is limited by the fact that most of the observed differences between nondiabetic and diabetic rats are nonspecific. Total prevention of diabetic glomerulopathy is possible by normalizing blood glucose levels in several experimental animal models of diabetes. Reversal of human diabetic glomerulopathy, however, has only been demonstrated in Abouna and associates' case report (vide supra), and in recurrent glomerulopathy in transplanted kidneys after subsequent pancreatic transplantation. Prospective clinical trials to establish or refute the "tight-control-will-prevent-vasculopathy" controversy are mandatory [41].

Conventional insulin treatment fails to interdict disabling and fatal complications in most type I diabetics [42].

Therapists who believe vasculopathic complications result from hyperglycemia hope that newer techniques of glucose regulation will permit euglycemia. Improved metabolic control is achievable today with fractional insulin doses, wearable pumps permitting continuous subcutaneous insulin infusion, or pancreatic transplants, any of which might alter the course of the microvascular disease associated with diabetes [43]. None of the "tight" control regimens available in 1985 are easy or uniformly successful.

Strategies for enhanced metabolic control are, however, likely to be vastly improved before this decade ends. Human islet transplant trials by Lacy [44], and an intensive exploration of the utility of cadaver donor pancreas transplants by Starzl [45] and others which are now under way may alter thinking about the ease of attaining "permanent" euglycemia. Until then, insulin administration by open loop pumps, or in fractional daily doses, demands of the patient that expensive and time-consuming multiple finger-stick blood glucose measurements be made each day. But, considering the high stakes involved in the gamble to permit suboptimal glucose regulation, it seems no longer rational to regard hyperglycemia as anymore acceptable in the diabetic than was "laudable pus" in the postoperative patient of yesteryear. Nearly constant euglycemia can be attained in many informed type I diabetics.

There are few complications of a tight control regimen, and patients feel better when their blood glucose level approaches the normal range most of the time. Should the long-term control versus complications trials now beginning show that the effort to maintain euglycemia was futile, little will have been lost. On the other hand, what will we say to the decade of diabetics allowed to progress to nephropathy and retinopathy which might have been prevented if the studies show the converse?

REFERENCES

1. Goodman MJ, Schung C. Diabetes mellitus: discrimination between single locus and multifactorial modes of inheritance. Clin Genet 8:66–74, 1975.
2. Mauer SM, Barbosa J, Vernier RL, et al. Development of diabetic vascular lesion in normal kidney transplanted into patients with diabetes mellitus. N Eng J Med 295:916–920, 1976.
3. Abouna GM, Al-Adnani MS, Kremer GD, Kumar SA, Daddah SK, Kusma G. Reversal of diabetic nephropathy in human kidneys after transplantation into non-diabetic recipients. Lancet 2:1274–1276, 1983.
4. Mogensen CE, Christensen CK. Predicting diabetic nephropathy in insulin-dependent patients. N Eng J Med 311:89–93, 1984.
5. Mogensen CE. Microalbuminuria predicts clinical proteinuria and early mortality in maturity-onset diabetes. N Eng J Med 310:356–360, 1984.
6. Friedman EA. Diabetic nephropathy: strategies in prevention and management. Kid Int 21:780–791, 1982.
7. Kimmelstiel P, Wilson C. Intercapillary lesions in glomeruli of kidney. Am J Pathol 12:83–105, 1936.
8. Ainsworth SK, Hirsh HZ, Brackett NC, et al. Diabetic glomerulonephropathy, histopathologic, immunofluorescent, and ultrastructural studies of 16 cases. Human Pathol 13:470–478, 1982.
9. Mauer SM, Steffes MW, Brown DM. The kidney in diabetes. Am J Med 70:603–612, 1981.
10. Mauer SM, Michael AF, Fish AJ, et al. Spontaneous immunoglobulin and complement deposition in glomeruli of diabetic rats. Lab Invest 27:488–494, 1972.
11. Mogensen CE, Andersen MJF. Increased kidney size and glomerular filtration rate in early juvenile diabetes. Diabetes 22:706–712, 1973.
12. McMillan D. Renal vascular changes in diabetes and their predicted effects. Endocrinol 97 (Suppl. 242): 26–28, 1981.
13. Viberti GC. Early functional and morphological changes in diabetic nephropathy. Clinical nephrology 12: 47–53, 1979.

14. Seyer-Hansen K. Renal hypertrophy in streptozotocin—diabetic rats. Clin Sci Mol Med 51:-551–555, 1976.
15. Seyer-Hansen K, Hansen J, Gundersen HJG. Renal hypertrophy in experimental diabetes: a morphometric metric study. Diabetologia 18:501–505, 1980.
16. Christiansen JS, Gammelgaard J, Frandsen M, et al. Increased kidney size, glomerular filtration rate and renal plasma flow in short-term insulin dependent diabetics. Diabetologia 20:451–456, 1981.
17. Fox M, Thier S, Rosenberg L, et al. Impaired renal tubular function induced by sugar infusion in man. J Clin Endocrinol Metab 24:1318–1322, 1964.
18. Brochner-Mortensen J. The glomerular filtration rate during moderate hyperglycemia in normal man. Acta Med Scand 194:31–37, 1973.
19. Ditzel J, Mortensen JB, Rodbro P. A combined disturbance in renal tubular handling of glucose and phosphate leads to increased glomerular filtration rate in diabetes mellitus: a new hypothesis. Acta Endocrinol 97 (Suppl. 242): 16–18, 1981.
20. Brenner BM, Hostetter TH, Olsen JL, et al. The role of glomerular hyperfiltration in the initiation and progression of diabetic nephropathy. Acta Endocrinol 97 (Suppl. 242): 7–10, 1981.
21. Viberti GC, Pickup JC, Phil D, et al. Effect of control of blood glucose on urinary excretion of albumin and B2 microglobulin in insulin-dependent diabetes. N Engl J Med 300:638–41, 1979.
22. Stephen RL, Maddock RK Jr., Kablitz C, Maxwell JG, Jacobson SC, Petelenz TJ. Stabilization and improvement of renal function in diabetic nephropathy. Diabetic nephropathy 1:8–13, 1982.
23. Keen H, Track ND, Sowry GSC. Arterial pressure in clinically apparent diabetics. Diabetes Metab 1:159–178, 1975.
24. Mogensen CE. Progression of nephropathy in long-term diabetics with proteinuria and effect of initial antihypertensive treatment. Scan J Clin Lab Invest 36:383–388, 1976.
25. Parving HH, Andersen AR, Smidt U, et al. The natural course of glomerular filtration rate and arterial blood pressure in diabetic nephropathy and the effect of antihypertensive treatment. Acta Endocrinol 97 (Suppl. 242): 39–40, 1981.
26. Christlieb AR, Kaldany A, D'Elia JA. Plasma renin activity and hypertension in diabetes mellitus. Diabetes 25:969–974, 1976.
27. Mogensen CE. Long-term antihypertensive treatment (over six years) inhibiting the progression of diabetic nephropathy. Acta Endocrinol 97 (Suppl. 242): 31–32, 1981.
28. Osterby R. Early phase in the development of diabetic glomerulopathy. Acta Med Scand 200 (Suppl. 574): 1–82, 1975.
29. Mauer SM, Brown DM, Steffes MW. Studies on the reversibility of kidney changes in experimental diabetes in the rat. Acta Endocrinol 97 (Suppl. 242): 29–30, 1981.
30. Rasch R. Prevention of diabetic glomerulopathy in streptozotocin diabetic rats by insulin treatment. Glomerular basement membrane thickness. Diabetologia 16:319–324, 1979.
31. Rasch R. Prevention of diabetic glomerulopathy in streptozotocin diabetic rats by insulin treatment, the mesangium region. Diabetologia 17:243–248, 1979.
32. Mauer SM, Steffes MW, Sutherland DER, et al. Studies of the rate of regression of the glomerular lesions in diabetic rats treated with pancreatic islet transplantation. Diabetes 24:-280–285, 1974.
33. Barbosa J. Diabetes: the science and the art. Arch Int Med 143:1118–1119, 1983.
34. Sutherland DER, Goetz FC, Najarian JS. Review of world's experience with pancreas and islet transplantation and results of intraperitoneal segmental pancreas transplantation from related and cadaver donors at Minnesota. Transplant Proc 13:291–297, 1981.
35. Goetz FC. Evaluating the benefit of human islet transplantation. Diabetes 29 (Suppl. 1): 52–55, 1980.
36. Traeger J, Dubernard JM, Touraine JL, et al. Pancreatic transplantation in man: a new method of pancreas preparation and results on diabetes correction. Transplant Proc 11:331–335, 1979.
37. Like AA, Rossini AA, Guberski DL, et al. Spontaneous diabetes mellitus—reversal and prevention in the BB/W rat with antiserum and rat lymphocyte. Science 206:1421–1423, 1979.
38. Laupacis A, Stiller CR, Gardell C, et al. Cyclosporine prevents diabetes in BB Wistar rats. Lancet 1 (8315): 10–12, 1983.
39. Lee SM, Bressler R. Prevention of diabetic nephropathy by diet control in the db/db mouse. Diabetes 30:106–111, 1981.
40. Rasch R. Studies on the prevention of glomerulopathy in diabetic rats. Acta Endocrinol 97 (Suppl 242): 43–44, 1981.

41. Mogensen CE, Steffes MW, Deckert TD, et al. Functional and morphological renal manifestations in diabetes mellitus. Diabetologia 21:89–93, 1981.
42. Deckert T, Poulsen JE, Larsen M. Progression of diabetes with onset before the age of thirty-one, II factors influencing the prognosis. Diabetologia 14:371–377, 1978.
43. Steno Study Group. Effect of 6 months of strict metabolic control on eye and kidney function in insulin dependent diabetics with background retinopathy. Lancet 8264:121–123, 1982.
44. Lacy PE. The feasibility of human islet transplants. In: Diabetic Renal-Retinal Syndrome 3: Therapy, Friedman EA, L'Esperance FA Jr. (eds). New York: Grune & Stratton, 1985, in press.
45. Starzl TE, Iwatsuk S, Shaw BW Jr., Gordon RD. A resurgence of interest in whole pancreas transplantation. In: Diabetic Renal-Retinal Syndrome 3: Therapy, Friedman EA, L'Esperance FA Jr. (eds). New York: Grune and Stratton, 1985, in press.

EPILOGUE

ELI A. FRIEDMAN

In terms of clinical commitment, epidemiologic understanding, and potential for prevention, 1984 will probably be remembered as "The Year of the Diabetic." For the first time, in 1984 some dialysis programs in urban America recorded a decline in the proportion of new patients who were diabetic. To explain this encouraging observation, it is tempting to suggest that the "message" of the importance—to the prevention of diabetic complications—of blood pressure reduction and maintenance of euglycemia is "getting through." Cumbersome regimens of fractional insulin dosing plus repeated daily finger-stick blood glucose testing may act as a "holding action" in slowing the progress of glomerulopathy and retinopathy in patients currently under care. For the next generation of diabetics, however, it may be anticipated, with confidence, that simplified routines for muting or eliminating hyperglycemia will be introduced before this decade ends. If it is true, as the author believes, that diabetic nephropathy is a hyperglycemic glomerulopathy, then the impact of induced euglycemia will be evident in a falling incidence of new cases of uremia (and blindness).

As shown in table E–1, in early 1985, several promising devices, approaches, and protocols are entering the stage of clinical trial. Should any of these prove efficacious, with minimal demand on patient energy, markedly enhanced metabolic control in type I diabetics will become the reference standard in therapy. Diabetatology has replaced syphilology, and later phthisiology, as the discipline to master if one wishes to be the consummate clinician. Providing an admixture of epidemiology, immunology, nutrition, endocrinology, gastroenterology, ne-

Table E–1. Promising approaches for sustaining euglycemia in diabetics

1. Closed loop insulin delivery devices (wearable, implantable)
2. Polymerized (depot) insulin injection (implantation)
3. Islet injection without rejection (cultured, irradiated, polymer-coated)
4. Hybrid organ implant with port for renewing cell charge (beta cells, insulinoma, islets)
5. Xenografted pancreas or islets
6. Stimulation of insulin receptor

phrology, specialized surgery, and psychiatry, the study and care of sick diabetics is both intellectually stimulating and emotionally rewarding. What makes the pursuit of an "answer" to diabetes even more exciting is the pragmatic reality that what we do today will shortly be relegated to medical history texts. The era of washing blood within (peritoneal dialysis) or outside of the body (hemodialysis), or assaulting a healthy person to remove a vital organ (kidney transplantation), will be replaced by a "brave" time of bionic and metabolic intervention, with minimal trauma and risk.

To appreciate how rapidly new ideas become current practice, the reader is urged to reflect on the necessity, only five years ago, for conferences convened to cope with a world supply of insulin dwindling while the number of diabetics rose. Teaching E. coli to synthesize human insulin ended that stress. An equally bold approach to preempting hyperglycemia and therefore vasculopathy in the diabetic may now be in early clinical trial. The future for both the diabetic patient and the student of diabetes is very bright indeed.

APPENDIX A: YOUR DIABETIC RENAL DIET

MILDRED FRIEDMAN

The purpose of this diet is to combine the currently used exchange lists for the diabetic with the controlled intake of sodium, potassium, and fluid of the dialysis patient. The exchange system is a way of measuring quantities of food so that the amount of nutrition in each portion is known. The diabetic must maintain a consistency of food intake in order to control blood sugar. The dialysis patient must (we are told) control the amounts of sodium, potassium, and fluid in his body in order to minimize the effect of insufficient kidney function.

Diet is prescribed individually and can be easily used in terms of the exchange units. Any item on one exchange list can be substituted for any other. You may have any crazy combination that suits you!

MEAL PLANNING

Diet: _____

Group	Serving Size			
	Breakfast	Lunch	Dinner	Snack
Milk				
Meat				
Bread				
Vegetable				
low–moderate potassium				
moderate po-tassium				

233

| Group | Serving Size | | | |
	Breakfast	Lunch	Dinner	Snack
Fruit	_____	_____	_____	_____
Fat	_____	_____	_____	_____
Fluid	_____	_____	_____	_____

LIST 1: MILK EXCHANGES

1 Exchange

1 cup whole milk
½ cup evaporated undiluted milk
1 cup skim milk (subtract 2 fat exchanges from your math or add 2 fat exchanges to what you eat)
½ cup evaporated skim undiluted milk (subtract 2 fat exchanges from your math or add 2 fat exchanges to what you eat)
1 cup 1% lowfat milk (subtract 1 ½ fat exchanges from your math or add 1 ½ fat exchanges to what you eat)
1 cup 2% lowfat milk (subtract 1 fat exchange from your math or add 1 fat exchange to what you eat)
1 cup yogurt (plain only)

1 Exchange

8 gms protein
12 gms carbohydrate
10 gms fat
120 mg sodium
352 mg potassium
170 calories

Avoid: milkshakes, malted milk, buttermilk, fruited yogurt, condensed milk, protein fortified skim milk or yogurt.
Note: Once per week you can have ½ cup plain flavored ice cream. It is not necessary to use dietetic ice cream. ½ cup ice cream is 1 bread exchange plus 2 fat exchanges for most people, but for some it is 2 fruit exchanges and 2 fat exchanges. This depends on your absorption of lactose and should be checked with your doctor.

LIST 2: FAT EXCHANGES

1 Exchange

1 tsp unsalted butter or margarine
1 tsp regular (salted) butter, margarine, or mayonnaise (contains 50 mg sodium)
1 tsp oil or cooking fat
1 tsp unsalted mayonnaise
Creams—limit to a maximum of 3 servings/day
1 tbsp heavy cream
2 tsp cream cheese
1 tbsp light cream

4 tsp sour cream
2 tsp whipping cream
2 tbsp coffee whiteners
4 tbsp nondairy whipped toppings
Note: You don't have to count protein, sodium, or potassium.

45 calories
5 gms fat

Avoid: avocados, bacon, bacon fat, bottled salad dressings, nuts, olives, salt pork, and cream sauces

LIST 3: MEAT EXCHANGES

1 Exchange

1 oz cooked beef, chicken, fish, veal, turkey, lamb, venison, rabbit, duck, fresh pork, organ meats (cooked size is 3″ × 2″ × ¼″)
¼ cup cottage, pot, or farmer cheese
1 oz hard cheese (not processed)—contains 200 mg sodium and less than 40 mg potassium
¼ cup tuna or salmon (canned, unsalted)
1 egg (65 mg potassium)
1 level tbsp peanut butter
5 small clams, oysters, scallops, shrimp (fresh only)
1 oz. shrimp, crab, lobster (fresh only)
3 sardines (low sodium only)

1 Exchange

7 gms. protein
5 gms. fat
30 mg. sodium
110 mg. potassium
73 calories (lean meat)

Avoid: dried, salted, spiced, smoked, pickled, or canned meats as bacon, corned beef, chipped and dried beef, frankfurters, hams, ham hocks, salt pork, "luncheon meats," pig knuckles, smoked neck bones, sausage, kidneys, calves liver, meat extracts and gravy, chinese food, *koshered meat,* shellfish (frozen, prepackaged, or boiled in salt water), frozen fish fillets, dried, salted, smoked, and canned fish, all cheeses except those allowed.

A HARD CHEESE LIST

1 Exchange is 1 oz.
The following cheeses contain up to 150 mg sodium and about 30 mg potassium: Mozzarella, Neufchatel, Brick, Monterey, Port de Salut, Gruyere, and Switzerland Swiss.
The following cheeses contain between 150 and 215 mg sodium and about 30 mg potassium: Caraway, Cheddar, Colby, Gjetost, Muenster, Tilsit, and Brie.
Gouda has 229 mg sodium.
Ricotta has 155 mg potassium.

LIST 4: BREAD EXCHANGES
Starred items indicate low sodium products which have 3 mg sodium.

1 Exchange

1 slice white, french, italian, rye, or whole wheat bread
¾ cup dry cereal
½ cup cooked cereal* or grits
½ matzoh (6" square)
4 pieces melba toast
6 small crackers (unsalted tops)
½ roll (hamburger, hot dog or hard, white)
1 small dinner roll
½ English muffin
½ small bagel
½ cup rice*
½ cup noodles,* spaghetti,* or macaroni*
3 cups popcorn, popped (unsalted)
2½ tbsp flour* or cornstarch
1 (2" diameter) muffin
½ large or 1 small pita
1½" cube sponge cake
6 vanilla wafers
5 Arrowroot biscuits
3 Lorna Doones
3 plain graham crackers (75 mg potassium)
1 small plain Pilot cracker
9 animal crackers
3 Uneedas
3 Zwieback
½ cup potatoes, mashed*
¼ cup sweet potato*
These last two should have their potassium lowered by:
1. Peeling and cubing them.
2. Soaking overnight in a large pot of water.
3. Dumping out the water and cooking them in fresh water.
This is called "dialyzing" the potatoes and is your only chance to fight back.

1 Exchange

2.5 gms protein
regular products—150 mg sodium
low sodium products—3 mg sodium
refined cereals—35 mg potassium
whole grains—75 mg potassium
68 calories

Avoid: instant and quick-cooking cereals, natural cereals containing nuts or any cereals with sugars or marshmallows, potato chips, cheese curls, salted crackers, salted popcorn, diet gelatin, pudding mixes, cakes, pies, tortilla chips, dried peas and beans, chick peas, lentils, wheat germ, commercially prepared soups, pumpernickel bread, cornbread, bran, pancakes, waffles, cookies, pretzels.

LIST 5: VEGETABLE EXCHANGES

1 Exchange is ½ cup cooked or raw vegetables. They may be fresh, frozen, or canned without salt, unless otherwise noted.

Low–moderate potassium

bean sprouts, beans (green or wax), cabbage (green, red, or chinese), carrots (canned only), cauliflower, celery (1 large stalk), chayote (½ medium), chicory, corn (canned only), cucumber (½ medium, no skin), eggplant (cooked, no skin), endive, escarole, lettuce, mustard greens (frozen only), onion, pepper (cooked), parsley (1 tbsp), radishes (5), romaine lettuce, scallion (2), squash (summer, yellow, zucchini—cooked), turnips (cooked), watercress

1 Exchange

1.5 gms protein
5 gms carbohydrate
10 mg sodium
110 mg potassium
25 calories

Moderate potassium:

asparagus, beets (cooked), broccoli (cooked), carrots (cooked), corn (1 small ear—4″), eggplant (raw), green pepper (raw), kale, kohlrabi (cooked), okra (cooked, 8–9 pods), peas, rutabaga (cooked)

1 Exchange:

1.5 gms protein
5 gms carbohydrate
10 mg sodium
180 mg potassium
25 calories

Avoid: artichokes, bamboo shoots, baked beans, beet greens, brussel sprouts, chick peas (garbanzos), collard greens, cowpeas, dandelion greens, dried peas and beans, kidney beans, lima beans, lentils, mushrooms, parsnips, pickles, plantains, potatoes, sauerkraut, sweet potatoes, tomatoes and tomato products, turnip greens, V-8 juice, winter squashes (acorn, butternut, hubbard), water chestnuts, yams, instant and powdered potatoes

LIST 6: FRUIT EXCHANGES

1 Exchange

If canned or frozen fruit is used be sure that it is not packed in sugar or syrup. Starred items have 125 mg potassium or less.

1 apple small*
⅓ cup apple juice*
½ cup applesauce (unsweetened)*
½ cup blackberries*
½ cup blueberries*
½ cup boysenberries*
½ cup or 10 large cherries
1 cup cranberries*
1 cup cranberry juice (diet)
1 medium fig (fresh or dried)
½ cup fruit cocktail (canned)
⅔ cup gooseberries
½ cup or 12 grapes (green or purple)*
¼ cup grape juice (frozen, diluted)*
½ medium grapefruit
3 medium kumquats
1 medium lemon or lime
⅔ cup lime juice
½ cup loganberries
½ small mango
1 small nectarine
½ cup orange segments (canned)
½ cup peaches (canned)
⅓ cup peach nectar
1 medium peach (raw)
2 halves pears (canned)*
½ pear (raw)
⅓ cup pear nectar
½ cup or 1 slice pineapple (raw or canned)*
⅓ cup pineapple juice*
2 medium purple plums (fresh or canned)
2 plums (green gage—canned)
2 medium prunes (dried)
1½ tbsp. raisins (packed)
½ cup raspberries*
¾ cup strawberries*
1 medium tangerine
1 cup watermelon (count as 140 cc's fluid)

1 Exchange

0.5 gms protein
10 gms carbohydrate
2 mg sodium
up to 200 mg potassium
40 calories

Avoid: apricots, avocado, banana, breadfruit, cantaloupe, cassaba melon, Damson plums, dates, fresh grapefruit juice, guava, honeydew melon, fresh orange, orange juice, papaya, persimmon, pomegranate, prune juice, rhubarb, tomato juice, and all dried fruits not listed such as apples, dates, etc.

Note: Remember to count juices as part of your fluid allowance.

A COUPLE OF HINTS

Use unsweetened and low sodium canned goods. Drain the liquid that fruits are packed in. Cooking vegetables in large amounts of water and draining off the liquid will lower their potassium content.

Perk up your meals with spices and herbs. Add ground spices to short-cooking dishes when salt would ordinarily be added. Add spices to long-cooking dishes near the end of the cooking period.

Seasonings allowed: allspice, almond extract, anise, basil, bay leaf, caraway, cardamon, chili powder, chives, cinnamon, cloves, coriander, cumin, curry powder, dill, fennel, garlic, ginger, horseradish (homemade), lemon juice or extract, lime juice, mace, maple extract, marjoram, mint, mustard (dry), nutmeg, onion, oregano, paprika, parsley (fresh), pepper, peppermint extract, poppyseed, poultry seasoning, rosemary, saffron, sage, savory, sesame seed, tarragon, thyme, turmeric, vanilla extract, vinegar, walnut extract

Avoid: alcoholic beverages, baking soda (sodium bicarbonate), Brewers yeast, candy, catsup, celery flakes, celery salt, chili sauce, Cocoa, chocolate, coconut, commercial dressing, commercial prepackaged gelatin desert, corn syrup, garlic salt, honey, prepared horseradish, ice cream, flavored ices, jam, jelly maple syrup, meat analogs, meat sauce and gravies, meat tenderizer, molasses, monosodium glutamate (Accent), prepared mustard, onion salt, pickles, relish and olives, salt, salt substitutes (unless recommended by physician), seasoned bread crumbs, seasoned coating mixes, seasoned rice mixes, seasoned noodle mixes, sherbet, soups and bouillon cubes, soy sauce, steak sauce, sugar (white or brown), TV dinners, and Worcestershire sauce

Treatment for insulin reaction

1 tbsp. honey, syrup, sugar or jelly
½ cup (120 cc's) regular sweetened soda
grape, apple, or cranberry juice
1 cup milk
6 jelly beans
5 Lifesavers

Remember to count any fluid intake as part of your allowance. Shortly afterwards have some carbohydrate, protein, and fat.

To convert fluids from one measuring system to the other:

cc	ozs	cups
15	½	—
30	1	—
120	4	½
240	8	1

Happy eating!

APPENDIX B: IDEAL WEIGHT TABLES

WEIGHT RANGE FOR WOMEN ACCORDING TO HEIGHT AND FRAME

Height for women		Weight (lb) in indoor clothing		
Ft	In	Small frame	Medium frame	Large frame
4	10	92–122	98–133	106–144
4	11	93–124	100–135	108–147
5	0	94–127	102–137	110–151
5	1	95–130	104–142	113–154
5	2	97–133	106–145	115–157
5	3	100–136	109–149	118–162
5	4	103–140	112–152	121–166
5	5	105–143	114–155	123–171
5	6	108–146	117–158	126–175
5	7	111–150	120–162	129–179
5	8	113–153	122–165	131–184
5	9	116–156	125–168	134–187
5	10	119–160	128–172	137–190
5	11	122–163	131–175	140–194
6	0	124–166	133–178	142–197

Weights at ages 25–59 based on lowest mortality.
Weight in pounds according to frame (in indoor clothing weighing 3 lbs, in shoes with 1″ heels).
The ranges have been extended an additional 10% at both the low and high ends to include a larger segment of the population.

To approximate frame size, extend your arm and bend the forearm upward at a 90° angle. Keep fingers straight, and turn the inside of your wrist toward your body. If you have a caliper, use it to measure the space between the two prominent bones on *either side* of your elbow. Without a caliper, place thumb and index finger of your other hand on these two bones. Measure the space between your fingers against a ruler or tape measure. Compare it with the table that lists elbow measurements for *medium frame*. Measurements lower than those listed indicate that you have a small frame. Higher measurements indicate a large frame.

Height in 1″ heels	Elbow breadth
4′10″–4′11″	2¼″–2½″
5′0″–5′3″	2¼″–2½″
5′4″–5′7″	2⅜″–2⅝″
5′8″–5′11″	2⅜″–2⅝″
6′0″	2½″–2¾″

WEIGHT RANGE FOR MEN ACCORDING TO HEIGHT AND FRAME

Height for men		Weight (lb) in indoor clothing		
Ft	In	Small frame	Medium frame	Large frame
5	2	115–147	118–155	124–165
5	3	117–150	120–157	126–168
5	4	119–152	122–160	128–172
5	5	121–154	123–163	130–176
5	6	122–156	125–166	131–180
5	7	124–160	128–169	134–185
5	8	126–163	131–173	137–189
5	9	128–166	133–176	140–194
5	10	130–169	136–179	142–198
5	11	131–173	139–183	145–202
6	0	134–176	141–187	148–207
6	1	137–180	144–191	151–211
6	2	140–185	148–196	155–217
6	3	142–190	150–200	158–222
6	4	146–194	154–206	163–228

Weights at ages 25–59 based on lowest mortality.
Weight in pounds according to frame (in indoor clothing weighing 5 lbs, in shoes with 1″ heels).
The ranges have been extended an additional 10% at both the low and high ends to include a larger segment of the population.

To approximate frame size, extend your arm and bend the forearm upward at a 90° angle. Keep fingers straight, and turn the inside of your wrist toward your body. If you have a caliper, use it to measure the space between the two prominent bones on *either side* of your elbow. Without a caliper, place thumb and index finger of your other hand on these two bones. Measure the space between your fingers against a ruler or tape measure. Compare it with the table that lists elbow measurements for *medium frame*. Measurements lower than those listed indicate that you have a small frame. Higher measurements indicate a large frame.

Height in 1″ heels	Elbow breadth
5′2″–5′3″	2½″–2⅞″
5′4″–5′7″	2⅝″–2⅞″
5′8″–5′11″	2¾″–3″
6′0″–6′3″	2¾″–3⅛″
6′4″	2⅞″–3¼″

APPENDIX C: PATIENT RESOURCES FOR ADDITIONAL HELP

American Kidney Fund
7315 Wisconsin Avenue
Bethesda, Maryland 20814 3266
Toll Free (800) 638-8299
Offers information and assistance to diabetics who have kidney failure. Financial aid available for patients who are unable to afford prescribed footwear, contact lenses, transportation, etc. Call or write for grant application.

American Foundation for the Blind
15 West 16th Street
New York, New York
The American Foundation for the Blind is a private, nonprofit agency providing services for the blind individual, the professional, and the public. The organization sells (at cost) aids that help blind persons live independently as well as publishing information about blindness and current research in the field. Free publications include the *Catalog of Publications, Catalog of Aids to Appliances,* and pamphlets on blindness and diabetes.

Vision Foundation, Inc.
770 Centre Street
Newton, Massachusetts 02158
Toll Free (800) 852-3029
(617) 965-5877

Provides information regarding benefits and services; how to find aids and devices; how to do things with less sight. Publishes a large-print directory, *Coping with Sight Loss: The Vision Resource Book*.

The Carroll Center for the Blind
770 Center Street
Newton, Massachusetts 02158
Publishes a quarterly review, *Aides and Appliances Review*. The purpose of the publication is to share with those involved in this field, experiences with new aids and appliances found to be useful for the blind and visually impaired.

National Association for Visually Handicapped
305 East 24th Street
New York, New York 10010
(212) 889-3141
Nonprofit, national organization devoted solely to the partially seeing. Offers: counseling, discussion groups, public and professional education, optical aids, information and referral services, and more.

Each state, by law, has services for the blind and visually impaired. Check with the social services department in your state.

Patient Organizations
National Association of Patients on Hemodialysis and Transplantation, Inc. (NAPHT)
156 William Street
New York, New York 10038
(212) 619-2727
Purpose: "Dedicated to promoting the interest and welfare of kidney patients." It functions in all areas of the renal field and educates both the public and patients about kidney disease, care, and rehabilitation.

Diabetic Renal Transplant Self Help Group
Downstate Medical Center
Box 52
450 Clarkson Avenue
Brooklyn, New York 11203
Purpose: To assist patients, their families, and newly referred uremic diabetics about to receive a transplant, with help in self-glucose monitoring, obtaining materials for the visually impaired, and dealing with the stresses of diabetic nephropathy.

INDEX

Albumin
    diabetic nephropathy with, 66, 67
    glomerulosclerosis pathology and, 69–70
    hypertension and, 225
Alcohol-induced diabetes, 8
Aldosterone, and hypertension, 78, 225
Alkaline phosphatase, and glucose control, 18
Amino acids, in continuous ambulatory peritoneal
    dialysis (CAPD), 114–115
Aminoglycosides, 200
Amitryptiline, and diabetic peripheral neuropathy,
    101
Amputation
    hemodialysis and, 98–100
    incidence of, 179
    renal transplantation and, 149
Angina, and hemodialysis, 100
Angiography, *see* Fluorescein angiography
Anticoagulation, and hemodialysis, 91
Antihypertensive drugs
    hypertensive management with, 77
    see also specific agents
Antilymphocyte globulin (ALG), in pancreas
    transplantation, 169
Argon laser photocoagulation, in diabetic
    retinopathy management, 47–48, 49
Aspirin, and fibrinogen survival, 16
Atherosclerosis, and renal transplantation, 142
Azathioprine
    infection risk and foot problems and, 179

pancreas transplantation with, 164–165, 169
    renal transplantation with, 144, 145, 179
Azotemia
    clinical manifestations of, 73–74
    hypertensive management in, 77
    radiocontrast media studies and, 79–80
    in type I diabetes, 73–74

Bacteremia, and hemodialysis, 101
Bacteruria, incidence of, 79
Beta blockers, and orthostatic hypotension, 116
Blindness
    continuous ambulatory peritoneal dialysis
        (CAPD) use in, 123–134
    hemodialysis causing, 97–98
    patient narrative of experience with, 215–
        216
Blood glucose tests
    diagnostician familiarity with, 8
    insulin therapy and, 28
    sensor device in insulin pumps for, 38–39
    see also Glucose tolerance test; Patient
        monitoring of blood glucose
Blood pressure
    nurse's role in monitoring, 200–201
    see also Hypertension; Hypotension
Bread exchanges, 236–237
Bright-flash electroretinography (ERG), in
    diabetic retinopathy evaluation, 43–44